SUDDEN CARDIAC DEATH

Developments in
Cardiovascular Medicine

VOLUME 110

The titles published in this series are listed at the end of this volume.

Sudden Cardiac Death

edited by

A. BAYÉS DE LUNA
Hospital de la Santa Creu i Sant Pau, Barcelona, Spain

P. BRUGADA
University Hospital, Maastricht, The Netherlands

J. COSIN AGUILAR
Hospital La Fe, Valencia, Spain

and

F. NAVARRO-LOPEZ
University of Barcelona, Hospital Clinic, Barcelona, Spain

Kluwer Academic Publishers
DORDRECHT / LONDON / BOSTON

Library of Congress Cataloging-in-Publication Data

Sudden cardiac death / edited by A. Bayés de Luna ... [et al.].
    p.   cm. — (Developments in cardiovascular medicine; v. 110)
   ISBN-13:978-94-010-6745-4   e-ISBN-13:978-94-009-0573-3
   DOI: 10.1007/978-94-009-0573-3

   1. Cardiac arrest. I. Bayés de Luna, Antonio. II. Series.
   [DNLM: 1. Arrhythmia. 2. Death, Sudden. 3. Heart Arrest. W1
DE997VME v. 110 / WG 205 S94 124]
RC685.C173S77   1990
616.1'23'025–dc20
DNLM/DLC
for library of Congress   90-4217
                                                                        CIP

ISBN-13:978-94-010-6745-4

Published by Kluwer Academic Publishers,
P.O. Box 17, 3300 AA Dordrecht, The Netherlands.

Kluwer Academic Publishers incorporates
the publishing programmes of
Martinus Nijhoff, Dr W. Junk, D. Reidel and MTP Press.

Sold and distributed in the U.S.A. and Canada
by Kluwer Academic Publishers,
101 Philip Drive, Norwell, MA 02061, U.S.A.

In all other countries, sold and distributed
by Kluwer Academic Publishers Group,
P.O. Box 322, 3300 AH Dordrecht, The Netherlands.

Printed on acid-free paper

Table of contents

Preface

Sudden death is probably the greatest challenge facing modern cardiology today. This is mainly due to the impact of its brusque appearance and the socioeconomic implications. The incidende is presently decreasing somewhat, mainly due to the decline in new cases of ischemic heart disease on one hand, and to better prevention in risk patients on the other. Nevertheless, the figures are still high and represent over 300.000 patients per year in the United States alone.

This book is an updating of the problem of sudden death from a multifactorial standpoint. It includes not only electrophysiologic data but also covers aspects ranging from epidemiology to prevention. Risk markers and triggering mechanicsms of sudden death are reviewed, with special emphasis on the role of electrical instability, ischemia and depressed ventricular function. The book includes the contributions from many experts, often pioneers in their respective fields.

It is our hope that the book serves as an updating for those cardiologist who are not specialized in these subjects, but may also be of interest to the expert.

We wish to express our sincerest gratitude to the authors for sending in their work so promptly, and also Kluwer Academic Publishers for their exactitude and perfection in this edition.

Barcelona, September 1990   The Editors

List of contributors

J. ALMENDRAL
Servico de Cardiología, Hospital Gral. 'Gregorio Marañón', Madrid, Spain
Chapter 14 co-author: A. ARENAL

A. BAYÉS DE LUNA
Department of Cardiology, Hospital de la Santa Creu i Sant Pau, University of Barcelona, Avda. San Antonio Maria Claret 167, Barcelona 08025, Spain
Chapter 1 co-authors: J. GUINDO, J. BARTOLUCCI, P. TORNER, M. DOMIN-GUEZ and R. OTER
Chapter 13 co-authors: J. GUINDO, S. GARCÍA-SÁNCHEZ, P. TORNER and R. OTER

J.Th. BIGGER, Jr.
Arrhythmia Control Unit, Columbia-Presbyterian Medical Center, 630 West 168th Street, New York, NY 10032 / 401 East 86th Street, New York, NY 10028, USA
Chapter 5

W.E. BODEN
Division of Cardiology, Department of Internal Medicine, Harper Hospital, 3990 John R. Street, Detroit, MI 48021, USA
Chapter 21: co-author: R.E. KLEIGER

G. BREITHARDT
Medizinische Klinik und Poliklinik, Innere Medizin C (Kardiologie, Angiologie), Westfälische Wilhelms-Universität, Albert-Schweitzer-Str. 33, D-4400 Münster, Germany
Chapter 19 co-authors: M. BORGGREFE and A. MARTÍNEZ-RUBIO

P. BRUGADA
Department of Cardiology, Academic Hospital, University of Limburg, P.O. Box 1918, 6201 BX Maastricht, The Netherlands
Chapter 17 co-authors: H. DE SWART, J.L.R.M. SMEETS and H.J.J WELLENS

R.W.F. CAMPBELL
Professor of Cardiology, University of Newcastle upon Tyne, Freeman Hospital,
Newcastle upon Tyne NE7 7DN, UK
Chapter 11

J. COSIN AGUILAR
Research Group Spanish Trail on Sudden Death, Hospital 'La Fe', Av de Cam-
panar 21, 46009 Valencia, Spain
Chapter 3

Ph. COUMEL
Hôpital Lariboisière, 2 rue Ambroise-Paré, F-75475 Paris, France
Chapter 18 co-author: J.-P. DESCHAMPS

G. FONTAINE
Hôpital Jean Rostand, 39–41 rue Jean Le Galleu, F-94200 Ivry, France
Chapter 16 co-authors: R. FRANK, J. TONET, I. ROUGIER, G. FARENQ, G.
LASCAULT and Y. GROSGOGEAT

F. FURLANELLO
Divisione di Cardiologia e Centro Aritmologico, Ospedale S. Chiara, 38100 Trento,
Italy
Chapter 9 co-authors: R. BETTINE, G. VERGARA, A. BERTOLDI, M. DEL
GRECO, G.B. DURANTE and L. FRISANCO

S. GARCÍA-SÁNCHEZ
Department of Cardiology, Sant Pau Hospital, Research Foundation Santa Creu i
Sant Pau, Barcelona, Spain
Chapter 7 co-authors: J. GUINDO and A. BAYÉS DE LUNA

J. GUINDO
Departamento de Cardiología, Hospital de la Santa Creu i Sant Pau, Universidad
Autónoma de Barcelona, Avda. San Antonio Maria Claret 167, Barcelona 08025,
Spain
Chapter 22 co-authors: A. BAYÉS DE LUNA, P. TORNER, J. BARTOLUCCI
and R. ESTIARTE

P.G. HUGENHOLTZ
Erasmus University, Rotterdam, The Netherlands
Chapter 23 co-author: J.R.T.C. ROELANDT

J.H. IP
Department of Medicine, Division of Cardiology, The Mount Sinai Medical Center,
One Gustave Levi Place, New York, NY 10029, USA
Chapter 4 co-author: V. FUSTER

H.E. KULBERTUS
Service de Cardiologie, CHU, Sart-Tilman B45, B-4000 Liège–1, Belgium
Chapter 12

J.-F. LECLERCQ
Department of Cardiology, Hôpital Lariboisière, 2rue Ambroise-Paré, F-75475, Paris, France
Chapter 10 co-author: Ph. COUMEL

A. MASERI
Sir John McMichael Professor of Cardiovascular Medicine, Royal Postgraduate Medical School, Director of Cardiology, Hammersmith Hospital, Ducane Road, London W12 ONN, UK
Chapter 8

A.J. MOSS
Heart Research Follow-up Program, University of Rochester Medical Center, Box 653, Rochester, NY 14642, USA
Chapter 2

F. NAVARRO-LOPEZ
Department of Cardiology and Coronary Care Unit, Hospital Clinico-University of Barcelona, Barcelona, Spain
Chapter 20

P. PUECH
Department of Cardiology, Hospital Saint Eloi, Montpellier, France
Chapter 25

N. REHNQVIST
Department of Medicine, Karolinska Institutet, Danderyds Sjukhus, S-182 88 Danderyd, Sweden
Chapter 6

H.-J. TRAPPE
Department of Cardiology, Hannover Medical School, Konstanty-Gutschow-Str. 8, D-3000 Hannover 61, Germany
Chapter 15 co-authors: H. KLEIN, G. FRANK, P. WENZLAFF and P.R. LICHTLEN

H.J.J. WELLENS
Academic Hospital of Maastricht, University of Limburg, Annadal 1, 6214 PA Maastricht, The Netherlands
Chapter 24 co-author: P. BRUGADA

1. Sudden cardiac death 1990: An update

A. BAYÉS DE LUNA, J. GUINDO, J. BARTOLUCCI, P. TORNER,
M. DOMINGUEZ and R. OTER

In most cases, over 80% in our experience (Figure 1) [1—4], ambulatory
sudden death (ASD) is due to the onset of malignant ventricular arrhythmia.
In 50% of these, ventricular fibrillation (VF) preceded by classic ventricular
tachycardia (VT) is responsible for ASD. In the remaining cases of malignant
ventricular arrhythmia, VF is of abrupt onset or is preceded by "torsades de
pointes". In the 20% not due to malignant ventricular arrhythmia, the cause
of ASD is bradyarrhythmia.

When the cause of sudden death is a bradyarrhythmia, the presence of
premature ventricular contractions (PVC) does not usually play an important
role, and ASD can often be attributed to a single mechanism (e.g., electromechanical dissociation in the acute phase of myocardial infarction). In contrast,

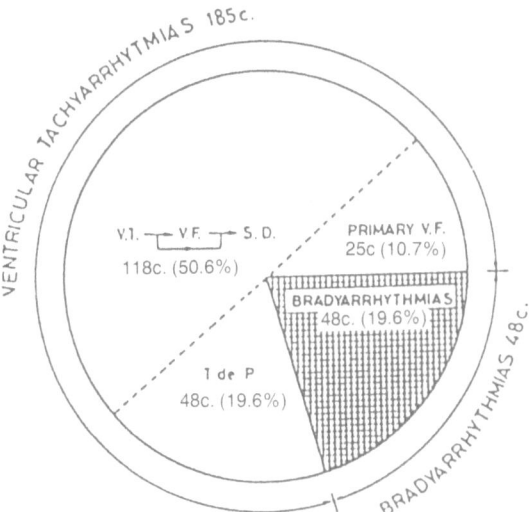

Figure 1. Distribution of different causes of ambulatory sudden death recorded by Holter
electrocardiography. VT = Ventricular tachycardia; VF = Ventricular fibrillation; PrVF =
Primary ventricular fibrillation; T de P = Torsades de pointes.

A. Bayés de Luna et al. (eds.): *Sudden Cardiac Death*, 1–11.
© 1991 Kluwer Academic Publishers, Dordrecht.

diverse factors intervene in the origin of malignant ventricular arrhythmia. It is a multifactorial problem, many of whose components are fairly familiar to us, but we do not know how the interaction between them triggers malignant ventricular arrhythmia. In this chapter we will discuss ASD mainly due to malignant ventricular arrhythmia.

In our opinion, a series of circumstances must coincide for sudden death to occur, as shown in Figure 2 [5]. PVC are necessary because, at the last moment, a PVC will trigger the malignant ventricular arrhythmia, independently of whether there are many or few in Holter recordings. The importance of PVC in the genesis of ASD was first stressed by Lown [6] and later confirmed by different studies [7—11], which have also shown that the importance of PVC as a marker of ASD increases in the presence of other factors.

A vulnerable myocardium, that is, an enhanced myocardial susceptibility to ventricular fibrillation, must also be present [7—12]. Diverse conditions can make a myocardium vulnerable: postinfarction scar, dilatation or ventricular hypertrophy, presence of an anomalous conduction pathway or prolonged repolarization, etc.

However, many patients after myocardial infarction, or with cardiomyopathy, arterial hypertension, Wolff-Parkinson-White syndrome or other abnormalities live for a long time, sometimes years, with a vulnerable myocardium and numerous, sometimes frequent, PVC, without presenting sudden death. For this event to take place, one or more additional modulating factors must act in a patient who presents these special conditions (PVC + vulnerable myocardium). These factors are (Figure 2):
1) alterations of the autonomic nervous system;
2) physical and/or psychic stress;
3) ischemic episodes;

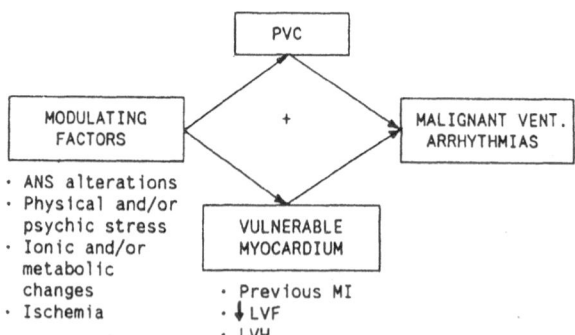

Figure 2. Physiopathology of malignant ventricular arrhythmias and sudden death in patients after myocardial infarction. PVC = Premature ventricular contractions; ANS = Autonomic nervous system; MI = Myocardial infarction; LVF = Left ventricular function; LVH = Left ventricular hypertrophy.

4) ionic and/or metabolic imbalance;
5) production of a rapid arrhythmia.

Often, as in the case of acute coronary insufficiency, decompensated cor pulmonale, electrolyte imbalance, ischemia, or ionic and/or metabolic disorders may also be responsible for the presentation of PVC or their increase and for producing or enhancing myocardial vulnerability.

We shall discuss the relative importance of these factors.

Importance of PVC

The presence of PVC in the ECG at rest in post-myocardial infarction patients almost doubles the risk of sudden death at 3 years (21% vs. 12%). More than 15 years ago, Lown and Wolf [6] established criteria for life-threatening PVC based on their number and characteristics. For these authors, the threshold between occasional and frequent PVC is 30 per hour. More recently, several authors [13, 14] have suggested that this threshold is lower; Bigger [15] has established between 1 and 10 per hour (Figure 3). The Lown scale, which is widely accepted, classifies levels of risk. Accordingly, the frequency of PVC is relatively unimportant (representing grades 1 and 2 of the scale), but the so-called complexity characteristic of PVC is more significant (multiform — grade 3, repetitive — grade 4, or R on T phenomena, which merits the maximum score — grade 5). Accordingly, patients with heart disease and frequent PVC have a 4-year mortality of 15—20% as compared to 30% for Lown types 4 and 5. The mortality of these patients without PVC would be about 10%.

Bigger and Weld [14] insist that there are important limitations in the

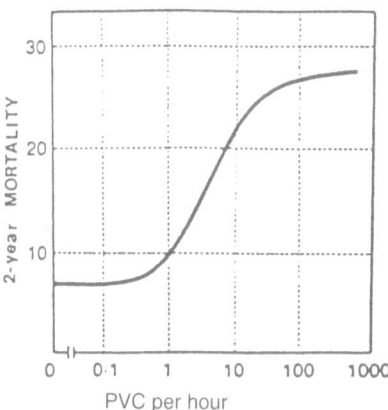

Figure 3. Mortality rate plotted against the incidence of ventricular premature impulses (VPI). When the number of PVC rises from 1 to 10 per hour the mortality increases appreciably (adapted from JT Bigger [13]).

Lown scale. Mortality varies widely for the same Lown criterion because it is also conditioned by other variables. For example, in the case of R on T type PVC, if this is the only complexity character found, the risk of mortality is eight times lower than if all four complexity criteria were present (polymorphism, couplets, runs and R on T), and six times lower than if couplets or runs of ventricular tachycardia were associated to R on T. On the other hand, the same Lown criteria (4a, 4b or 5) reflect a much more threatening situation when there are more than 10 PVC per hour. Bigger *et al.* [13] affirm that mortality in the first year after infarction is higher in patients with PVC $\geqslant$ 10/hr or repetitive forms than in those who present R on T phenomena or polymorphism (Table 1). Anderson [16] also found a more elevated mortality rate — more than double — in patients with ventricular tachycardia, but these figures were not statistically significant.

The papers of Ruberman *et al.* [7] and others [8—10] have also stressed the independent importance of PVC as a marker for global and sudden death, although emphasizing that the risk is greater in the presence of abnormal left ventricular function. It has recently been demonstrated in the BHAT Study Group [17] that patients receiving placebo who present PVC have a worse prognosis. Nevertheless it appears that in 1990 the mortality rate of postmyocardial infarction patients in decreasing considerably due to different reasons.

Importance of vulnerable myocardium

For PVC to trigger a malignant ventricular arrhythmia under the influence of a certain modulanting factor, the presence of a vulnerable myocardium is required. This means that the myocardium must have a lower than normal fibrillation threshold or a greater capacity for generating sustained ventricular tachycardia. On the other hand, postinfarction scars make the myocardium vulnerable because they facilitate the appearance of sustained ventricular tachycardia due to re-entry.

Ventricular function has important prognostic implications, because

Table 1. Relationship of complex PVC features to one year cardiac death after myocardial infarction (n = 430). (From Bigger *et al.* [8]).

Characteristics	Patients		Mortality	
	No.	%	No.	%
PVCs $\geqslant$ 10/hr	111	26	30	27
Multiform PVCs	224	52	42	19
Couplets	129	30	36	28
Ventricular tachycardia	50	12	19	38
R on T	130	30	28	22

depressed function also makes the myocardium vulnerable. In effect, aside from the PVC characteristics just commented, which are an independent factor that partially conditions the prognosis of patients with heart disease, particularly postinfarction patients, the prognosis is also known to be independently related to ventricular function, as evaluated by clinical procedures (presence of the 3rd heart sound or ventricular failure, for example) or by ejection fraction. Recent multicentric studies have established that the ejection fraction is an independent marker of total and cardiac sudden death [9, 10], but the combination of characteristic PVC and left ventricular function provides additional prognostic information. As such, patients with a low ejection fraction (less than 40—50%) and frequent PVC (3—10 per hour), or repetitive PVC, have a higher incidence of sudden death and mortality. Recently [12] it has been suggested that an ejection fraction of less than 45% in postinfarction patients, used as the sole criterion, is more sensitive (62% vs. 39%) but less specific (64% vs. 84%) for total 1-year cardiac mortality than an ejection fraction of 45% plus complex PVC. According to these authors, the ejection fraction alone is more useful than combined criteria in stratifying postinfarction patients.

Other circumstances can contribute to the myocardium becoming vulnerable. One of them is left ventricular enlargement, which accounts for the myocardial vulnerability of patients with hypertension, cardiomyopathy, valvular disease and some of those with coronary disease [18]. In patients with hypertrophic cardiomyopathy, vulnerability can also be conditioned by the special disposition of the myocardial fibers [19].

In patients with Wolff-Parkinson-White syndrome, the myocardium is vulnerable due to the presence of anomalous conduction pathways. In these cases atrial fibrillation can conduct many atrial impulses to the ventricles. The risk is that a very early atrial impulse can reach the ventricular myocardium, in the vulnerable phase, and trigger malignant ventricular arrhythmia, specially in the presence of heart disease or atrial fibrillation with very rapid ventricular conduction (modulating factors) [20—21].

The case of long QT syndrome is similar; prolonged and irregular repolarization (vulnerable myocardium) facilitates the appearance of malignant ventricular arrhythmias, particularly in patients with physical or psychic stress (modulating factors) [22—24]. Finally, ionic and/or metabolic alterations can act as modulating factors in the presence of vulnerable myocardium (see below), but sometimes they can also make a normal myocardium in a vulnerable one.

Importance of modulating factors

Alterations in the autonomic nervous system

It has been demonstrated that the heart rate often accelerates before the fatal arrhythmia in patients who die suddenly. Leclerq *et al.* [25] have found a statistically significant increase in sinus heart rate or the onset of a rapid supraventricular arrhythmia in the hour before the fatal arrhythmia. This is also observed in our review of 233 patients who died wearing a Holter device [2]. On other occasions, the malignant ventricular arrhythmia seems to

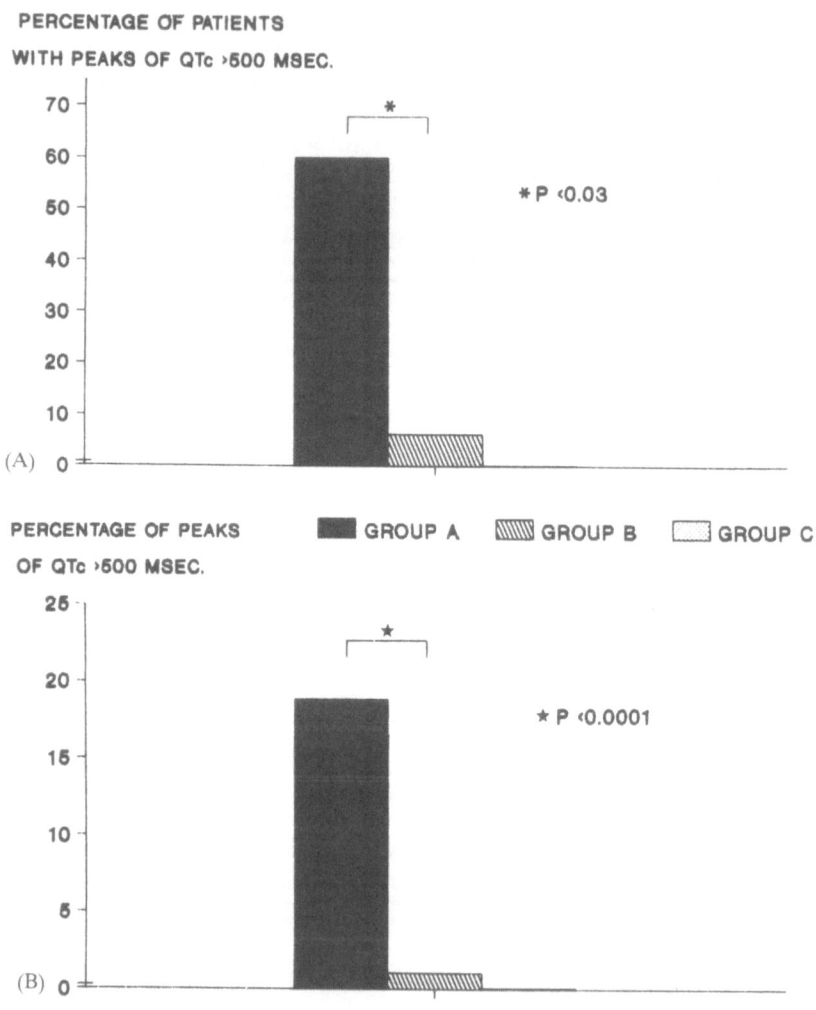

Figure 4. (A) Percentage of patients with peaks of QTc greater than 500 ms; group A: postmyocardial infarction patients with malignant ventricular arrhythmias; group B: postmyocardial infarction patients without malignant ventricular arrhythmias; group C: patients without heart disease. Note in group A there are more patients than in group B with peaks of QTc greater than 500 ms (p < 0.03) and none in group C. (B) Percentage of peaks of QTc greater than 500 ms in relation to the total hours of Holter monitoring. Patients from group A presented more peaks of QTc greater than 500 ms than those in group B (p < 0.0001). Patients from group C did not present any peak of QTc above this value.

be induced by a PVC that appears after a long pause generated by a previous PVC [26].

There is evidence that other parameters that are modulated by the autonomic nervous system, such as the variability of the R-R interval and the dynamic behaviour of the QT interval, also play a role in the onset of sudden death. Kleiger *et al.* [27] have demonstrated that postinfarction patients with scant R-R interval variability have a worse prognosis, and we [28] have observed that postinfarction patients who present malignant ventricular arrhythmias have more QTc peaks over 500 ms on 24-hour recordings (Figure 4).

Other modulating factors

There is no doubt that in certain circumstances physical effort and psychic stress are factors that induce malignant ventricular arrhythmia. This occurs frequently in patients with long QT syndrome [24], but it has also been seen in coronary patients and in other heart diseases (Figure 5). Nor should we overlook the cases of athletes who die suddenly, frequently in relation to their athletic activity [29].

The direct relationship between ischemia and sudden death is not clear, although it is certain that the incidence of sudden death is very high in the acute phase of myocardial infarction [30] and that, experimentally, acute prolonged ischemia provokes the appearance of malignant ventricular arrhythmias [31—32]. However, outside these situations of prolonged and intense ischemia, the relationship between ischemia (angina and silent) and sudden death is less evident, and there are arguments for and against this. We

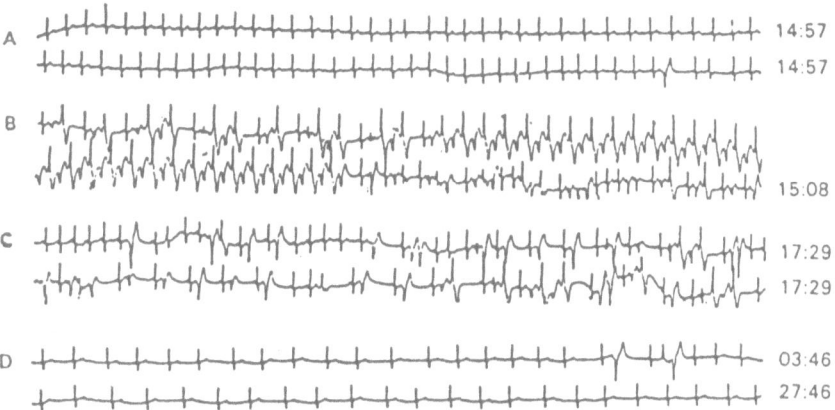

Figure 5. Induction of bidirectional ventricular tachycardia during a psychological stress test (B) and hours later on recounting the test to friends (C). (A) Basal recording. (D) Post-stress recording.

will comment on some of these. In some isolated cases there is evidence of a direct link between crises of angina or silent ischemia and sudden death [33]. Nevertheless, malignant ventricular arrhythmia rarely occurs during attacks of variant angina [34], even though PVC are often originated and despite marked ST elevation [34] (Figure 6). This is probably due to the fact that the ischemia, although severe, in these circumstances is not prolonged.

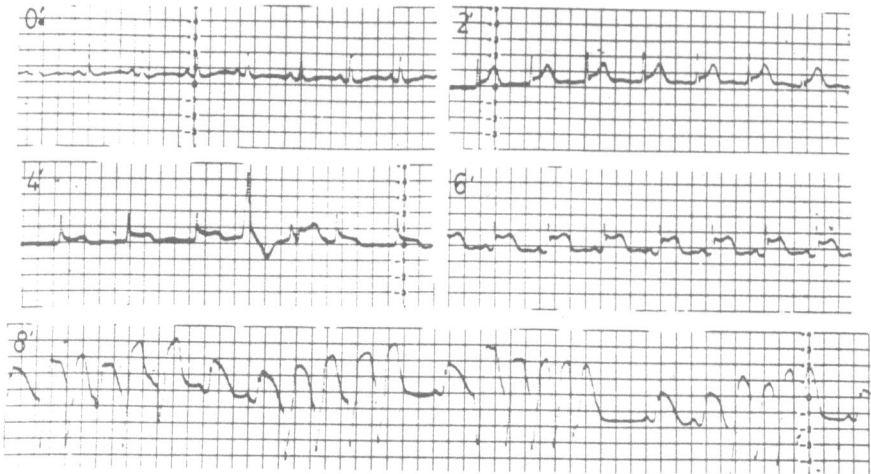

Figure 6. Sequence of an attack of Prinzmetal angina with the appearance of ventricular tachycardia runs at the moment of maximum ST elevation.

It is also evident that the presence of a positive effort test, with or without angina, after myocardial infarction is a marker of bad prognosis over the next months [35], and it has been demonstrated that patients resuscitated from out-of-hospital cardiac arrest have often a positive effort test [36].

Only 12.5% of the cases of ASD we have studied [1—4] showed evidence of a new ischemic attack, as manifested by a change in the ST segment prior to the fatal arrhythmia.

The relationship between the presence of silent ST depression on Holter recordings and increased incidence of ventricular arrhythmias and sudden death is not so evident [33, 37—40]. Neither Graboys [41] nor ourselves [42] encountered in patients with silent ischemia an increase in PVC incidence in episodes of asymptomatic ST depression on Holter recording, although the ST depression in our study was not very intense. On the contrary, Rocco *et al.* [43] have demonstrated in a group of patients with positive effort test that complications (not including sudden death) appear more frequently in patients who have asymptomatic ST depression on Holter recordings.

In our opinion, the problem of determining the true importance of ischemia in ASD is still unresolved, particularly for silent ischemia detected by Holter ECG. It is difficult for us to explain why ST depression is seen so often on the Holter recording without originating malignant ventricular arrthythmias and, on the other hand, why these are frequently not accompanied by any previous depression of the ST segment.

Ionic and/or metabolic alterations can also play an important role in inducing malignant ventricular arrhythmia, particularly of the "torsade de pointes" type, whether produced by indiscriminate drug administration or due to processes that originate ionic or metabolic imbalance (alcoholism, kidney failure, cor pulmonale, etc.) [1—4].

Finally, the onset of a rapid tachyarrythmia can be an inductive factor, both in postinfarction patients [2] and in the Wolff-Parkinson-White syndrome (see above). In effect, in all the cases studied by P. Torner [20] sudden death appeared as the consequence of ventricular fibrillation in the course of rapid supraventricular tachycardia (39% atrial fibrillation and 9% atrial glutter).

Using the algorithm in Figure 2 we can explain most, if not all, of the situations that lead to sudden death due to ventricular tachyarrhythmia. In each specific case, the characteristics of the PVC, vulnerable myocardium and modulating factors can vary, but in any given case death is due to an interaction of these three phenomena (PVC + vulnerable myocardium + modulating factors) which induces malignant ventricular arrhythmia, the immediate cause of more than 80% of cases of ASD. What we still do not know is the exact contribution of each of these factors to the complex phenomenon of ASD. Probably in the future we will be able to know which patients are at risk of sudden death using a scale based on the clinical evaluation of the patient and on the results of different non-invasive techniques to study different parameters:
1) Holter ECG (arrhythmias, ST, QT, RR variability),
2) effort test (arrhythmias, ST),
3) late potentials,
4) left ventricular fraction (isotopic studies).
With all these data we will have a lot of information about the three phenomena (PVC, vulnerable myocardium and modulating factors) that will probably be very useful in stratifying patients at risk of sudden death. In fact, some papers studying these different parameters have already been published with encouraging results.

References

1. Bayés de Luna A, Coumel Ph, Leclercq JF. Ambulatory sudden death: mechanisms of production of fatal arrhythmia on the basis of data from 157 cases. Am Heart J 1989; 117: 154.
2. Bayés de Luna A, Guindo J, Rivera J. Ambulatory sudden death: Holter monitoring 1989.

3. Rivera I, Bayés de Luna A, Martinez MD, Iturralde P. Muerte súbita ambulatoria. In Bayés de Luna. Programa de Formación continuada in Cardiología. Avances en Electrocardiología. Ed. Doyma 1987; p. 128.
4. Bayés de Luna A, Torner P, Guindo J, Soler M, Oca F. Holter ECG study of ambulatory sudden death. Review of 158 published cases. New Trends in Arrhythmias 1985; 1(3): 293.
5. Bayés de Luna A, Guindo Soldevila J. Sudden Cardiac Death. Ed. MCR. Barcelona 1989.
6. Lown B, Wolf M. Approaches to sudden death from coronary heart disease. Circulation 1971; 44: 330.
7. Ruberman W, Wienblatt E, Golberg J. Ventricular premature complexes and sudden death after myocardial infarction. Circulation 1981; 64: 297.
8. Bigger J, Weld F, Rolnitzky L. Which postinfarction ventricular arrhythmias should be treated. Am Heart J 1982; 103: 660.
9. Moss AJ, Davis HT, DeCamilla J, Bayer LW. Ventricular ectopic beats and their relation to sudden and non-sudden cardiac death after myocardial infarction. Circulation 1979; 60: 998.
10. Bigger JT, Fleiss JL, Kleiger R. Miller P, Kolnitzky. The relationships among ventricular arrhythmias, left ventricular dysfunction, and mortality in the 2 years after myocardial infarction. Circulation 1984; 69: 250.
11. Mukharji J, Rude RE, Poole WK *et al*. The MILIS study Group. Risk factors sudden death after acute myocardial infarction: Two year follow-up. Am J Cardiol 1984; 54: 31—36.
12. Ahnve S, Gilpin E, Henninng H, Curtis G, Ross J Jr. Limitations and advantages of the ejection fraction for defining high risk after acute myocardial infarction. Am J Cardiol 1986: 58: 872.
13. Bigger JT. Relation between left ventricular dysfunction and ventricular arrhythmias after myocardial infarction. Am J Cardiol 1986; 57: 8B—14B.
14. Bigger JT Jr, Weld FM. Shortcomings of the Lown grading for observational of experimental studies in ischemic heart disease. Am Heart J 1980; 100: 1.081.
15. Bigger JT Jr, Weld FM, Coromilas J. Prevalence and significance of arrhythmias in 24 hour ECG recordings made within one month of acute myocardial infarction. In: Kulbertus HE, Wellens H, eds. The first year after a myocardial infarction. New York, Futura 1983.
16. Anderson KP, De Camila J, Moss AJ. Clinical significance of ventricular tachycardia (3 beats longer) detected during ambulatory monitoring after myocardial infarction. Circulation 1977; 57: 890—897.
17. Lichteins E, Morganroth J, Harriests R, Hubble E for the BHAT Study Group. Effect of propranolol on ventricular arrhythmia. The Beta-Blocker Heart Attach Trial experience. Circulation 1983; 67(Suppl I): 5—10.
18. McLenachan JM, Henderson E, Karen I, Morris, Dargie HJ. Ventricular arrhythmias with hypertensive left ventricular hypertrophy. N Engl J of Med 1987; 317 (13): 787.
19. Maron BJ, Anan TJ, Roberst WC. Quantitative analysis of the distribution of cardiac muscle cell disorganisation in the left ventricular wall of patients with hypertrophic cardiomyopathy. Circulation 1981; 63: 882—894.
20. Torner P, Brugada P, Smeets J, Talajic M, Della P, Lezaun R, Dool A, Wellens H, Bayés de Luna A, Oter R, Breithardt G, Borggrefe M, Klein H, Kuck K, Kunze K, Coumel P, Leclercq JF, Chouty F, Frank R, Fontaine G. Ventricular fibrillation in the Wolff-Parkinson-White syndrome. Eur Heart J (in press).
21. Klein GJ, Bashore TM, Sellers TD, Pritchett ELC, Smith WM, Gallagher JJ. Ventricular fibrillation in the Wolff-Parkinson-White syndrome. N Engl J Med. 1979; 301: 1080.
22. García Sánchez S, Guindo J, Bayés de Luna A. Arritmias y estrés psíquico. In Bayés de Luna A. Avances en Electrocardiología. Ed. Doyma. Barcelona 1987.
23. Brackett CD, Powell LH. Psychosocial and physiological predictors of sudden cardiac death after healing of Acute myocardial infarction. Am J Cardiol 1988; 61: 979.

24. Schwartz PJ. The idiopathic long QT syndrome: the need for a prospective registry. Eur Heart J 1983; 4: 529.
25. Leclercq JF, Coumel Ph, Maison-Blanche F *et al.* Mise en evidence des mechanismes determinants de la mort subite. Enquête cooperative portant sur 69 cas enregistrés par le méthode de Holter. Arch Mal Cœur 1986; 79: 1.024.
26. Leclercq JF, Maison Blanche P, Caucheme B, Coumel P. Mechanisms of sudden death during Holter monitoring: a study of 74 cases. In Cosin J, Bayés de Luna A, García Civera R, Cabades A. Cardiac Arrhythmias. Pergamon Press, Oxford 1988.
27. Kleiger RE, Miller J Ph, Bigger JT, Moss AJ. Decreased heart rate variability and its association with increased mortality after acute myocardial infarction. Am J Cardiol 1987; 59: 256.
28. Martí V, Bayés de Luna A. Arriola J. Songa V, Guindo J, Domínguez de Rozas J, *et al.* Value of dynamic QTc in arrhythmology. 8th International Congress: The New Frontier of Arrhythmias. New Trends in Arrhythmia 1988; 4: 683.
29. Maron BJ, Epstein SE, Roberts WC. Causes of sudden death in competitive athletes. J Am Coll Cardiol 1986; 7: 204.
30. Rosenthal ME, Oseran DS, Gang E, Peter T. Sudden cardiac death following acute myocardial infarction. Am Heart J 1985; 109: 865.
31. Janse MJ, Kleber AG, Capucci A, *et al.* Electrophysiological basis for arrhythmias caused by acute ischemia. Role of the subendocardium. J Mol Cell Cardiol 1986; 18: 339—355.
32. Janse MJ. Arrhythmias in the early ischemic period. Rosen MR, Palti Y. En: Lethal arrhythmias resulting from myocardial ischemia and infarction. Ed. Kluwer Academic Publishers. Massachussetts 1989.
33. Meinertz Th. Zehener M, Hohnloser S, Just H. Prevalence of Ventricular arrhythmias during silent myocardial ischemia. CVR & supplement 1988; p. 34.
34. Bayés de Luna A, Carreras F, Cladellas M, Oca F, Sagués F, García Moll M. Holter ECG study of the electrocardiographyc phenomena in Prinzmetal angina attacks with enfasis on the study of ventricular arrhythmias. J Electrocardiol 1985; 18: 267.
35. Théroux P, Waters DD, Halphen C *et al.* Prognostic value of exercised testing soon after myocardial infarction. N Engl J Med 1979; 301: 341.
36. Sharma B, Asinger R, Francis G, *et al.* Demonstration of exercise-induced painless myocardial ischemia in survivors of out-of-hospital ventricular fibrillation. Am J Cardiol 1987; 59: 740.
37. Amsterdam E. Silent myocardial ischemia, arrhythmias and sudden death: Are they related? Am J Cardiol 1987; 59: 740.
38. Meissner M, Morganroth J. Silent myocardial ischemia as a mechanism of sudden cardiac death. Cardiol clin 1986; 4: 593.
39. Bayés de Luna A, Guindo J, Ballester M, Obrador D, Oriol A, Crexells C, Augé JM, Arriola J, Martí V. Sudden death in patients with silent myocardial ischemia. CVR & R Supplement 1988; p. 40.
40. Hong R, Bhandari A, McKay C, *et al.* Life-threatening ventricular tachycardia and fibrillation induced by painless myocardial ischemia during exercise test. JAMA 1987; 257: 1937.
41. Graboys TB, Stein IM, Cueni L, *et al*: Is the prevalence of silent ischemia associated with the provocation of ventricular arrhythmia? (Abstr). Circulation 1987; 76 (Suppl IV): IV-365.
42. Bayés de Luna A, Camacho AM, Guindo J, Torner P, Martinez-Duncker D, *et al.* Is there a relationship between crises of silent ischemia and appearance of ventricular arrhythmias? Abstract. Rev. Lat Cardiol 1989; 10: II-33.
43. Rocco MB, Nabel EG, Campbell S, Goldman L, Barry J, Mead K, Selwyn AP. Prognostic significance of myocardial ischemia detected by ambulatory monitoring in patients with stable coronary artery disease. Circulation 1988; 78: 877.

2. Epidemiology of sudden cardiac death

ARTHUR J. MOSS

Epidemiology is the branch of medial science which deals with incidence, distribution, and control of disease in a population. An epidemiologic approach to the problem of sudden cardiac death should help identify risk groups and risk factors responsible for the disorder, and it should provide insight into the risk mechanisms. The knowledge gained from these population and subgroup studies should provide the foundation for preventive strategies. Epidemiologic data demonstrate that almost 50% of cardiac deaths are sudden, and the annual incidence of sudden cardiac death is more than 300,000 victims in the United States alone. Sudden cardiac death almost always occurs in patients who have underlying heart disease, although a large percentage of the sudden cardiac death occurs in individuals without prior symptoms or signs of an underlying cardiac problem.

Although many chronologic definitions have been used to define the suddenness of cardiac death, for the purposes of this review the 1-hour definition will be utilized. The International Society of Cardiology and the American Heart Association have proposed a 24-hour definition for sudden cardiac death [1], but such a broad temporal definition decreases the percentage of patients with a cardiac cause of death. A 1-hour definition results in a more homogeneous population, and it emphasizes the out-of-hospital occurrence of these sudden cardiac events. Sudden cardiac death also implies that the terminal cardiac event is a primary arrhythmia. In over 90% of the cases the electrical disorder is ventricular fibrillation.

In this review, the epidemiology of sudden cardiac death will be compared and contrasted in children and adults. Three questions come to mind when the problem is approached in this manner. First, what can we learn from the pediatric experience where there is a preponderance of congenital cardiac disorders responsible for sudden cardiac death? Secondly, is there a common thread which links the occurrence of sudden cardiac death in children and adults? And thirdly, are the fundamental cardiac risk factors similar or different in these two populations?

A. Bayés de Luna et al. (eds.): *Sudden Cardiac Death*, 13–17.
© 1991 Kluwer Academic Publishers, Dordrecht.

Sudden cardiac death in children

Epidemiologic studies of sudden cardiac death in children indicate that 75% of the deaths occur in children with known cardiovascular disease who have not had cardiac surgery, 15% in patients who have had prior cardiovascular surgery for congenital or acquired abnormalities, but the death was unrelated to the surgery, and 10% of the sudden cardiac deaths occur during the one-month period following correction or palliation of complex cardiovascular disorders [2]. Approximately 7% of sudden cardiac deaths are unexpected and the children were thought to be well. However, post-mortem examinations almost always uncover an unsuspected cardiac disorder. Approximately half of the sudden cardiac deaths in children occur when the individual is awake but not active, a quarter of the events occur during sports or athletic activities, and a similar quarter of the events occur during sleep.

The pediatric cardiologist sees a different spectrum of causes of sudden cardiac death, then does the general pediatric physician. For example, in a recent report from a leading pediatric cardiology unit, unoperated and operated congenital heart disease accounted for almost 75% of all sudden cardiac death events [3]. The remaining 25% of sudden cardiac deaths occurred in patients who had had a surgical palliation procedure for complex congenital heart disease, acquired heart disease, the long QT syndrome, and a miscellaneous spectrum of rare disease entities. In contrast, the general pediatrician may observe in his practice over the course of many years a few cases of sudden unexpected death in children who were thought to have been well. An analysis of these unexpected events almost always includes hypertrophic obstructive cardiomyopathy, acute myocarditis, coronary anomaly, the long QT syndrome, mitral value prolapse, and the Wolff-Parkinson-White syndrome [4].

Table 1. Classification of sudden cardiac death in children

1. Congenital malformations (90%)
   a. Aortic stenosis or subaortic stenosis
   b. Eisenmenger's syndrome
   c. Ebstein's anomaly
   d. Corrected transposition
   e. Post-op congenital heart disease
   f. Coronary artery anomaly
2. Myocardial disease (7%)
   a. Myocarditis
   b. Hypertrophic cardiomyopathy
   c. Dilated cardiomyopathy
   d. Neuromuscular disorders
   e. Endocardial fibroelastosis
3. Primary electrical disorders (2%)
   a. Long QT syndrome
   b. Wolff-Parkinson White syndrome
   c. Mitral valve prolapse
   d. Heart block
   e. Sinus node dysfunction
4. Other conditions (1%)
   a. Primary pulmonary hypertension
   b. Myocardial tumor
   c. Cocaine
   d. Kawasaki's coronary aneurysms
   e. Medication

A classification of sudden cardiac death in children is presented in Table 1. The eight most common causes of sudden cardiac death in children include, in descending order, surgical palliation for cyanotic congenital heart disease, left to right shunt with Eisenmenger's syndrome, post operative correction of tetralogy of fallot, unoperated tetralogy of fallot, cardiomyopathy, post-op atrio-ventricular canal repair, post-operative Mustard operation for transposition, and the long QT syndrome. This list emphasizes the complex interrelationship between disordered structure, altered blood flow, and malignant arrhythmias.

Sudden cardiac death in adults

A review of the epidemiology of sudden cardiac death in adults indicates that over 90% of such events occur in patients who have underlying coronary heart disease [5, 6]. In addition, almost half of the patients who die suddenly have underlying cardiomegaly and/or left ventricular hypertrophy. Ventricular fibrillation occurs in approximately 25% of patients who sustain acute myocardial infarction. Overt precipitating factors such as vigorous exertion are rarely responsible for the occurrence of sudden cardiac death. Currently, the rate of sudden cardiac death due to coronary disease is declining in parallel with that of total cardiac mortality. A classification of sudden cardiac death in adults is presented in Table 2.

During the past several years, our research group has been involved in the study of patients following myocardial infarction, and we have had the opportunity to look into the problem of sudden cardiac death in this subset [7]. Holter recordings in this patient population have identified an association between the frequency and repetitiveness of ventricular premature beats and

Table 2. Classification of sudden cardiac death in adults

1. Coronary heart disease (90%) a. Acute myocardial infarction b. Post-hospital phase of myocardial infarction c. Ventricular aneurysm d. Ischemic cardiomyopathy	4. Primary electrical disorders (0.5%) a. Long QT syndrome b. Wolff-Parkinson White syndrome c. Mitral valve prolapse
2. Cardiomyopathy (7%) a. Hypertrophic — obstructive and non-obstructive types b. Dilated	5. Other conditions (0.5%) a. Primary pulmonary hypertension b. Cocaine c. Medication
3. Aortic stenosis (2%) a. Rheumatic b. Congenital bicuspid	

the subsequent occurrence of sudden cardiac death. However, this association is not very robust, and the presence of frequent and repetitive ventricular premature beats are associated with a relative risk of sudden cardiac death that is only twice that of patients without these ventricular premature beat features. Myocardial ischemia as opposed to acute myocardial infarction does not seem to contribute a major risk. In contrast, patients with left ventricular dysfunction are at a considerably increased risk for both sudden and non-sudden cardiac death. There is increasing evidence that increased sympathetic nervous system activity contributes to electrical instability [8], especially in patients with disordered left ventricular function. Finally, therapy with beta blockers but not calcium channel blockers is associated with a reduction in sudden cardiac death in the posthospital phase of myocardial infarction.

Epidemiologic conclusions

It should be emphasized that the heart is remarkably resilient to electrical instability. Over the course of a lifetime, one ventricular fibrillation event may occur after three billion heart beats. Secondly, the underlying substrate for sudden cardiac death involves major alteration in cardiac structure and function. In both children and adults, there is usually evidence of extensive myocardial damage and/or ventricular hypertrophy. The pro-arrhythmic effect of certain medications suggests that myocellular membrane dysfunction contributes to electrical instability. Electrophysiologic studies have demonstrated the presence of re-entry circuits in patients with recurrent ventricular tachycardia. Animal studies suggest that the autonomic nervous system plays an important role in altering the threshold for excitability and probably for ventricular fibrillation in patients with underlying myocardial disease.

The trigger responsible for ventricular fibrillation remains elusive. It is unclear why patients develop ventricular fibrillation in the absence of any discernable percipitating factors. It is obvious that subclinical alterations in homeostatic mechanisms must be playing a role. It is reasonable to speculate that exaggerated fluctuations in myocellular membrane currents and un-damped oscillations in the sympathetic and parasympathetic traffic to the heart may be triggering mechanisms for malignant ventricular arrhythmias in the vulnerable heart. Our current fund of knowledge in this area is quite sparse, and additional investigation is needed.

As physicians, we tend to focus on secondary prevention. Such an approach will require improved physiologic risk stratifcation and focused therapy for the disordered physiology. In the adult, a significant reduction in the incidence of sudden cardiac death will be achieved when primary preventive strategies are effective in inhibiting the development of coronary artery artery disease.

References

1. Paul O, Schatz M. On sudden death. Circulation 1971; 43: 7—10.
2. Lambert EC, Menon VA, Wagner HR, Vlad P. Sudden unexpected death from cardiovascular disease in children. Am J Cardiol 1974; 34: 89—96.
3. Garson A Jr. Sudden death in a pediatric cardiology population, 1958—1983. In: Sudden Cardiac Death. Grune & Stratton, Inc. 1985.
4. Manning JA. Sudden, unexpected death in children. Am I Dis Child 1977; 131: 1201—2.
5. Kuller LH. Sudden death-definition and epidemiologic considerations. Prog Cardiovas Dis 1980; 23: 1—12.
6. Liberthson PR, Nagel EL, Hirichman JC, Nussenfeld SR, Blackbourn BD, Davis JR. Pathophysiologic observations in prehospital ventricular fibrillation and sudden death. Circulation 1974; 49: 790—8.
7. Moss AJ, Bigger JT Jr, Odoroff CL. Post-infarct risk stratification. Prog Cardivoas Dis 1987; 29L 389—412.
8. Schwartz PJ, Stone HL. The role of the autonomic nervous system in sudden coronary death. In: Sudden Coronary Death. Annals New York Acad Sciences 1982; 382: 162—180.

3. Out-of-hospital sudden death in Spain

J. COSIN AGUILAR
Research Group Spanish Trial on Sudden Death

Introduction

The Spanish study on sudden death [1] contains three different projects. Project A examines epidemiological aspects of sudden deaths that occur in Spain's non-hospitalized general population. It is impossible in our country to ascertain the SD mortality rate, personal and familiar pathological background, risk factors and general circumstances (place, time, witnesses, etc.) of the SD through official documents like death certificates or hospital records.

The only way, in fact, to detect cases of sudden death was to survey the families of SD victims in the cemetery. The data obtained from this survey could not be compared with data on the general living population collected by direct observation. For this reason parallel to the survey of SD victims, a survey of the families of non-sudden death (NSD) victims was also made. This latter survey provided us with a comparison group.

Project A was begun in the City of Valencia in February, 1986. Other areas of Spain that were incorporated into the project at a later data are: Santiago de Compostela, Vic, Manlleu, Gandia, Xativa and Girona. The statistical analysis of the results from the study of the City of Valencia, the largest population examined, is now near completion. The Santiago study has been completed, and the others are at various different stages of development. The results presented here refer primarily to the City of Valencia (Table 1).

Methods

The epidemiological survey used contained 54 questions, and in all cases the closest suitable of the deceased person was interviewed directly by a physician. The initial study covered 4,718 deaths in the City of Valencia over a one-year period.

The survey was done daily by medical personnel in the Municipal Cemetery of the City of Valencia (which gets 97% of all the burials in this

A. Bayés de Luna et al. (eds.): *Sudden Cardiac Death*, 19–30.

Table 1. Project A. Epidemiology of sudden death in Spain

	Data collection	Data analysis	Population
Vic-Manlleu	Finalized	—	45,593
Santiago	Finalized	Finalized	453,857
Girona	In progress	—	454,042
Xativa	In progress	—	24,427
Gandia	In progress	—	50,094
Valencia	Finalized	In progress	729,419

city). In the other towns studied, data were collected in an equivalent way (from the local registry office in Gandia, Xativa and Girona; from the funeral parlours in Vic and Manlleu; and from the physicians who signed the death certificates in Santiago de Compostela).

The surveys were completed in various ways depending on the circumstances of each case (by telephone, mail, home visit, etc.).

A second phase of the study (in progress at the moment) involves checking the case histories of the SD subjects on our list in the Area Hospitals. In addition an effort is being made to obtain anatomopathological information on the sudden death cases in wich autopsies are done.

Sudden death: Concepts

Sure sudden death (SSD): natural, unexpected and fast (60 minutes with witnesses; 12 hours without witnesses). *Possible sudden death* (PoSD): cases in wich the death certificate suggests SD but it is not known if the terms of the preceding definition are fulfilled. In the present report, all results refer to SSD.

Results

Figure 1 shows the geographical location of the areas under study. Sudden deaths represent between 2.6% (Santiago de Compostela) and 10.2% (Vic and Manlleu) of the total number of deaths in these areas. The sudden death mortality rates in the different areas are very similar, ranging from 24.1/ 100,000 inhabitants/year in Vic and Manlleu and 38.9/100,000 inhabitants/ year in Valencia. The distribution by sex was also very similar in the different studies: in general, 1/3 corresponded to females and 2/3 to males.

The following results refer to the City of Valencia [2]. Table 2 shows the

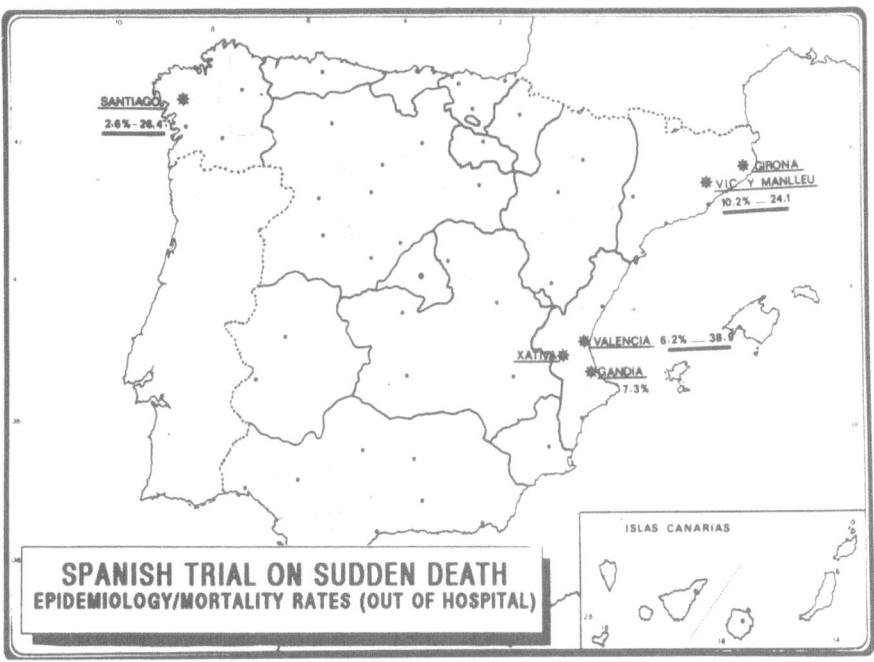

Figure 1. You can see the distribution of sudden death in the cities where it has been studied. The first number means the percentage of sudden death on total death population and the second the sudden death mortality rate per 100,000 inhabitants and per year.

mortality rates by age and sex. In Valencia it was 62.83/100,000 inhabitants/ year for males and 19.54/100,000 inhabitants/year for females.

Age of SD victims

Sudden death is a premature death, and it is more premature in men than in women (Figure 2). The average SD age was 65 for males and 74 for females, whereas the NSD average age was 71 (males) and 76 (females). As can be seen in Figure 2, most deaths among males who are under the age of about 65 are SD, whereas among women there is no age at which SD is prevalent over natural death.

Family history of SD

In 23% of the male SD cases, the victim's immediate family had a history of SD (p < 0.001), whereas this was true of only 12% of female SD victims. Although the latter percentage is higher than that of NSD (9%), it is not

Table 2. SSD mortality rates by age and sex

Age groups	Population	SSD	Incidence
Males			
0—4	20,162	1	4.95
5—9	28,634	—	—
10—14	31,705	—	—
15—19	31,536	1	3.17
20—24	30,124	—	—
25—29	26,427	1	3.78
30—34	23,117	—	—
35—39	23,222	2	8.61
40—44	20,975	4	19.07
45—49	19,880	18	90.54
50—54	20,511	14	68.25
55—59	19,542	16	81.87
60—64	17,402	29	166.64
65—69	12,751	26	203.90
70—74	10,208	27	264.49
+74	11,447	52	454.26
Total	347,643	191	54.94
Females			
0—4	19,069	—	—
5—9	26,965	—	—
10—14	30,212	—	—
15—19	30,080	—	—
20—24	29,308	—	—
25—29	27,178	1	3.67
30—34	25,338	—	—
35—39	25,203	—	—
40—44	22,865	2	8.74
45—49	21,768	1	4.59
50—54	23,072	3	13.00
55—59	23,254	6	25.80
60—64	21,557	2	9.27
65—69	17,966	11	61.22
70—74	15,230	11	72.22
+74	22,711	53	233.36
Total	381,776	90	23.57

statistically significant. Parents (41%), brothers and sisters (46%) are most frequently the relatives who have died of SD (Figure 3).

Personal medical history of SD victims

SD males show increased incidence of ischemic cardiopathy (p < 0.001)

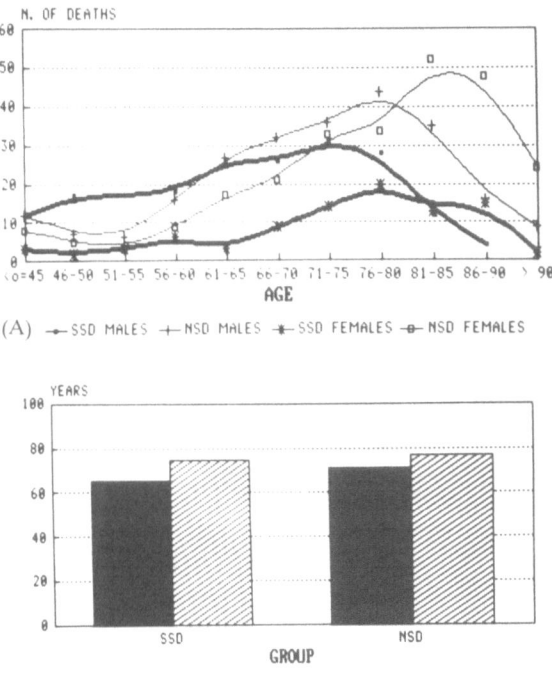

Figure 2. (A) Age of death SSD/NSD (by sex); (B) SSD/NSD mean age (by sex; males: p <
0.001; females: p < 0.001). Abreviations: SSD: Sure Sudden Death; NSD: Non Sudden Death.

and syncope (p < 0.05). A similar pattern is found in females, but in their
case the incidence of syncope is higher (p < 0.001) (Figure 4).

Risk factors in SD

Hypertension (p < 0.001) was the most markedly increased risk factor in
SD victims of both sexes. Dyslipemia was also high both in males (p <
0.001) and females (p < 0.01). The risk involved in smoking was no greater
than in NSD, regardless of the sex of the victim or the amount of tobacco
smoked. Perhaps, tobacco could be considered a risk factor for SD among
young males in our study (Figure 5). Diabetes also did not prove to be a
significant risk factor in SD [3, 4].

SD without antecedents

In 38% of the males and 35% of the females we were able to ascertain that

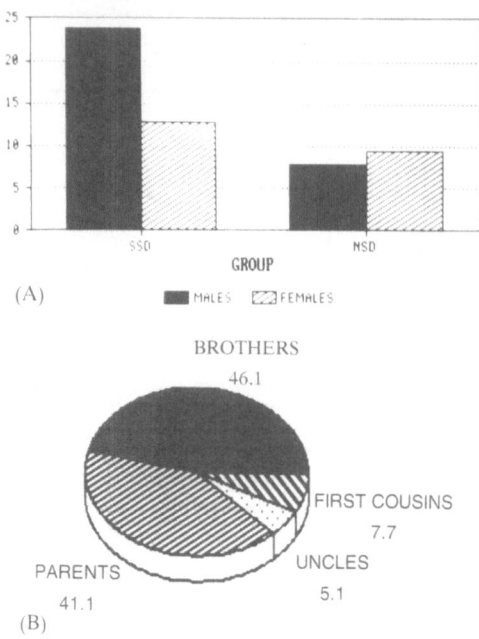

Figure 3. (A) Previous families SD (by sex; males: p < 0.001; females: NS); (B) SD ancestors.

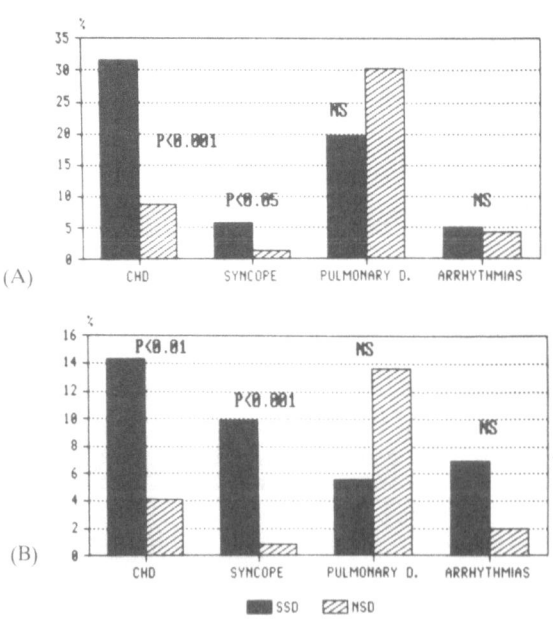

Figure 4. Previous diseases: (A) males; (B) females. Abreviation: CHD: Coronary Heart Disease.

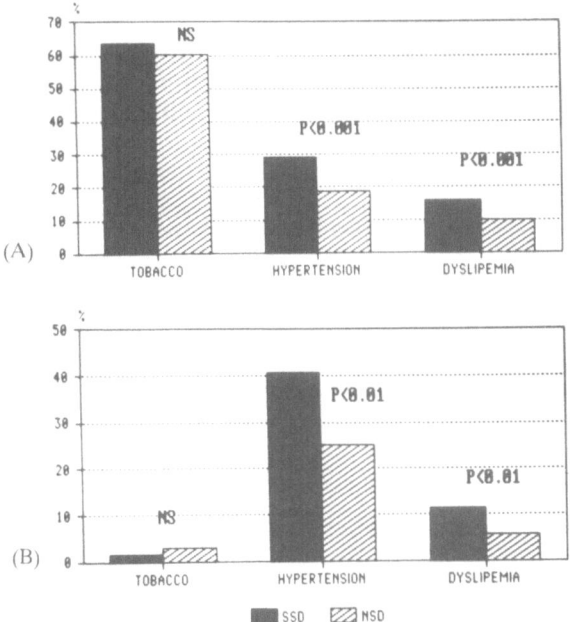

Figure 5. Risk factors: (A) males; (B) females.

no member of the family had died of SD. 43% of the males and 48% of the females had no family history of ischemic cardiopathy (angina or infarction). 9% of the males and 20% of the females had none of the risk factors included in this study. During 15 days prior to SD, 44% of the males and 36% of the females gave no sign of any health problem (Figure 6).

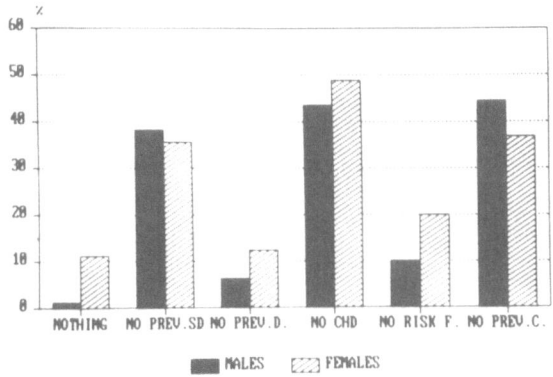

Figure 6. SD-antecedents. Abreviations: *No Prev. SD*: No previous sudden death in family; *No Prev. D*: No previous disease; *No CHD*: No coronary heart disease; *No Risk F*: No risk factors; *No Prev. C*: No previous complaints.

Time of SD

When SD cases were plotted along a period of a year, it was observed that there was an increase between September and January (Figure 7). This datum will have to be verified in future studies.

Most deaths, both sudden and non sudden, occur in the morning or early afternoon (Figure 7).

Place of SD

87% of SD occurred at home (34% in bed) and only 8% in the street or at the victim's place of work. SD outside the home was more common in individuals with a history of syncope (30%). In contrast, NSD usually

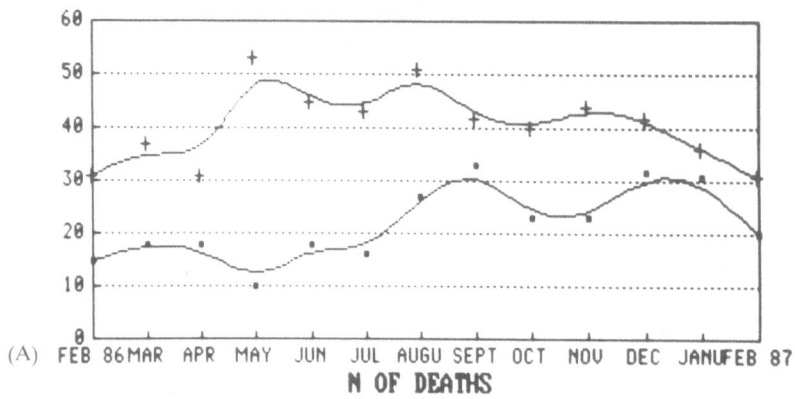

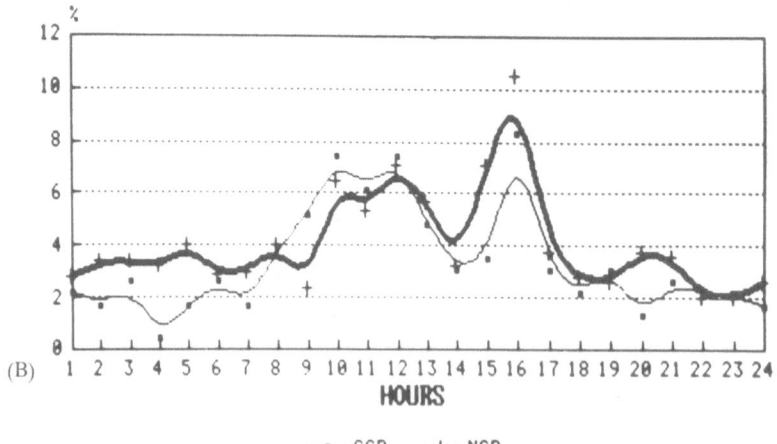

Figure 7. (A) SSD/NSD distribution (months); (B) time of death (SSD/NSD).

occurred in a hospital (62%), while only 37% of NSD died at home (15% in bed), and no NSD occurred in the street, in transport or in the victim's place of work (Figure 8).

These statistics do not include sudden deaths that occurred in a hospital.

Activity at the moment of SD

SD occurs most frequently when the victim is resting (70%). 37% of SD occur when the individual is sleeping, 7% during exercise and 2% while the victim is working. Nevertheless, non sudden deaths never occur during work or exercise. 32% of SD cases with a history of syncope die while doing some kind of exercise; this group cited above that dies outside the home (Figure 9).

Witnesses of SD and resuscitation maneuvers

In 81% of the cases, SD occurred in the presence of witnesses; in 35% of these deaths the witness was the spouse, whereas in 16% the victim's sons and daughters were the witnesses. Resuscitation techniques were applied in only 35% of the cases and they were applied by medical or paramedical personnel in only 26% of the cases. There were no reports of resuscitation being attempted by persons trained specifically in cardiac resuscitation (Figure 10).

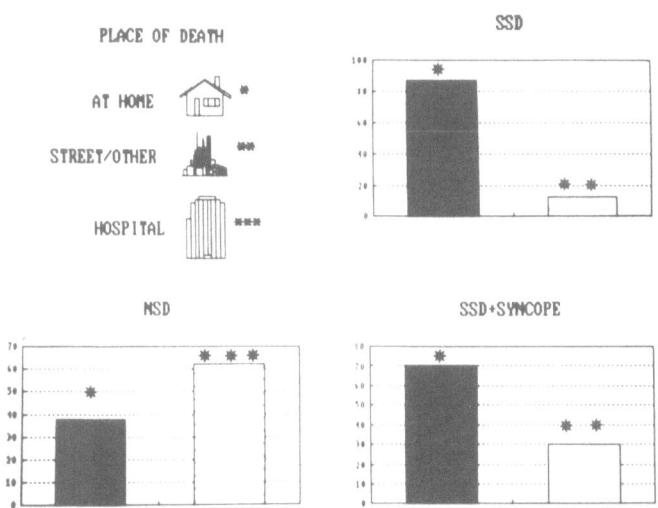

Figure 8. Place of death for people who die, of sure sudden death (SSD), of non sudden death (NSD) and of sure sudden death and before have suffered of syncope.

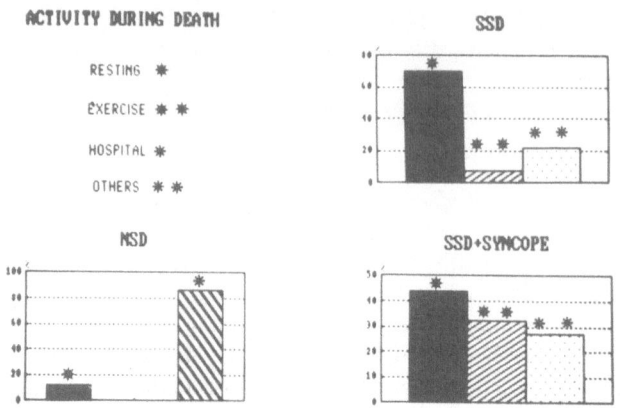

Figure 9. Activity during death in the same grou₊s than in figure number 8. See text.

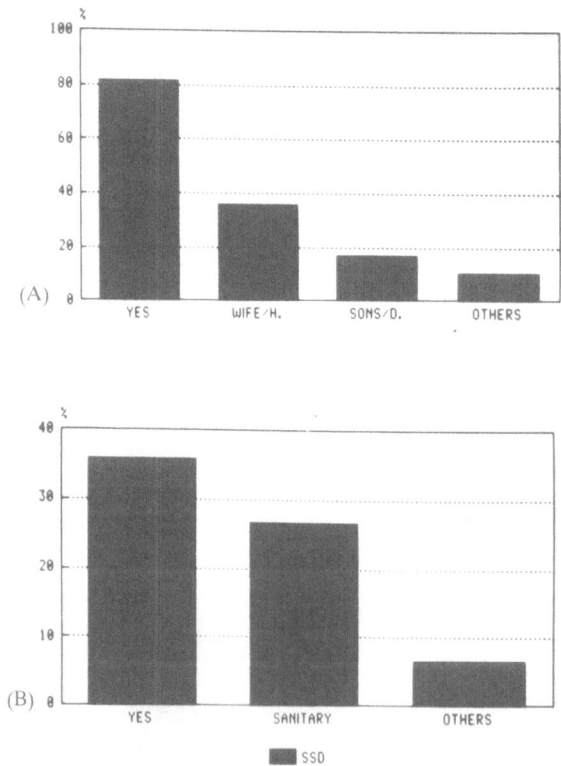

Figure 10. (A) SD witness, (B) attempted resuscitation. Abreviations: Wife/H: Wife or Husband; Sons/D: Sons or Daughters.

Death certificates in SD cases

There are no significant differences between the immediate causes of sudden and non sudden death. In both cases and in both sexes, 70% of the deaths can be attributed to cardiac arrest and cardiac failure (Figure 11).

As far as the underlying cause of death is concerned, in SD the predominance of ischemic cardiopathy is significant, while in NSD cancer is the main underlying cause. This is true of both sexes (Figure 12).

Conclusions

The SD out-of-hospital mortality rates in Valencia, calculated in terms of age and sex, are: 62.8/100,000/year for males 19.5/100,000/year for females.

The total SD mortality rate in Valencia is 42.5/100,000/year.

The incidence of a family history of SD is significanly increased in SD males.

Ischemic cardiopathy and syncope are more frequent in SD than in NSD.

Hypertension and dyslipemia are two risk factors that show a significant increase in the SD population.

Both SD and NSD occur most frequently in the morning or early afternoon.

SD most frequently occurs at home while the subject is resting and in the presence of witnesses. The witnesses are usually the wife and sons.

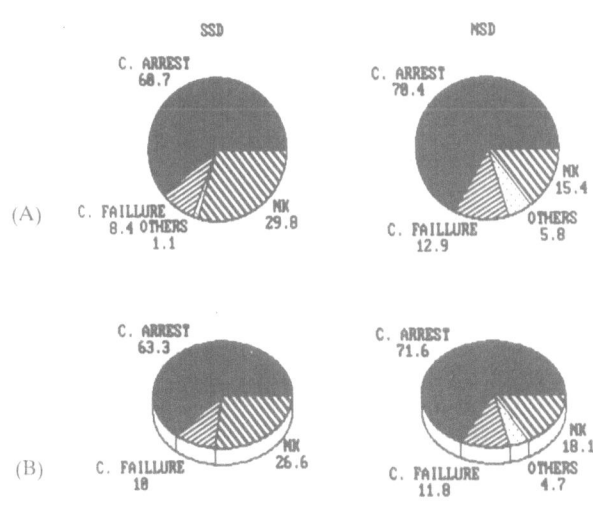

Figure 11. Diagram on death certificates immediate cause: (A) males; (B) females. Abreviations: *C. Arrest*: Cardiac arrest; *C. Failure*: Cardiac failure; *NK*: Non known.

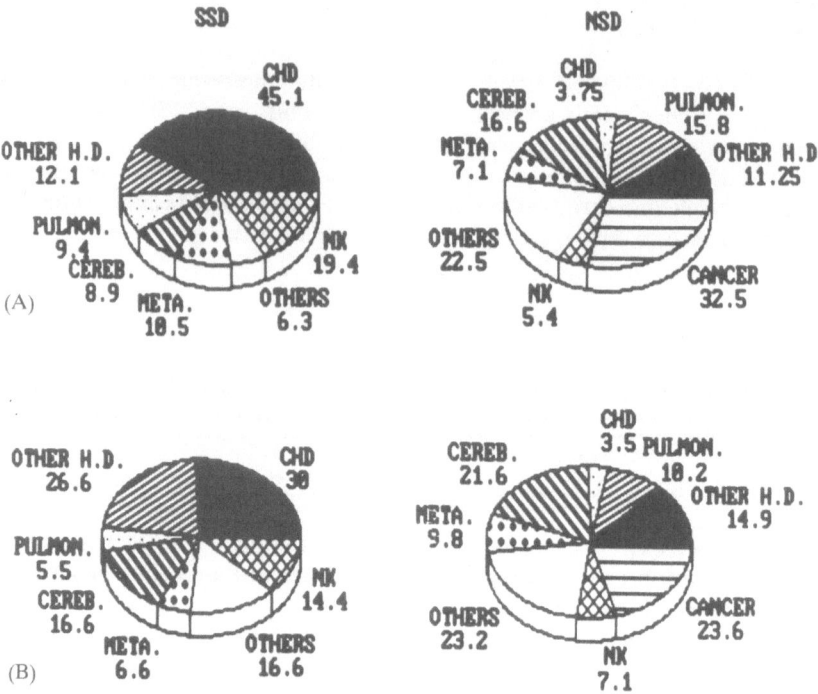

Figure 12: Diagram on death certificates underlying cause: (A) males; (B) females. Abbreviations: *CHD*: Coronary heart disease; *Cereb*: Neurological diseases; *Meta*: Metabolic diseases; *Pulmon*: Pulmonary diseases; *Other HD*: Other heart diseases.

When the subject has a history of syncope, SD often occurs away from home and during exercise.

Our study indicates that resuscitation measures were seldom applied.

References

1. Grupo Investigador del Estudio Español sobre Muerte Súbita. Bayés de Luna A, Cosín Aguilar J (coordinadores): Ensayo clínico multicéntrico sobre la prevención de la muerte súbita con agentes antiarrítmicos en el postinfarto de miocardio. Rev Esp Cardiol 1989; 42: 77—83.
2. Andrés F, Cosín J, Hernándiz A, Caffarena T, Solaz J, Botella P, Seguí J: Características de la muerte subita en la Ciudad de Valencia. XXi Congreso Nacional de Cardiología. Rev Esp Cardiol 1988; 41 (suppl. 1): 87.
3. Hernándiz A, Cosín J, Caffarena T, Solaz J, Andrés F, Botella P: Antecedentes en los muertos súbitos. Rev Esp Cardiol 1989; 42: 84—87.
4. Andrés F, Cosín J, Hernándiz A, Caffarena T, Solaz J, García Civera R, Ruiz R: Muerto súbito-muerto no súbito: características diferenciales. XXI Congreso Nacional de Cardiologia. Rev Esp Cardiol 1988; 41 (suppl. 1): 126.

4. Thrombosis, antithrombotic therapy and sudden death

JOHN H. IP and VALENTIN FUSTER

Emerging pathological and clinical data has allowed us to formulate an evolving concept regarding thrombosis and sudden death. Several fundamental relevant issues need to be addressed before we go on. First, cardiac death is always sudden since it is generally the result of an abrupt electrical phenomenon. The question is when it occurs in term of timing. Four different stages of sudden death can be identified. Second, emphasis on the pathogenic mechanism of sudden death has always been placed on the primary electrical component of the heart related to ventricular function (substrate), accumulating evidence suggests that acute thrombosis and ischemia (isichemia) may also play an important role in sudden death; depending on the stages of sudden death, one or both of these pathogenic mechanisms predominate. Third, in most antithrombotic trials, sudden cardiac death is not properly defined in terms of timing nor in terms of mechanisms. Nevertheless, there is enough information to provide us with the relevant hypothesis. With this background, we will discuss the four different stages of sudden death, the pathogenic mechanisms, and the role of antithrombotic therapy in each stage of sudden death (Table 1).

Stages of sudden cardiac death

Based on the Framingham study, middle aged men have an incidence of clinical coronary artery disease of about 1% per year, sudden death is the first manifestation of the disease accounting for about 13% of these patients [1]. As we will indicate later, such instantaneous and unexpected sudden death — Stage I is, in a majority of these patients, probably ischemic in origin (ischemia). The remaining 87% of the patients have their first manifestation of coronary artery disease as either stable angina, unstable angina or myocardial infarction. We define Stage II sudden death as the event that occurs within the first 4 weeks of the onset of an acute coronary syndrome, more specifically, myocardial infarction or unstable angina. As we will be discussing later, the mechanisms appear to be related to the degree of left

A. Bayés de Luna et al. (eds.): *Sudden Cardiac Death*, 31–40.

Table 1. Antithrombotic therapy in the stages of sudden cardiac death

Stages	Risk of SD	Mechanism	Evolving antithrombotic therapy		
			ASA	A/C	ASA + A/C
I	Low	Ischemia	± [1]	—	—
II	High	Ischemia and substrate	+	+	?
III	Medium	Substrate and ischemia	+ [2]	+	—
IV	Medium	Ischemia	+ [2]	+	—

SD: sudden death, ASA-aspirin, A/C-anticoagulant.
Stage I: No history of coronary artery disease.
Stage II: Unstable angina and myocardial infarction (< 2 months).
Stage III: Myocardial infarction (< 2 years).
Stage IV: Myocardial infarction (> 2 years) and stable coronary disease.
1: High risk males over age of 50.
2: ASA preferred over A/C for long term use because of similar benefit and less risk.

ventricular dysfunction (substrate), the status of the infarct related artery (open or closed) and the risk of re-occlusion (ischemia). Stage III sudden death relates to event that occurs within the first 2 years following myocardial infarction, and as we will discuss later, appears to be related to the functional status of the left ventricle, i.e. absence or presence of SCAR and/ or aneursym (substrate) or to sudden recurrence of acute ischemia or re-infarction (ischemia). Finally, Stage IV relates to patients with coronary artery disease who either have old infarct of more than 2 years or stable coronary artery disease. These patients usually have good ventricular function and the cause of sudden death, as we will discuss later, is probably ischemic in origin (ischemia).

Mechanism of sudden death.

a. *Stage I sudden death.* This stage relates to the syndrome of instantaneous or unexpected sudden death of individuals who did not have known previous manifestations of coronary artery disease. We speculate that this event occurs in the setting of an acute coronary occlusion, usually thrombotic, leading to electrical instability and depending on the availability of microvascular collaterals, subsequent development of fatal arrhythmia can occur. In this context, it is of interest that, animals with good coronary collateral system do not develop ventricular fibrillation following an acute coronary occlusion, but rather an infarction that is not necessarily extensive. Alternately, those with poor collateral circulation, easily manifest ventricular arrhythmia and sudden death following ischemia or an extensive infarction [2].

The single most impressive data that led us to speculate that an acute thrombotic episode accounts for this stage of sudden death derives from several autopsy studies that demonstrate the presence of coronary thrombi in the majority of patients who have this fatal event as their first presentation [3—5]. For example, Davies and coworkers reported in 168 cases of sudden cardiac death; over 72% of the patients had evidence of either mural or occlusive thrombi and plaque rupture in the coronary tree [3]. Interestingly, the presence of old infarcts and severe triple vessel disease in autopsy were associated with the absence of acute coronary events and coronary thrombosis. This suggests that in Stage III sudden death, as will be discussed later, pathogenic factors other than acute thrombosis, i.e. left ventricular function, may play the predominate role. Several other lines of clinical data also provide supportive evidence concerning the role of an acute ischemic event in Stage I sudden death. First, a prominent circadian rhythm in the frequency of sudden death, remarkably similar to that of nonfatal myocardial infarction, have recently been demonstrated [6, 7]. This similarity may suggest that these individuals may have a common pathogenic process, namely plaque rupture and coronary thrombosis. Second, there are 4 major studies demonstrating that over 50% of patients whom were resuscitated from sudden death had Q waves and/or significant cardiac enzymes elevation suggestive of an acute myocardial infarction [8—11]. Third, according to thirteen published secondary prevention trials using aspirin in patients with cerebral vascular disease, thus at high risk of coronary disease, the incidence of sudden death was decreased by 15% while the incidence of nonfatal myocardial infarction was decreased by 35% [12]. This fact points out, again, that sudden death in this population probably has an important thrombotic-ischemic origin. In this context, the recently published Physicians' Health Study demonstrated that the use of aspirin produced a significant 44% reduction in the risk of myocardial infarction in male patients over the age of 50 [13]. Although the incidence of sudden death in this study was very low and the effect of aspirin could not be demonstrated, according to all of the above information, the use of aspirin in high risk asymptomatic male patients over the age of 50 may be justified [14].

b. *Stage II sudden death.* Stage II sudden death relates to the event occurring within the acute phase (< 8 weeks) of an acute coronary syndrome, namely acute myocardial infarction or unstable angina. In the context of an acute myocardial infarction, this period is of particular importance because over 50% of all sudden deaths within the first year of the infarction occur in this period [15]. Three pathogenic factors have been identified and appear to play important roles in stage II sudden death: left ventricular function, the patency of the infarct related artery and the risk of re-occlusion. Left ventricular function is one of the most important independent prognostic indicators for both short and long term survival. Mukharji and coworkers demonstrated that the incidence of sudden death early after acute myocardial infarction was 18% in patients with poor left ventricular function (ejection fraction < 0.4), which is 11 times that of patients with normal function [15]. Similar data has been reported by other groups [16]. The benefit of timely thrombolytic therapy on improving survival in acute myocardial infarction has been unequivocally demonstrated by many large clinical trials. The decrease in early mortality apparently is related, in part, to preservation of left ventricular function. For example, in the European trials such as GISSI-1 and ISIS-2 with more than 15,000 study patients demonstrated a 15–20% improvement in ejection fraction at 4 weeks after myocardial infarction as compared to placebo group while the cardiac mortality decreased by 18–20% [17, 18]. Similarly, trials using TPA showed a comparable improvement in left ventricular function and survival rate [19—21].

Several observations, however, suggest that successful reperfusion may provide beneficial effect even in the absence of improvement of left ventricular function. In the Western Washington trial comparing intra-coronary streptokinase with placebo, reperfusion was achieved in an average of 5 hours after the onset of symptoms. Despite the achievement of successful reperfusion in the majority of the treated patients, this was not associated with improvement of left ventricular function or decrease in infarct size, probably secondary to the relatively late onset of therapy. However, patients who have successful reperfusion demonstrated a lower mortality than those who did not [22]. The improved survival in the treated group appears to be related to whether the infarct-related artery is patent or not. Indeed, patency of the infarct-related vessel has been suggested to be an important independent predictor of survival [23, 24]. It has been demonstrated that, early mortality of patients with anterior wall infarction treated with streptokinase with complete reperfusion of infarct-related artery was only 5% as compared to a mortality of 36% with partial or no reperfusion [23]. Similarly, in the German Multicenter trial of Anisylated Plasminogen Streptokinase Activator Complex (APSAC), the mortality was reduced from 12.6% in the control group to 5.6% in the APSAC-treated patients without an effect on the global left ventricular function [25]. Van de Werf and coworkers also reported that the early mortality was reduced from 5.8% in placebo group to 2.7% in those receiving TPA, yet improvement of left ventricular function was only slight and would not appear to account for the marked reduction in early mortality [21]. The mechanism accounting for the benefical effect of successful reperfusion other than limiting infarct size and the associated deterioration of left ventricular function is not entirely clear. One possibility, as suggested by animal data and clinical observation, is that reperfusion may limit infarct expansion and prevent the resultant left ventricular dilatation and aneurysm formation [26, 27]. Another possibility is that reperfusion may improve electrical stability of the heart. In this context, it has been shown that successful thrombolysis reduces the incidence of ventricular late potentials and early ventricular fibrillation and thus may prevent sudden death following myocardial infarction [28, 29, 30].

Another factor that may play a role in the pathogenesis of Stage II sudden death is coronary re-occlusion following myocardial infarction. Coronary re-occlusion occurs in 10—15% of patients receiving thrombolytic therapy and usually within the first 2 weeks following myocardial infarction and accounts for re-infarction and sudden death [31, 32]. The mechanism of re-occlusion appears to be related to the severity of residual luminal narrowing following thrombolysis and the presence of residual thrombus, a potent thrombogenic surface [31, 32, 33]. Prevention requires inhibition of mechanisms involved in rethrombosis and includes 2 basic principles: 1. thorough lysis, 2. antithrombotic therapy. The first principle involves the use of newer generation and synergistic combination of thrombolytic agents and is beyond the scope of discussion of this chapter. The second principle involves the use of anticoagulants and/or antiplatelet drugs following thrombolysis. The use of anticoagulants in this stage is logical and rountinely used in clinical practice. Although as of the time of this writing, there is no definitive study of the effect of heparin on re-occlusion rate following thrombolysis, several retrospective studies have indicated that the use of anticoagulants during the first month following myocardial infarction may reduce in-hospital mortality [34, 35, 36]. Indeed, a recently published prospective, randomized trial demonstrated the use of high dose subcutaneous heparin and intravenous streptokinase in patients with acute myocardial infarction produced a 50% reduction of in-hospital cardiac mortality as compared with the use of streptokinase alone [37]. The use of aspirin following thrombolysis also appears to be of benefit. In the ISIS-2 study, there was a higher reduction in 5-week mortality in patients allocated to streptokinase plus aspirin than in patients allocated either to streptokinase or aspirin alone [18]. Although there are no data on the association of aspirin administration and the prevention of re-occlusion, the results of this study may reflect a beneficial effect of aspirin in preventing platelet activation and probably re-occlusion.

In patients with acute myocardial infarction but were not given thrombolytic therapy, the use of antithrombotic agents have also been demonstrated to be of benefit. In the pre-thrombolysis era, Chalmers and coworkers performed a meta-analysis of 6 randomized trials and demonstrated that the use of anticoagulants in patients with acute myocardial infarction reduced cardiac mortality by 21% [38]. Similarly, in a recent analysis of pooled data of several clinical trials, the use of aspirin and/or an anticoagulant reduced vascular death by 16%, nonfatal re-infarction by 22%, and stroke by 51% (Personal communication, P. Sleight). In addition, in the ISIS-2 trial, patients with suspected myocardial infarction treated within 24 hours of onset with aspirin alone had a 23% reduction in 5-week vascular mortality compared with those given placebo [18]. This dramatic effect was possibly related to prevention of re-infarction in patients with spontaneous vessel re-canalization. Indeed, aspirin reduced the rate of re-infarction by almost half [18]. Finally, in the most recently published Italian study, the use of high dose subcutaneous heparin in patients who did not receive thrombolysis reduced cardiac mortality by 34% as compared to placebo [37].

In the context of unstable angina, the beneficial effect of antithrombotic therapy in reducing sudden death in this group of patients is well defined. The Veterans Adminstration Cooperative Study found a 51% collective reduction in mortality and nonfatal myocardial infarction with aspirin during a period of 12 weeks [39]. The Canadian multicenter trial corroborated these findings using higher aspirin dosage for a mean of 18 months. An identical 51% reduction of myocardial infarction and cardiac death was found [40]. The use of anticoagulants in unstable angina is equally advocated based on the similar beneficial effects obtained in the reduction of cardiac mortality [41, 42]. Nevertheless, a substantial proportion of these patients develop myocardial infarction despite treatment with one agent or the other, there is a pressing need to test combinations of antiplatelet agents and anticoagulant which may offer better protection.

In summary, the pathogenic mechanisms of stage II sudden death appear to be related to the functional status of left ventricular function (substrate), the patency of the infarct-related vessel (substrate and ischemia), and the risk of re-occlusion (ischemia). Based on emerging clinical evidence, the use of low dose aspirin is justified within the first 4 weeks of an acute myocardial infarction. The use of anticoagulants in this stage may add additional benefit, however due to the higher risk of bleeding complications, the combined use of aspirin and anticoagulants cannot be advocated at this time. Similarly, in patients with unstable angina, the combined use of antiplatelet agent and anticoagulant is probably better then either agent alone, but further clinical trials are needed to define the risk and benefit ratio.

c. *Stage III sudden death.* Stage III sudden death relates to the event occurring within the first 2 years of myocardial infarction. Within this period, the most important risk factor for occurrance of sudden death is left ventricular dysfunction. However, acute ischemia secondary to thrombosis also may play a role in this stage of sudden death, as illustrated by the result of the recently published meta-analysis of more than 10 randomized trials involving platelet inhibitors in patients with prior myocardial infarction [12]. Despite the inherent problems of pooled data, this overview concluded that among survivors of myocardial infarction, platelet inhibitors reduced vascular mortality by 13%, nonfatal re-infarction by 31%, nonfatal stroke by 42%. Of interest, the use of anticoagulant also reduces the incidence of sudden death in this group of patients as demonstrated by a resent randomized, placebo-controlled, long term follow-up trial showing a 35% reduction of cardiac mortality and a 41% reduction of re-infarction rate in patients receiving coumadin as compared to placebo [43]. Until more data are available, the use of aspirin may offer several advantages over long term anticoagulants in cost, ease of administration, and side effect. The use of combined antiplatelet agents and anticoagulants is probably not advised at this time because of the significant incidence of bleeding complications.

d. *Stage IV sudden death.* Stage IV sudden death relates to the event occurring in patients with remote history of myocardial infarction and good ventricular function and in patients with chronic coronary artery disease with also good ventricular function. Sudden deaths in these cases are probably ischemic in origin and related to thrombotic occlusion. Most studies of platelet inhibitors in survivors of myocardial infarction have shown a beneficial trend toward lower mortality, which became significant only when the data derived from all trials are pooled [12]. As for anticoagulant therapy, the Sixty-Plus Reinfarction study demonstrated a 26% reduction in cardiac mortality and a 55% reduction in re-infarction in patients receiving coumadin as compared to placebo [44]. Although no randomized trial of antithrombotic therapy in chronic stable angina has been published, the sustained beneficial effects of aspirin in patients with unstable angina suggest a role for aspirin in stable angina. Indeed, preliminary evidence from an angiographic study in patients with stable angina demonstrated that platelet inhibitors reduced the incidence of myocardial infarction and new atheromatous lesion formation [45]. Probably one can conclude that for the prevention of stage IV sudden death, aspirin and anticoagulant have the same beneficial effect. Although the combination of both would probably be of antithrombotic advantage, this cannot be advised because of the higher rate of bleeding complications seen during long term administration of this combination.

Antithrombotic therapy

For the understanding of the pathogenesis and prevention of sudden death in patients with coronary artery disease, it is important to distinguish four stages of sudden death because each have different pathogenesis in terms of ischemia, substrate or the the combination of both as the primary cause.

In stage I sudden death, which relates to event occurring in individuals without a prior history of cardiac disease, the use of aspirin in previously asymptomatic high risk male patients over the age of 50 is probably justified. Anticoagulant at low dose is presently being tested on a large British study.

In stage II sudden death, which relates to event occurring within 4 weeks of an acute coronary syndrome, specifically acute myocardial infarction, the combined use of thrombolytic agents early in the course along with aspirin during the first month appears to be mandatory. In addition, there is increasing evidence that the concommitant use of an anticoagulant during this period may be of additional benefit, but we cannot advocate the use at this time because of the high risk of bleeding complication. In the subset of patients with acute myocardial infarction who did not receive thrombolytic therapy, the use of antiplatelet agents or anticoagulants is advised. Similarly, in patients with unstable angina, the combined use of antiplatelet agent and anticoagulant may be better than either one alone, but we continue to advise the use of either one agent until the long term risk is more defined.

In stage III sudden death, which entails the first two years following myocardial infarction, the degree of left ventricular dysfunction secondary to scarring plays the most important role. However, there is evidence that the use of aspirin may be of benefit in the proportion of sudden deaths that are due to ischemia. Anticoagulants appear to be of similar benefit but they have a higher risk of bleeding complications and for this reason, the combined use of aspirin and anticoagulant for this long term therapy is not warranted.

In stage IV sudden death, which relates to event occurring in patients with a remote history of myocardial infarction or with chronic stable coronary artery disease, the use of aspirin or anticoagulant appear to be of similar benefit and the use of aspirin alone is advised because of a lower incidence of bleeding.

In summary, an evolving concept of cardiac sudden death has emerged. 4 stages of sudden death with respect to different timing and pathogenic mechanisms can be identified. Recognition of the role of myocardial substrate, ischemia (particularly thrombosis) or both in the pathogenesis of each stage of sudden death has allowed us to formulate a strategy, that outlines the specific use of antithrombotic therapy, in the prevention of sudden death.

Reference

1. Kannel WB, Feinlieb M: The natural history of angina pectoris in the Framingham study. Am J Cardiol 1972; 29: 154—163.
2. White FC, Bloor CM: Coronary collateral circulation in the pig: correlation of collateral flow with coronary bed size. Basic Res Cardiol 1981; 76: 189—196.
3. Davies MJ, Bland JM, Hangartner RW, Angelini A, Thomas AC: Factors influencing the presence or absence of acute coronary thrombi in sudden ischemic death. Eur Heart J 1989; 10: 203—208.
4. Fawal MA, Berg GA, Wheatley DJ, Harland WA: Sudden coronary death in Glasgow: nature and frequency of acute coronary lesions. Br Heart J 1987; 57: 329—335.
5. Davies MJ, Thomas AC: Thrombosis and acute coronary artery lesions in sudden cardiac ischemic death. N Engl J Med 1984; 310: 1137—1140.
6. Muller JE, Ludmer PL, Willich SN, Tofler GH, Aylmer G, Klangos I, Stone P: Circadian variation in the frequency of sudden cardiac death. Circulation 1987; 75: 131—138.
7. Miller JE, Stone PH, Turi ZG: Circadian variation in the frequency of onset of acute myocardial infarction. N Eng J Med 1985; 313: 1315—1322.
8. Myerburg RJ, Conde CA, Sung RJ: Clinical, electrophysiological and hemodynamic profile of patients resuscitated from pre-hospital cardiac arrest. Am J Med 1980; 68: 568—576.
9. Baum RS, Alvarez H, Cobb LA: Survival after resuscitation from out-of-hospital ventricular fibrillation. Circulation 1974; 50: 1231—1235.
10. Liberthson PR, Nagel EL, Hirshman JC, Nussenfeld SR, Blackbourne BD, Davis JH: Pathophysiologic observations in prehospital ventricular fibrillation and sudden cardiac death. Circulation 1974; 49: 790—798.
11. Goldstein S, Landis JR, Leighton R: Characteristics of the resuscitated out-of-hospital cardiac arrest victims with coronary heart disease. Circulation 1981; 64: 977—984.
12. Antiplatelet Trialists' Collaboration: Secondary prevention of vascular disease by prolonged antiplatelet treatment. Br Heart J 1988; 192: 320—332.
13. Steering Committee of the Physicians' Health Study Research Group: Final report on the

aspirin component of the ongoing Physicians' Health Study. N Engl J Med 1989; 321: 129—135.

14. Fuster V, Cohen MC, Halperin J: Aspirin in the prevention of coronary disease. N Engl J Med 1989; 321: 183—185.

15. Mukharji J, Rude RE, Poole K, Gustafson N, Thomas LJ, Strauss WH, Muller J, Roberts R, Raabe DS, Croft CH, Passamani E, Braunwald E, Willerson JT and the MILIS Study Group: Risk factors for sudden death after acute myocardial infarction: two year follow-up. Am J Cardiol 1984; 54: 31—36.

16. Schulze RA, Strauss WH, Pitt B: Sudden death in the year following myocardial infarction. Am J Med 1977; 62: 191—199.

17. Gruppo Italiano per lo Studio della Streptochinasi nell' Infarto Miocardica (GISSI): Long term effects of intravenous thrombolysis in acute myocardial infarction: final report of the GISSI study. Lancet 1987; 2: 871—874.

18. ISIS-2 (Second International Study of Infarct Survival) collaborative group: Randomized trial of intravenous streptokinase, oral aspirin, both or neither among 17, 187 cases of suspected acute myocardial infarction: ISSIS-2. Lancet 1988; 2: 349—356.

19. O'Rourke M, Baron D, Keogh A: Limitation of myocardial infarction by early infusion of recombinant tissue-type plasminogen activator. Circulation 1988; 77: 1311—1315.

20. National Heart Foundation of Australia Coronary Thrombolysis Group: Coronary thrombolysis and myocardial salvage by tissue-type plasminogen activator given up to 4 hours after onset of myocardial infarction. Lancet 1988; 1: 203—207.

21. Van de Werf F, Arnold AEF and the European Cooperative Study Group for Recombinant Tissue-type Plasminogen Activator: Intravenous tissue type plasminogen activator and size of infarct, left ventricular function and survival in acute myocardial infarction. Br Med J 1988; 297: 1374—1379.

22. Kennedy JW, Ritchie JL, Davis KB: The Western Washington Randomized trial of intracoronary streptokinase in acute myocardial infarction. A 12 month follow-up report. N Engl J Med 1985; 312: 1073—1078.

23. Stadius ML, Davis KB, Maynard C, Ritchie JL, Kennedy JW: Risk stratification for 1 year survival based on characteristics identified in the early hours of acute myocardial infarction. Circulation 1986; 74: 703—711.

24. Braunwald E: Myocardial reperfusion, limitation of infarct size, reduction of left ventricular dysfunction, and improved survival. Should the paradigm be expanded? Circulation 1989; 79: 441—444.

25. Meinertz T, Kasper W, Schumacher M, Just H and APSAC Multicenter Trial Group: The German multicenter trail of anisylated plasminogen streptokinase activator complex versus heparin for acute myocardial infarction. Am J Cardiol 1988; 62: 347—351.

26. Hochman JS, Choo H: Limitation of myocardial infarct expansion by reperfusion independant of myocardial savage. Circulation 1987; 75: 299—306.

27. Pfeffer MA, Lases GA, Vaughan DE, Parisi AF, Braunwald E: Progressive ventricular dilatation following anterior myocardial infarction: effects of captopril. N Engl J Med 1988; 319: 186—201.

28. Gang E, Hong M, Wong M, Velasquez I, Nalos P, Myers M, Lew AS: Does reperfusion influence the incidence of ventricular late potentials in acute myocardial infarction (abstract). Circulation 1987; 76 (suppl IV): 342.

29. Vermeer F, Simoons ML, Lubsen J: Reduced frequency of ventricular fibrillation after early thrombolysis in myocardial infarction. Lancet 1986: 1: 1147—1148.

30. Gang Es, Lew AS, Hong M, Wang FZ, Sielbert CA, Peter T: Decreased incidence of ventricular late potential after successful thrombolytic therapy for acute myocardial infarction. N Engl J Med 1989; 321: 712—716.

31. Heras M, Chesebro JH, Thompson PL, Fuster V: Prevention of early and late rethrombosis and further strategies after coronary reperfusion. In: Thrombolysis in Cardiovascular Disease. Julian D, Kubler W, Norris RM, Swan HJC, Collen D, Verstraete M (eds). Dekker, New York 1989, pp. 203—231.

32. Fuster V, Stein B, Badimon L, Chesebro JH: Antithrombotic therapy after myocardial reperfusion in acute myocardial infarction. J Am Coll Cardiol 1988; 12 (suppl A): 78A—84A.
33. Grines CL, Topol EJ, Bates ER, Juri JE, Walton JA, O'Nell WW: Infarct vessel status after intravenous tissue plasminogen activator and acute coronary angioplasty: prediction of clinical outcome. Am Heart J 1988; 115: 1—7.
34. Modan B, Shani M, Schor S: Reduction of hospital mortality from acute myocardial infarction by anticoagulant therapy. N Engl J Med 1975; 292: 1359—1362.
35. Tonascia J, Gordis L, Schmerler H: Retrospective evidence favoring the use of anticoagulants for myocardial infarction. N Engl J Med 1975; 292: 1362—1367.
36. Szkla M, Tonascia JA, Goldberg R: Additional data favoring the use of anticoagulant therapy in myocardial infarction. JAMA 1979; 242: 1261—1267.
37. The SCATI Group: Randomized controlled trial of subcutaneous calcium-heparin in acute myocardial infarction. Lancet 1989; 2: 182—186.
38. Chalmere TC, Matta RJ, Smith H Jr: Evidence favoring the use of anticoagulants in the hospital phase of acute myocardial infarction. N Engl J Med 1977; 297: 1091—1096.
39. Lewis HD, Davis JW, Archiband DG, Steinke WE, Smitherman TC, Doherty JE, Schapper HW, LeWinter MM, Linares E, Pouget JM, Sabbarwal SC, Chester E, DeMots H: Protective effects of aspirin against myocardial infarction and death in men with unstable angina. Results of a Veteran Adminstration Cooperative Study. N Engl J Med 1983; 309: 396-403.
40. Cairns JA, Gent M, Singer J, Finnie KL, Froggatt GM, Holder DA, Jablonsky G, Koster WJ, Melendez LJ, Myers MG, Sackett DL, Sealy BJ, Tanser PH: Aspirin, sulfinpyrazone, or both in unstable angina. N Engl J Med 1985; 31: 1369—1375.
41. Theroux P, Ouimet H, McCans J, Latour JG, Joly P, Levy G, Pelletier E, deCruise P, Pelletier GB, Rinzler D, Waters DD: Aspirin, heparin, or both to treat acute unstable angina. N Engl J Med 1988; 319: 1105—1111.
42. Telford AM, Wilson C: Trial of heparin versus atenolol in prevention of myocardial infarction in intermediate coronary syndrome. Lancet 1981; 1: 1225—1228.
43. Smith P, Arnesen H: Oral anticoagulants reduce mortality, reinfarction and cerebral vascular events after myocardial infarction. WARIS Study (abstract). Eur Heart J 1989; 264.
44. Report of the Sixty Plus Reinfarction Study Research Group: A double blind trial to assess long term oral anticoagulant therapy in elderly patients after myocardial infarction. Lancet 1980; 2: 989—993.
45. Chesebro JH, Webster MW, Smith HL, Frye RL, Holmes DR, Reeder GS, Nishimera RA, Clements I, Bardsley WI, Grill DE, Fuster V: Antiplatelet therapy in coronary disease progression: reduced infarction and new lesion formation (abstract). Circulation 1989; 80 (suppl II): II-266.

5. The potential for antiarrhythmic drugs to reduce mortality from sudden cardiac death

J. THOMAS BIGGER, JR.

In this article, we will discuss the evidence that antiarrhythmic drug treatment improves outcome, (i.e., prevents symptomatic ventricular arrhythmias and sudden cardiac death) and how to evaluate antiarrhythmic drug therapy for patients with malignant ventricular arrhythmias. Then, we will discuss previously completed and ongoing trials of antiarrhythmic drug treatment in patients with potentially malignant ventricular arrhythmias. We will not discuss the potential of beta adrenergic blocking drugs to prevent sudden cardiac death because Dr. Van Durme has discussed this in detail elsewhere [55] We will separate the ventricular arrhythmias into malignant and potentially malignant (see Morganroth [22]).

Prediction of antiarrhythmic drug efficacy in patients with malignant ventricular arrhythmias

There have been a number of studies to show that drugs that prevent initiation of ventricular tachycardia (VT) or ventricular fibrillation during programmed ventricular stimulation have a high degree of efficacy during long-term follow-up whereas those that do not prevent sustained ventricular arrhythmias are associated with a much higher rate of arrhythmia recurrence and sudden death during long-term follow-up [1—12]. One group has reported that a programmatic evaluation using ECG monitoring, 24-hour ECG recording, and exercise testing also has predictive accuracy for long-term efficacy of drug therapy for malignant ventricular arrhythmias [13—17].

Selection of long-term drug treatment for malignant ventricular arrhythmias

The efficacy of antiarrhythmic drug treatment has been demonstrated for patients with malignant ventricular arrhythmias, i.e., sustained VT or cardiac arrest due to ventricular fibrillation. More and more patients with malignant ventricular arrhythmias are salvaged from their initial event by prehospital emergency medical systems. Patients who are resuscitated after an episode of

A. Bayés de Luna et al. (eds.): *Sudden Cardiac Death*, 41–62.
© 1991 Kluwer Academic Publishers, Dordrecht.

sustained VT have a recurrence rate for sustained ventricular arrhythmias of
25—50% per year and many recurrences are fatal. Thus, these patients
require aggressive treatment. The first approach to treatment is antiarrhythmic drugs. Arbitrary drug therapy, i.e., giving a patient an antiarrhythmic
drug without evaluation of efficacy is associated with high recurrence and
with fatality rates and is therefore unacceptable. Drug/dose finding in
patients with malignant ventricular arrhythmias should be evaluated with
rigorous methods shown to have excellent predictive accuracy for a good
long-term clinical response. Patients with malignant ventricular arrhythmias
are admitted to hospital and monitored continuously while a search is made
for a reversible or temporary cause for the arrhythmia, e.g., myocardial
infarction, electrolyte derangement, or drug toxicity. If no reversible cause
is found, further workup should proceed under the assumption that the
arrhythmia will recur. Antiarrhythmic drugs should be discontinued and
baseline evaluation done that includes 48 hours of continuous ECG recording, exercise testing, and an electrophysiologic study. In addition, left ventricular function and coronary anatomy should be evaluated. If sustained
ventricular tachycardia is recurring several times a day, then treatment
should be guided with ECG recordings and exercise testing. This situation is
rare. If ventricular ectopic activity is infrequent, e.g., averages less than 10
VPD per hour over the 48 hour recording period, treatment should be
guided by electrophysiologic studies. This situation is common. The standard
method for drug/dose finding is endocardial electrical stimulation (programmed ventricular stimulation) [1—12]. Recent studies suggest that a
programmatic non-invasive approach using 24-hour continuous ECG recordings and exercise tests also can be used to evaluate treatment of
malignant ventricular arrhythmias [13—17].

Sequencing tests and drugs for malignant ventricular arrhythmias

The rationale and process of evaluating drug efficacy in malignant ventricular
arrhythmias is similar for the non-invasive method and the invasive electrophysiologic method [4, 5, 13, 18]. With either method, the patient is
stabilized and baseline drug-free studies are done to determine the biologic
nature of the arrhythmia and the techniques that can be used to evaluate the
patient. Patients who are not evaluable by one method are evaluated by the
alternate method or are treated empirically. Patients who are evaluable are
then tested with a series of drugs until the efficacy criteria are satisfied. For
the non-invasive method, efficacy usually is defined as a 50 to 80% reduction
in VPD frequency, 80—90% reduction in paired VPD and a 90—100%
reduction in runs of unsustained ventricular tachycardia (3 or more consecutive VPDs) [13, 18]. When a drug or drug combination is predicted to be
successful by these criteria, the patient is discharged on this regimen and
followed.

The criterion for efficacy using programmed ventricular stimulation is conversion of inducible, sustained ventricular tachycardia to unsustained or no ventricular tachycardia. There is some variability in the definition of ventricular tachycardia among clinical electrophysiology laboratories: >10 complexes, >100 complexes, >15 seconds, and >30 seconds have all been used. At present, there is no theoretical or experimental basis for choosing among these definitions. Excellent long-term results can be expected when a drug renders ventricular arrhythmias uninducible. Some other electrophysiologic endpoints have been used to define drug efficacy e.g., increased difficulty in inducing sustained ventricular tachycardia [19], or induction of a slower, better tolerated ventricular tachyarrhythmia [11, 12].

The most convincing evidence that changing the characteristics of the induced VT can be used as a predictor of favorable long-term outcome was reported by Waller *et al.* who studied 258 patients who had inducible sustained VT or ventricular fibrillation. [12]. The two most common etiologic forms of heart disease were coronary heart disease, 210 patients (81%), and cardiomyopathy, 19 patients (11%). At the baseline study, the induced arrhythmia was sustained VT in 221 patients (86%) and ventricular fibrillation in 37 patients (14%). Severe symptoms were present in 241 patients (93%) during tachycardia in the baseline study. These authors found that slowing of the ventricular arrhythmia (an increase in cycle length $\geqslant 100$ msec) and lack of severe symptoms during the induced arrhythmia predicted a good long-term outcome. For patients with ventricular fibrillation, the absolute cycle length of the VT had to be 300 msec or greater during drug treatment. Severe symptoms were defined as syncope, near syncope, dizziness, angina, or dyspnea. Using these responses, the patients were divided into three groups:

1) those who were rendered uninducible (n = 103);
2) those who remained inducible but had a response considered beneficial (n = 51); and
3) those who had no benefit predicted (n = 104).

Patients were followed up to three years (mean of 21 months).

Table 1 shows the follow-up findings in the three groups. The patients

Table 1. Response to electrophysiologic drug testing and outcome (from Waller *et al.* [12])

Drug response	N	Recurrence of sustained ventricular arrhythmia	Total mortality	Sudden cardiac death*
Uninducible	103	7%	13%	3%
Beneficial	51	39%	12%	4%
No benefit	104	50%	39%	34%

* Unexpected, witnessed death occurring within one hour of the onset of symptoms not otherwise explained. Patients who were resuscitated from cardiac arrest also were considered as sudden cardiac deaths. These events occurred during an average follow-up of 21 months.

who became non-inducible had a low rate of recurrence of VT and a low mortality rate. Patients who were inducible but showed a beneficial response had a high rate of recurrence of VT, but a low mortality rate. Patients who showed no beneficial response had a high rate of recurrence of VT and a high mortality rate. Half of the patients were treated with amiodarone alone, 37% with a drug with class I action alone, and the remainder with drug combinations or other classes of drugs. The response to programmed ventricular stimulation was as predictive for amiodarone as for other drugs. It is interesting that neither the increase in VT cycle length nor the change in severity of symptoms during tachycardia alone was predictive of clinical outcome. Thus, the combined endpoint seemed necessary for accurate prediction. The recommendation made on the basis of these findings is that patients who remain inducible on drugs and do not have a beneficial response should be treated with an automatic implantable cardioverter defibrillator or with surgical ablation. Patients who remain inducible but have a beneficial drug response can be treated with the drug that slows their tachycardia and renders them asymptomatic. However, half of these patients will experience a non-fatal recurrence of their tachycardia within one year. The follow-up results reported by Waller *et al.* [12] for the softer efficacy endpoints are promising but need additional study and independent validation.

The usual sequence for drugs that are tested in patients with malignant ventricular arrhythmias is substantially different from the sequence used in benign or potentially malignant ventricular arrhythmias [20]. For malignant ventricular arrhythmias, the following sequence is as follows:

sotalol or class IA → class IA + IB → class IC → amiodarone.

Typically, sotalol or quinidine is followed by a combination like quinidine and mexiletine, followed by encainide, flecainide, or propafenone, and, finally, amiodarone. dl-Sotalol is an interesting drug that will be marketed in the United States in the near future. This drug has class II (beta blockade) and class III antiarrhythmic action [21]. It is more likely than either class I drugs or amiodarone to render patients with malignant ventricular arrhythmias uninducible; it will convert about 40% versus about 20%. Drugs with class IC action are used later in the treatment sequence in patients with malignant ventricular arrhythmias because, although they are more efficacious than IA drugs, they also are more likely to aggravate the arrhythmia and left ventricular dysfunction [22, 23]. These latter adverse effects are disease related. For patients with benign arrhythmias or patients with potentially malignant ventricular arrhythmias without severe left ventricular dysfunction, drugs with class IC action are least likely to aggravate ventricular arrhythmias. For patients with benign ventricular arrhythmias and for most patients with potentially malignant ventricular arrhythmias, aggravation of left ventricular dysfunction is not an issue. Amiodarone is used last because of its frequent and severe toxicity [24].

Patients in whom drugs cannot be evaluated

About 10% of patients with malignant ventricular arrhythmias are not evaluable with either non-invasive or electrophysiologic methods, i.e., have low frequency of spontaneous ventricular ectopic activity and are not inducible by programmed ventricular stimulation [25, 26]. This situation is much more common in survivors of cardiac arrest due to ventricular fibrillation than in patients who have had recurrent, sustained ventricular tachycardia. Patients who are not evaluable by either the Holter/exercise method or the electrophysiologic method present difficult judgements. Patients who have ischemia demonstrated on exercise/perfusion studies should be revascularized aggressively with percutaneous transluminal coronary angioplasty (PTCA) or coronary artery bypass graft surgery on the likelihood that an ischemic episode may have been responsible for the cardiac arrest. This approach is encouraged further if ischemic symptoms preceded the cardiac arrest and left ventricular function is good. Patients with previous myocardial infarction, poor left ventricular function, and, particularly those with left ventricular aneurysms, are more likely to have had a scar-related sustained ventricular arrhythmia. Additional attempts should be made to induce them, including stimulation of left ventricular sites and use of maneuvers that increase cardiac sympathetic activity, e.g., isoproterenol infusion [27]. If none of these maneuvers elicits a sustained arrhythmia, the most effective empirical treatment should be selected. For patients with coronary heart and previous myocardial infarction, this usually is the automatic implantable cardioverter defibrillator. Currently, this is not an approved indication for the device, but it should be.

Are all drugs evaluable by acute drug testing?

The concern has been raised that some drugs may not be evaluable by the tests that are used currently to predict efficacy, i.e., that the predictive value of either 24-hour continuous ECG recordings or electrophysiologic studies is lower for some drugs. Thus, the drug may fail during long-term treatment even though success is predicted by acute drug testing. Conversely, the drug may succeed during long-term treatment even though failure is predicted by acute drug testing. Amiodarone is a prominent example of this latter concern. Early reports suggested that a negative electrophysiologic test in patients with malignant ventricular arrhythmias, had low predictive accuracy, i.e., patients who were still inducible on amiodarone did well during follow-up. There are a number of possible explanations for this finding. First, the test may have been done improperly. Amiodarone has bizarre pharmacokinetic properties, accumulating in the body over many weeks. It is possible therefore that a test done too early could be uninformative. Second, without a control group, it is difficult to conclude whether or not a drug is altering the natural history of an arrhythmia. In many patients, recurrences of sustained ventricular arrhythmias are so infrequent that ineffective drugs give a false impression of efficacy. No controlled studies were ever done to evaluate amiodarone treatment of malignant ventricular arrhythmias.

Contrary to early opinion, recent studies show that electrophysiologic studies have excellent predictive accuracy for amiodarone [9, 11, 28—33]. The largest study is that of Horowitz *et al.* [5] who studied 100 patients with coronary heart disease, 97 of whom had experienced a previous myocardial infarction [24]. All of the patients were inducible, i.e., had sustained ventricular arrhythmias in response to programmed ventricular stimulation during their baseline electrophysiologic study. Patients were studied about two weeks after a 10 to 13 gram loading dose of amiodarone had been administered. In 20 patients, the ventricular tachyarrhythmia was no longer inducible after amiodarone; no recurrent arrhythmia occurred in this group during an average follow-up period of 18 $\pm$ 10 months. In 80 patients, the arrhythmia remained inducible after amiodarone; 38 of these patients (48%) had arrhythmia recurrence during a follow-up of 12 $\pm$ 9 months. The dose of amiodarone at the time of recurrence was 600 mg per day in 21 patients, 400 mg per day in 14 patients, and < 400 mg per day in 3 patients. The dose and plasma concentration of amiodarone was higher in the group of patients with recurrences during follow-up than in those without recurrences. Additional prognostic information was obtained from analysis of the rate of the sustained ventricular arrhythmia induced by programmed ventricular stimulation and the symptoms experienced during the tachyarrhythmia. Of 24 patients who had cardiovascular collapse or other severe symptoms during electrophysiologic study after amiodarone treatment, 12 died suddenly during follow-up. Of 56 patients who had moderate symptoms during the induced ventricular arrhythmia, 26 (46%) had a spontaneous sustained arrhythmia during follow-up, but there were no fatal arrhythmias or sudden cardiac deaths in this group. This study showed that electrophysiologic testing provides clinical guidance and predicts prognosis in patients treated with amiodarone as it does for the evaluation of other antiarrhythmic agents. These findings suggest that patients who develop rapid symptomatic ventricular arrhythmias during an electrophysiologic evaluation of amiodarone should be taken off this drug and managed with another treatment, e.g., implantation of an automatic cardioverter defibrillator or surgical ablation.

Direct comparison of non-invasive methods and invasive electrophysiologic studies

Until head-to-head comparisons of electrophysiologic studies and non-invasive methods are done, we will not know which method is preferable for drug evaluation in patients with malignant ventricular arrhythmias. These two methods need to be compared for predictive accuracy, efficiency and cost. Only two such comparisons have been done, a recently completed small study done by investigators in Calgary, Canada [34] and an ongoing multicenter study called ESVEM [18]. Some of the major features of these two important trials are given in Table 2.

The Calgary trial

Between February 1983 and April 1986, Mitchell *et al.* in Calgary, Canada randomized patients with symptomatic potentially malignant or malignant ventricular arrhythmias to therapy selected either with non-invasive (Holter recordings and exercise tests) or with electrophysiologic studies [34]. During the study period, 124 patients presented of whom 105 survived, were not excluded, and consented to participate. After consent was signed, baseline studies were done off of antiarrhythmic drugs. The baseline studies included a 24-hour continous ECG recording, exercise test, electrophysiologic study, and radionuclide ventriculogram. For the non-invasive evaluation, patients had to average $\geqslant 30$ VPD/hour or have reproducible exercise induced VT (i.e., $\geqslant 5$ consecutive VPD at a rate > 120/min). For the invasive evaluation, patients had to have VT ($\geqslant 5$ consecutive VPD at a rate > 120/min) resembling their clinical arrhythmia induced by programmed ventricular stimulation. Of the 105 patients who enrolled, 57 qualified for both non-invasive evaluation and invasive evaluation, 30 qualified for only the invasive evaluation, 14 for only the non-invasive evaluation, and 4 qualified for neither method of evaluation (see Figure 1). Of the 57 patients who qualified for both methods of evaluation, 29 were randomized to the non-invasive approach and 28 to the invasive approach. Randomization was stratified on left ventricular ejection fraction ($< 40\%$ versus $\geqslant 40\%$) and on the type of VT induced by programmed ventricular stimulation (5 consecutive complexes to 30 sec versus > 30 sec). The two groups of patients were well matched on age, sex, etiologic heart disease, and ventricular arrhythmia frequency. The group assigned to non-invasive assessment had lower left ventricular ejection fractions, $34 \pm 13\%$, compared with the group assigned to electrophysiologic assessment, $39 \pm 16\%$.

The drug sequence in the Calgary study usually was:

class IA or IB (mexiletine) $\rightarrow$ IA + IB $\rightarrow$ II $\rightarrow$ sotalol.

Table 2. Comparison of the Calgary study and ESVEM

	Calgary Study [34]	ESVEM [18]*
Presented with clinical arrhythmia	124	1114
Not excluded	105	779
Randomized	57	232
No drug found effective	13	63
Discharged on drug predicted effective	44	136

* As of April 30, 1988

When no drug predicted to be effective was found, patients were given amiodarone and followed. Efficacy in the non-invasive approach was defined as an 80% decrease in VPD frequency, 90% decrease in paired VPD, and 100% decrease in repetitive VPD of ≥ 3 complexes plus absence of ≥ 2 repetitive VPD during the exercise test. A drug treatment predicted to be efficacious was found for all 29 patients (100%) assigned to the non-invasive approach; none were given amiodarone. However, 7 patients in the non-invasive limb were switched to amiodarone during follow-up. Efficacy in the invasive approach was defined as fewer than 6 consecutive VPD induced by programmed ventricular stimulation. A drug treatment predicted to be efficacious was found for 15 patients (54%) assigned to the invasive approach; 13 patients (46%) were given amiodarone. Electrophysiologic testing done on amiodarone showed that all patients treated with this drug had inducible, sustained VT. When patients developed intolerable adverse effects of their drug treatment, they were rehospitalized for the selection of an alternate therapy using the approach to which they were originally randomized.

The average follow-up for the Calgary study was 27 ± 13 months. The primary endpoints for the study were the occurence of symptomatic, sustained ventricular tachycardia or sudden cardiac death. Deaths that were not sudden were censored. The results are shown in Table 2. During follow-up, 11 patients in the non-invasive limb and 6 in the invasive limb were rehospitalized for the selection of an alternate therapy. Sustained VT occurred in 45% of the non-invasive group and 18% of the invasive group. Sudden death occurred in two patients in the non-invasive group and in one of the invasive group. The total mortality was 19% in both groups. Thus, this small study showed fewer non-fatal recurrences of VT in the group whose therapy was selected by programmed ventricular stimulation, but their was no difference in sudden death or total mortality between the groups. It remains for larger studies to confirm the lower VT recurrence rates seen in the group evaluated by electrophysiologic studies in the Calgary study and to determine the association with mortality rate.

The trend toward less frequent recurrence of symptomatic sustained VT in the group treated with drugs selected by programmed ventricular stimulation was not due to treatment with amiodarone. As predicted by their electrophysiologic assessment, the patients in the invasive group treated with amiodarone actually tended to have more recurrences than those in the same group treated with other antiarrhythmic drugs predicted by programmed ventricular stimulation to be effective.

Electrophysiologic Study versus Electrocardiographic Monitoring (ESVEM)

ESVEM is a 13 center trial supported by the National Heart, Lung, and Blood Institute to determine if electrophysiologic studies or non-invasive methods (24-hour continuous ECG recordings and exercise tests) give more accurate predictions of efficacy for antiarrhythmic drug treatment in patients who have survived one or more episodes of cardiac arrest or sustained VT [18]. ESVEM began enrolling on October 1, 1985 and follow-up is scheduled to be completed in 1991. The number of patients to be enrolled in the ESVEM trial is predicted on the assertion that a 60% difference in the median time to arrhythmia occurence between the two methods of selecting antiarrhythmic drugs will be found. About 70 patients with arrhythmia recurrence will provide a power $(1 - \beta)$ of 0.80 to detect a 60% difference at a significance (α) level of 0.05. Estimating the annual recurrence rate to be 25%, it was calculated that 285 patients will have to be enrolled, randomized, discharged on a drug predicted to be successful, and followed an average of 2.5 years. Patients who have sustained, uniform ventricular tachycardia in response to programmed ventricular stimulation and average at least 10 VPD/hour during a 48-hour baseline recording period are randomized to be evaluated either by non-invasive methods or by programmed ventricular stimulation (see Figure 1). Drugs from a set of six are

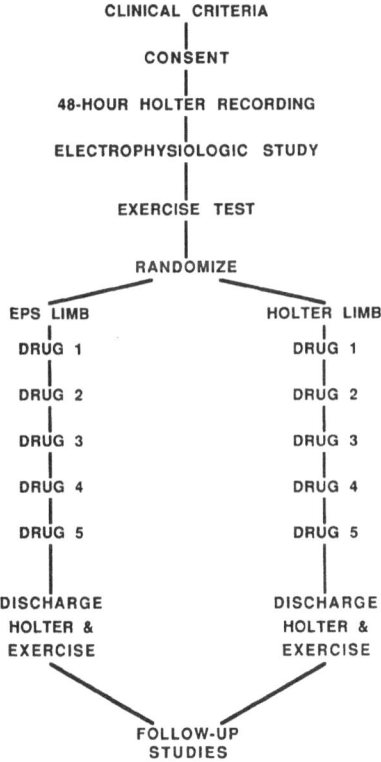

Figure 1. The design of Electrophysiologic Studies versus Electrocardiographic Monitoring (ESVEM). EPS = electrophysiologic studies. The drugs are assigned in random order.

randomly assigned one at the time; the investigator does not know which drug will be assigned next until the evaluation of the current drug is completed. Efficacy in the electrophysiologic limb is defined as failure to induce a run of VT longer than 15 consecutive complexes. Efficacy in the non-invasive limb is a $\geqslant 70\%$ reduction in VPD frequency, $\geqslant 80\%$ reduction in paired VPD, $\geqslant 90\%$ reduction in unsustained VT, and 100% reduction in runs of VT > 15 complexes. When analysis of 24-hour ECG recordings indicates the efficacy of an antiarrhythmic drug, a treadmill exercise test is done using the Bruce protocol. If a run of VT > 15 complexes occurs during exercise, the drug is declared a failure and titration resumes. When an effective drug is found, the patient is discharged and followed until an endpoint or the end of the study occurs.

Follow-up visits are scheduled at an ESVEM enrolling center at 1, 3, 6, and 12 months and then every 6 months until the end of study is reached. Study drug doses can be adjusted during follow-up to control adverse effects or to bring the plasma concentration into the target range. The endpoint criteria for evaluation of patients in this comparison study is the occurrence of sudden death or the recurrence of symptomatic sustained ventricular arrhythmias during follow-up. The primary analysis will be an actuarial analysis of the accuracy of drug efficacy predictions based on the "intention to teat" principle. Secondary analyses will include comparisons of the two methods for frequency of declaring efficacy, time to find a drug predicted to be effective, safety, and cost. Also, the relative efficacy of the study drugs and the accuracy of the methods for predicting the outcome with each drug will be evaluated.

The Calgary study and ESVEM will produce important information about the sequencing of tests and treatments. If drugs predicted to fail by non-invasive methods were always predicted to fail by electrophysiologic studies, then, electrophysiologic studies can be reserved for patients who have non-invasive criteria predicting drug success.

Observational studies to determine the association between ventricular arrhythmias and mortality independent of left ventricular dysfunction

By 1981, several studies had established a statistically significant and reasonably strong association between ventricular arrhythmias detected between 7 and 90 days after myocardial infarction and subsequent mortality [35—38]. These studies also indicated that the prediction of mortality by ventricular arrhythmias was independent of clinical manifestations of heart failure. However, these studies did not clarify definitively the relationships among ventricular arrhythmias, left ventricular dysfunction and mortality after myocardial infarction. These relationships were clarified by two large multicenter studies that did 24-hour continuous ECG recordings and radio-nuclide ventriculograms prior to discharge from hospital after myocardial infarction.

The Multicenter Post Infarction Program (MPIP)

MPIP was an observational study conducted by four university cardiology groups that attempted to enroll all patients less than age 70 with myocardial infarction in nine affiliated hospitals, located in New York City, Rochester, N.Y., St. Louis, and Tucson [39]. Three special tests, i.e., radionuclide ejection fraction, 24-hour continous ECG recording, and exercise test were performed prior to hospital discharge. The objective of these tests was to assess the relationships among three functional risk factors (left ventricular systolic function, ventricular arrhythmias, and myocardial ischemia) and total or cause-specific mortality.

Of the 867 patients enrolled, 820 had a 24-hour ECG recording and 767 patients had both a 24-hour ECG recording and a radionuclide ventriculogram. The group who got both tests permitted analyses to determine the relationships among ventricular arrhythmias, left ventricular dysfunction, and mortality during follow-up.

During the 31 month average follow-up, 144 patients died on or before December 31, 1982. The classification by Hinkle and Thaler was used to assign a mechanism to each death [40]. The major categories in this classification are arrhythmic death, death due to circulatory failure and deaths that are not classifiable into either of the other two categories. MPIP found that frequent and/or repetitive ventricular arrhythmias were associated with total, sudden and arrhythmic mortality. Ventricular arrhythmias had a stronger association with arrhythmic death than with non-arrhythmic death [41]. Low values of left ventricular ejection fraction also were associated with total, sudden, and arrhythmic mortality [42, 43]; the association of left ventricular ejection fraction with arrhythmic death was substantially stronger than with non-arrhythmic death [42, 43]. There was only a weak association between left ventricular ejection fraction and ventricular arrhythmias after myocardial infarction. For example, 70% of the patients with ventricular tachycardia had left ventricular ejection fraction $\geqslant 30\%$ [41, 42]. There was no interaction between ventricular arrhythmias and left ventricular dysfunction with respect to their mortality effects [41, 44]. Table 3 shows that the fractional step up in mortality rate in patients with ventricular arrhythmias is identical for those with low and high left ventricular ejection fraction indicating a lack of a statistical interaction between ventricular arrhythmias and left ventricular dysfunction with respect to subsequent mortality.

The Multicenter Investigation of the Limitation of Infarct Size (MILIS)

Population. MILIS was a randomized, placebo-controlled trial to determine whether hyaluronidase or propranolol treatment given within 18 hours of the onset of myocardial infarction could limit the extent of myocardial necrosis [45]. MILIS was conducted in 5 hospitals: Barnes Hospital; Brigham and Women's Hospital; Massachusetts General Hospital; Medical Center Hos-

Table 3. Relationship among left ventriuclar dysfunction, ventricular arrhythmias, and mortality rate in the MPIP observational study and for the MILIS trial

Left ventricular ejection fraction	Ventricular[a] arrhythmias	MPIP[b]		MILIS[c]	
		Number	Mortality rate	Number	Mortality rate
<40%	Present	72	41%	40	18%
	Absent	184	20%	141	10%
≥40%	Present	78	16%	30	8%
	Absent	433	8%	314	2%

[a] VPD frequency ≥ 10/hour.
[b] Kaplan-Meier estimate of 30 month mortality rate.
[c] Average follow-up 18 months.

pital of Vermont; and Parkland Memorial Hospital. Patients below age 75 with myocardial infarction within 18 hours were enrolled. Radionuclide ventriculograms and 24-hour continuous ECG recordings were obtained prior to hospital discharge about 10 days after myocardial infarction and the results were used to evaluate the relationships among ventricular arrhythmias, left ventricular ejection fraction, and sudden cardiac death [45]. The average follow-up in the MILIS report was 18 months. Of the 66 deaths in MILIS, 29 were judged to be sudden, defined as death occurring within 1 hour of terminal symptoms (n = 16), patients found dead in bed (n = 9), or patients who collapsed at home (n = 4).

The patients were divided into four groups based on ventricular arrhythmias (VPD < 10 per hour versus ≥ 10 per hour) and left ventricular ejection fraction (≥ 40% versus > 40%) [45]. The results obtained in the MILIS sample are shown in Table 3. The step up in mortality rate attributable to ventricular arrhythmias is not significantly different in the two left ventricular ejection fraction groups. These results agree with those of MPIP that ventricular arrhythmias are related to mortality independent of any relationship with left ventricular ejection fraction. MPIP and MILIS considerably strengthened the scientific rationale for a large-scale clinical trial to determine if treatment of ventricular arrhythmias after myocardial infarction would reduce sudden cardiac death.

Previous long-term clinical trials with antiarrhythmic drugs after myocardial infarction

In the 1970's, several trials were conducted in patients with recent myocardial infarction. All of these trials must be considered to be feasibility studies since none had a sample size that provided any chance of detecting a realistic drug effect. The hypothesis tested seems to have been: a small fixed dose of antiarrhythmic drug given to all patients after myocardial infarction (with or without the presence of spontaneous arrhythmias) will reduce mortality by about 80%.

May *et al.* and Furberg [46] reviewed the long-term clinical trials of antiarrhythmic drug therapy after myocardial infarction that met the following criteria:

1) 100 or more patients were enrolled in the trial;
2) subjects were randomly assigned to treatment or control groups;
3) all-cause mortality was reported [46, 47].

Although a sample size of 100 is far too small to show a definitive effect on mortality, it was hoped that a trend might be observed in studies this small. Table 4 summarizes several important features of eight long-term clinical trials with antiarrhythmic drugs after myocardial infarction [48—56]. Six of the eight studies used an antiarrhythmic drug with class IB action, i.e., phenytoin, tocainide, or mexiletine and the other two used aprindine, a drug that is not marketed in the United States. All of the studies were much too small to have the power to detect treatment effects of reasonable magnitude, e.g., a 25% reduction in total mortality. Only the aprindine studies required that patients have ventricular arrhythmias to be eligible for enrollment in the clinical trial [55, 56]. Since only 20% or less of patients have significant ventricular arrhythmias after myocardial infarction, the other six studies are, for practical purposes, one-fifth as large as their total number of patients, i.e., none of these six studies has more than 200 patients with spontaneous ventricular arrhythmias. Also, the drugs with class IB action are not likely to suppress ventricular arrhythmias markedly in patients with a recent myocardial infarction, especially when used in a fixed dose. Only the aprindine studies modified the dose of the active study drug in the attempt to suppress ventricular arrhythmias [55, 56]. and none of the eight studies permitted a change of active drug to achieve suppression of ventricular arrhythmias or avoid adverse effects. The drop-out rates were high in these trials, ranging from 20 to 30% even though the follow-up period was relatively short, one year or less in seven of the eight trials. The number of deaths was small in all of the studies and, therefore, the precision of the estimates of mortality rates is very low. For what they are worth, three of the studies had almost identical mortality rates in the control and active treatment groups, three studies showed a mortality rate that was 32 to 58% higher in the group treated with antiarrhythmic drug, and the aprindine studies showed a 40 and 23% lower mortality rate in the groups treated with antiarrhythmic drug. It is interesting that the two studies that showed encouraging results only enrolled patients who had ventricular arrhythmias and attempted to suppress ventricular arrhythmias by dose ranging with the active treatment [55, 56].

The results of the eight small studies summarized in Table 4 fail to suggest any benefit of treatment with antiarrhythmic drugs in unselected patients after myocardial infarction. It may be that treatment with antiarrhythmic

Table 4. Long-term randomized trials of antiarrhythmic treatment after myocardial infarction[a]

Drug	Dose (mg/day)	No of patients	Placebo control	Double blind	Arrhythmia required to enroll	Dose titrated to suppress arrhythmia	Months of follow-up	Percent mortality Controls (%)	Percent mortality Treated (%)
Phenyton [48]	300—400	568	No (low-dose phenytoin)	Yes	No	No	12	9.1	8.1
Phenytoin [49]	—[b]	150	No (usual therapy)	No (open)	No	No	24	18.4	24.3
Tocainide [50]	1200	112	Yes	Yes	No	No	6	8.9	8.9
Tocainide [51]	600	146	Yes	Yes	No	No	6	4.1	5.6
Mexiletine [52]	600—750	344	Yes	Yes	No	No	4	11.7	13.3
Mexiletine [53, 54]	720	630	Yes	Yes	No	No	12	4.8	7.6
Aprindine [55]	100—200[c]	300	Yes	Yes	Yes	Yes	12	12.1	7.3
Aprindine [56]	100—200[c]	143	Yes	Yes	Yes	Yes	12	22.2	17.1

a All studies enrolled patients within 3 weeks of the index myocardial infarction.
b Dose adjusted to achieve plasma concentration of 40—80 μmol/L.
c Dose adjusted to achieve suppression of ventricular arrhythmias.

drugs does not improve survival. However, since the studies done so far do not have nearly enough power to detect a treatment effect, a negative conclusion is not warranted. All the previous studies were far too small to make statements about lack of benefit and they must be regarded as preliminary. No long-term post infarction study of over 1,000 patients with ventricular arrhythmias has been performed to date. Also, fixed dose studies are likely to have lower efficacy and higher adverse effects and drop-out rates than studies that permit dose changes. Only one previous study attempted to document suppression of ventricular arrhythmias. Unfortunately, therefore, previous studies do not tell us whether it is feasible to suppress ventricular arrhythmias after myocardial infarction under clinical trial conditions. Both efficacy and drop outs due to adverse effects should improve if changes in drugs and doses are permitted in the study protocol. Because of large inter-patient variability in response to treatment, flexibility in dosing with antiarrhythmic drugs is important to achieve a high level of arrhythmia suppression and to avoid drop out due to adverse effects in a study that plans to treat a group of patients. Finally, previous studies were done before the problems of drug-induced proarrhythmia and aggravation of heart failure were widely appreciated so that these potentially negative effects of treatment were not carefully detected and controlled. For a variety of reasons, previous studies of antiarrhythmic treatment after myocardial infarction do not shed much light on the efficacy or adverse effect rates.

Interestingly, in the United States, fewer and fewer patients with asymptomatic ventricular arrhythmias after myocardial infarction are being treated each year. This increasingly conservative attitude probably results from the lack of any preliminary evidence to suggest that antiarrhythmic drug treatment improves survival. If this is, in fact, the case, then there is no point in treating an asymptomatic patient because no benefit would offset the risk of drug adverse effects, or the inconvenience, and cost of treatment.

The Cardiac Arrhythmia Pilot Study (CAPS)

Previous studies of antiarrhythmic treatment after myocardial infarction do not establish the feasibility of doing a full-scale trial to determine whether treatment or suppression of ventricular arrhythmias after myocardial infarction with antiarrhythmic drugs will improve survival. Previous studies also failed to provide some of the essential information on how to design a full-scale trial to evaluate either a treatment hypothesis or a suppression hypothesis. Therefore, the National Heart, Lung, and Blood Institute initiated the Cardiac Arrhythmia Pilot Study (CAPS) in July 1983 to establish the feasibility of doing a full-scale trial and to provide information on how to design such a trial [57]. Ten enrolling centers and 27 hospitals participated.

To be eligible, patients had to be < 75 years of age, have acute myocardial infarction, have ≥ 10 VPD per hour in a 24-hour ECG recording made

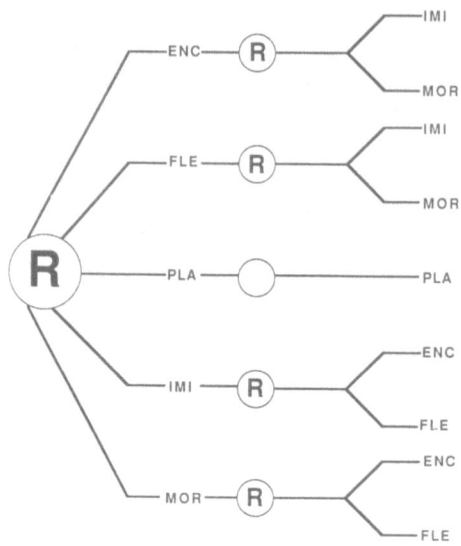

Figure 2. The design of the Cardiac Arrhythmia Pilot Study. **R** = randomization, ENC = encainide, FLE = flecainide, PLA = placebo, IMI = imipramine, MOR = moricizine. Note that patients originally assigned to drugs with class IC action crossed over to drugs with class IA action and vice versa.

between 6 and 60 days after myocardial infarction, have a left ventricular ejection fraction (LVEF) $\geq 20\%$, and sign a written informed consent. The enrollment goal of 500 patients was achieved; 502 patients (418 men and 84 women with mean age of 59 $\pm$ 9) were randomized an average of 31 days after myocardial infarction [58].

CAPS participants were randomized to one of the five treatment 'tracks' (shown in Figure 2) 100 patients to each track [57]. The placebo track provided a comparison with the active treatment strategies and a control for spontaneous VPD variability. The four active drug treatments were selected on the basis of: potential efficacy, safety, and the prospect of developing new information for planning a full-scale trial [57]. Based on these considerations, encainide, moricizine, flecainide, and imipramine were selected for CAPS.

CAPS permitted drug and dose changes in the attempt to suppress ventricular arrhythmias without adverse effects. The criteria for efficacy were: a 70% reduction in VPD frequency, and a 90% reduction in runs of VT. Each of the four active treatment tracks permitted up to three doses of two drugs to be evaluated (see Table 5). If the first drug failed to achieve efficacy or caused intolerable adverse effects, the patient was crossed over to the second drug in the track. Encainide and flecainide, always crossed over to drugs with class IA action, imipramine and moricizine, and vice versa. Thus, encainide and flecainide, or imipramine and moricizine were never compared in the same patient. If efficacy was reached, the patient was treated for the rest of the year on that drug and dose. The efficacy achieved at the end of the drug/dose selection phase and at the end of the year of CAPS follow-up are shown in Table 6.

Table 5. Doses of drugs used in CAPS.

Drug	Dose as Mg three times a day		
	Low	Medium	High
Encainide	35	50	60
Flecainide	67	100	133
Imipramine	50	75	125
Moricizine	200	250	300

Table 6. Efficacy of treatment during CAPS

Drug	% Efficacious and tolerated	
	At the end of drug titration	At the end of 1 year
Encainide	79	76
Flecainide	83	77
Imipramine	52	54
Moricizine	66	61
Placebo	37	28

Adverse effects

Patients were hospitalized and carefully monitored for at least the first 48 hours of each treatment [59]. There were no differences between active treatments and placebo with respect to adverse events. Serious adverse effects were rare and no early deaths were ascribed to CAPS treatment. At the beginning of follow-up, the assignments to drug treatment were: encainide, 108; flecainide, 119; imipramine, 57; moricizine, 77; and placebo, 87 [59]. About 75% of the patients remained on their assigned drug for the year of follow-up. Disqualifying ventricular tachycardia, proarrhythmic effect, or syncope that occurred during the follow-up phase, prompted withdrawal from CAPS drug, and disappeared during drug washout was seen in 9% of the patients on placebo, 7% on encainide, 7% on flecainide, 2% on imipramine, and 6% on moricizine. The actuarial one-year incidence of heart failure was 25%. There was no statistically significant difference in the incidence of heart failure between the active treatments and placebo [59]. The discontinuation rates during follow-up were: placebo, 7%; encainide, 2%; flecainide, 3%; moricizine, 6%; and imipramine, 18% [59].

Summary of CAPS findings

CAPS showed that:
1) it is possible to identify and recruit suitable subjects for a definitive trial to test the hypotheses that either treatment or suppression of ventricular arrhythmias after myocardial infarction will significantly improve survival;
2) several antiarrhythmic agents were found to be well tolerated and highly efficacious for suppressing ventricular arrhythmias after myocardial infarction;
3) dose titration with multiple drugs is feasible under clinical trial conditions and improves the chance of finding effective, well-tolerated treatment;
4) two doses perform as well as three doses of encainide, flecainide or moricizine during titration;
5) patient compliance and follow-up can be maintained for at least a year in a post infarction cohort [59].

Cautionary note. It is important to recognize that because of the exclusion criteria used in CAPS, one cannot extrapolate the results to the entire post myocardial infarction population. CAPS excluded patients with VT ≥ 10 complexes, and left ventricular ejection fraction $\leq 20\%$. Aggravation of heart failure or proarrhythmia might occur more frequently if patients with left ventricular ejection fraction $\leq 20\%$ or sustained ventricular tachycardia were exposed to these drugs [22, 23].

Full-scale clinical trials to assess antiarrhythmic drug treatment after myocardial infarction

Two full-scale clinical trials of antiarrhythmic drug treatment of asymptomatic ventricular arrhythmias after myocardial infarction are underway — the Cardiac Arrhythmia Suppression Trial (CAST) [60] and the Spanish Sudden Death Trial. These two important trials are described in detail elsewhere in this volume. CAST will provide a definitive answer about the efficacy and safety of drugs with class I antiarrhythmic action and the Spanish trial will provide definitive information about the efficacy and safety of amiodarone. A pilot trial with amiodarone has been done in Canada and a full-scale trial is tentatively planned to follow. Hopefully, the results of these controlled clinical trials will provide us with badly needed information that will guide the treatment of post infarction ventricular arrhythmias in the future.

Acknowledgements

Supported in part by contracts HV-28006 and HC-65048 from the National Heart, Lung, and Blood Institute, National Institutes of Health, Bethesda,

MD; in part by Grants HL-22982, HL-70204, HL-41552 from the National
Heart, Lung, and Blood Institute, and RR-00645, from the Research
Resources Administration, National Institutes of Health, Bethesda, MD; and
in part by a grant from the Henry and Shirlee Benach Foundation, New
York, New York.

References

1. Fisher JD, Cohen HL, Mehra R, Altschuler H, Escher DJW, Furman S: Cardiac pacing and pacemakers, II. Serial electrophsiologic-pharmacologic testing for control of recurrent tachyarrhythmias. Am Heart J 1997; 93: 658—68.
2. Horowitz LN, Josephson ME, Farshidi A, Spielman SR, Michaelson EL, Greenspan AM: Recurrent sustained ventricular tachycardia. 3: Role of the electrophysiologic study in selection of antiarrhythmic regimens. Circulation 1978; 58: 986—97.
3. Mason JW, Winkle RA: Electrode-catheter arrhythmia induction in the selection and assessment of antiarrhythmic drug therapy for recurrent ventricular tachycardia. Circulation 1978; 58: 971—85.
4. Mason JW, Winkle RA: Accuracy of the ventricular tachycardia induction study for predicting long-term efficacy and inefficacy of antiarrhythmic drugs. N Engl J Med 1980; 303: 1073—7.
5. Horowitz LN, Josephson ME, Kastor JA: Intracardiac electrophysiologic studies as a method for the optimization of drug therapy in chronic ventricular arrhythmia. Prog Cardiovasc Dis 1980; 23: 81—98.
6. Ruskin JN, DiMarco JP, Garan H: Out-of-hospital cardiac arrest: electrophysiologic observations and selection of long-term antiarrhythmic therapy. N Engl J Med 1980; 303: 707—13.
7. Swerdlow CD, Winkle RA, Mason JW: Determinants of survival in patients with ventricular tachyarrhythmias. N Engl J Med 1983; 308: 1436—42.
8. Benditt DG, Benson DW, Klein GJ, Pritzker MR, Kriett JM, Anderson RW: Prevention of recurrent sudden cardiac arrest: role of provocative electropharmacologic testing. J Am Coll Cardiol 1983; 2: 418—25.
9. McGovern B, Garan H, Malacoff RF, DiMarco JP, Grant G, Sellers TD, Ruskin JN: Long term clinical out-come of ventricular tachycardia or fibrillation treated with amiodarone. Am J Cardiol 1984; 53: 1558—63.
10. Rae AP, Greenspan AM, Spielman SR, Sokoloff NM, Webb CR, Kay HR, Horowitz LN: Antiarrhythmic drug efficacy for ventricular tachyarrhythmias associated with coronary artery disease as assessed by electrophysiologic studies. Am J Cardiol 1985; 55: 1494—9.
11. Horowitz LN, Greenspan AM, Spielman SR, Webb CR, Morganroth J, Rotmensch H, Sokoloff NM, Rae AP, Segal BL, Kay HR: Usefulness of electrophysiologic testing in evaluation of amiodarone therapy for sustained ventricular tachyarrhythmias associated with coronary heart disease. Am J Cardiol 1985; 55: 367—372.
12. Waller TJ, Kay HR, Spielman SR, Kutlaek SP, Greenspan AM, Horowitz LN: Reduction in sudden death and total mortality by antiarrhythmic therapy evaluated by electrophysiologic drug testing: criteria of efficacy in patients with sustained ventricular tachyarrhythmia. J Am Coll Cardiol 1987; 10: 83—9.
13. Graboys TB, Lown B, Podrid PJ, DeSilva R: Long-term survival of patients with malignant ventricular arrhythmia treated with antiarrhythmic drugs. Am J Cardiol 1982; 50: 437—43.
14. Hoffman A, Schutz E, White R, Follath F, Burckhardt D: Suppression of high-grade ventricular ectopic activity by antiarrhythmic drug treatment as a marker for survival in patients with chronic coronary artery disease. Am Heart J 1984; 107: 1103—1108.

15. Vlay SC, Kallman LH, Reid PR: Prognostic assessment of survivors of ventricular tachycardia and ventricular fibrillation with ambulatory monitoring. Am J Cardiol 1984; 54: 87—90.
16. Hohnloser SN, Raeder EA, Podrid PJ, Graboys TB, Lown B: Predictors of antiarrhythmic drug efficacy in patients with malignant ventricular tachyarrhythmias. Am Heart J 1987; 114: 1—7.
17. Lampert S, Lown B, Graboys TB, Podrid PJ, Blatt CM: Determinants of survival in patients with malignant ventricular arrhythmias associated with coronary artery disease. Am J Cardiol 1988; 61: 791—7.
18. Bigger JT Jr: Holter/exercise and electrophysiologic methods for evaluating drug therapy for malignant ventricular arrhythmias: do we need both models? In: Cardiac Arrhythmias: New Therapeutic Drugs and Devices, Morganroth J Moore EN eds, Martinus Nijhoff, Boston, 1985, 211—221. Am J Cardiol 1988; 61: 501—9.
19. Breithardt G, Borggrefe M, Seipel L: Selection of optimal drug treatment of ventricular tachycardia by programmed electrical stimulation of the heart. In: Clinical Aspects of Life-Threatening Arrhythmias, Greenberg HM, Kulbertus HE, Moss AJ, Schwartz PJ eds, Ann NY Acad Sci 1984; 427: 49—65.
20. Bigger JT Jr: Cardiac arrhythmias. Chapter 45 in Cecil's Textbook of Medicine, Wyngaarden JB and Smith HK eds, W.B. Saunders Co., Philadelphia, 1988, pp. 250—274.
21. Kienzle MG, Martins JB, Wendt DJ, Constantin L, Hopson R, McCue ML: Enhanced efficacy of oral sotalol for sustained ventricular tachycardia refractory to type I antiarrhythmic drugs. Am J Cardiol 1988; 61: 1012—7.
22. Morganroth J, Anderson JL, Gentzkow GD: Classification by type of ventricular arrhythmia predicts frequency of adverse cardiac events from flecainide. J Am Coll Cardiol 1986; 8: 607—615.
23. de Paola AAV, Horowitz LN, Morganroth J, Senior S, Spielman SR, Greenspan AM, Kay HR: Influence of left ventricular dysfunction on flecainide therapy. J Am Coll Cardiol 1987; 9: 163—168.
24. Mason JW: Amiodarone. N Engl J Med 1987; 316: 455—66.
25. Swerdlow CD, Pederson, J: Prospective comparison of Holter monitoring and electrophysiologic study in patients with coronary artery disease and sustained ventricular tachyarrhythmias. Am J Cardiol 1985; 56: 577—80.
26. Kim SG, Seiden SW, Felder SD, Waspe LE, Fisher JD: Is programmed stimulation of value in predicting the long-term success of antiarrhythmic therapy for ventricular tachycardias? N Engl J Med 1986; 315: 356—362.
27. Freedman RA, Swerdlow CD, Echt DS, Winkle RA, Soderholm Difatte V, Mason JW: Facilitation of ventricular tachyarrhythmia induction by isoproterenol. Am J Cardiol 1984; 54: 756—70.
28. McGovern B, Ruskin JN: The efficacy of amiodarone for ventricular arrhythmias can be predicted with clinical electrophysiologic studies. Int J Cardiol 1983; 3: 71—76.
29. Borggrefe M, Breithardt G: Predictive value of electrophysiologic testing in the treatment of drug-refractory ventricular arrhythmias with amiodarone. Eur Heart J 1986; 7: 735—742.
30. Naccarelli GV, Fineberg NS, Zipes DP, Heger JJ, Duncan G, Prystowsky EN: Amiodarone: risk factors for recurrence of symptomatic ventricular tachycardia identified at electrophysiologic study. J Am Coll Cardiol 1985; 6: 814—821.
31. Fisher JD, Kim SG, Waspe LE, Johnston DR: Amiodarone: value of programmed electrical stimulation and Holter monitoring. (review) PACE 1986; 9: 422—435.
32. Kadish AH, Buxton AE, Waxman HL, Flores B, Josephson ME, Marchlinski FE: Usefulness of electrophysiologic study to determine the clinical tolerance of arrhythmia recurrences during amiodarone therapy. J Am Coll Cardiol 1987; 10: 90—96.
33. Schmitt C, Brachmann J, Waldecker B, Rizos I, Senges J, Kubler W: Amiodarone in

patients with recurrent sustained ventricular tachyarrhythmias: results of programmed electrical stimulation and long-term clinical outcome in chronic treatment. Am Heart J 1987; 114: 279—283.

34. Mitchell LB, Duff HJ, Manyari DE, Wyse DG: A randomized clinical trial of the noninvasive and invasive approaches to drug therapy of ventricular tachycardia. N Engl J Med 1987; 317: 1681—1687.

35. Ruberman W, Weinblatt E, Goldberg JD, Frank CW, Shapiro S: Ventricular premature beats and mortality after myocardial infarction. N Engl J Med 1977; 297: 750—757.

36. Moss AJ, Davis HT, DeCamilla J, Bayer LW: Ventricular ectopic beats and their relation to sudden and nonsudden cardiac death after myocardial infarction. Circulation 1978; 60: 998—1003.

37. Bigger JT Jr, Weld FM, Rolnitzky LM: The prevalence and significance of ventricular tachycardia detected by ambulatory ECG recording in the late hospital phase of acute myocardial infarction. Am J Cardiol. 1981; 48: 815—823.

38. Kleiger RE, Miller JP, Thanavaro S, Marin TF, Province MA, Oliver GC: Relationship between clinical features of acute myocardial infarction and ventricular runs two weeks to one year following infarction. Circulation 1981; 63: 64—70.

39. The Multicenter Postinfarction Research Group: Risk stratification and survival after myocardial infarction. N Engl J Med 1983; 309: 331—336.

40. Hinkle LE, Thaler JT: Clinical classification of cardiac deaths. Circulation 1982; 65: 457—464.

41. Bigger JT Jr, Fleiss JL, Kleiger R, Miller JP, Rolnitzky LM and The Multicenter Post-Infarction Group: The relationship between ventricular arrhythmias, left ventricular dysfunction and mortality in the 2 years after myocardial infarction. Circulation 1984; 69: 250—258.

42. Bigger JT Jr, Fleiss JL, Kleiger, RE, Miller JP, Rolnitzky LM, and The Multicenter Post Infarction Research Group: Prevalence, characteristics and significance of ventricular tachycardia detected by 24-hour continuous electrocardiographic recordings in the late hospital phase of acute myocardial infarction. Am J Cardiol 1986; 58: 1151—1160.

43. Marcus FI, Cobb LA, Edwards JE, Kuller L, Moss AJ, Bigger JT Jr, Fleiss JL, Rolnitzky LM, Serokman R, and the Multicenter Postinfarction Research Group: Mechanism of death and prevalence of myocardial ischemic symptoms in the terminal event after acute myocardial infarction. Am J Cardiol 1988; 61: 8—15.

44. Bigger JT Jr: Relation between left ventricular dysfunction and ventricular arrhythmias after myocardial infarction. Am J Cardiol 1986; 57: 8b—14b.

45. Mukharji J, Rude RE, Poole WK, Gustafson N, Thomas LJ Jr, Strauss HW, Jaffe AS, Muller JE, Roberts R, Raabe DS Jr, Croft CH, Passamani E, Braunwald E, Willerson JT and the MILIS Study Group: Risk factors for sudden death after acute myocardial infarction: two years follow-up. Am J Cardiol 1984; 54: 31—6.

46. May GS, Eberlein KA, Furberg CD, Passamani ER, DeMets DL: Secondary prevention after myocardial infarction: a review of long-term trials. Prog Cardiovasc Dis 1982; 24: 331—52.

47. Furberg CD: Effect of antiarrhythmic drugs on mortality after myocardial infarction. Am J Cardiol 1983; 52: 32C—36C.

48. Collaborative Group: Phenytoin after recovery from myocardial infarction. Controlled trial in 568 patients. Lancet 1971; 2: 1055—57.

49. Peter T, Ross D, Duffield A, Luxton M, Harper R, Hunt D, Sloman G: Effect on survival after myocardial infarction of long-term treatment with phenytoin. Br Heart J 1978; 40: 1356—60.

50. Ryden L, Arnman K, Conradson TB, Hofvendahl S, Mortensen O, Smedgard P: Prophylaxis of ventricular tachyarrhythmias with intravenous and oral tocainide in patients with and recovering from acute myocardial infarction. Am Heart J 1980; 1006—12.

51. Bastian BC, Macfarlane PW, McLauchlan JH, Ballantyne D, Clark R, Hillis WS, Rae AP,

Hutton I: A prospective randomized trial of tocainide in patients following myocardial infarction. Am Heart J 1980; 100: 1017—22.

52. Chamberlain DA, Jewitt DE, Julian DG, Campbell RWF, Boyle DMcC, Shanks RG: Oral mexiletine in high-risk patients after myocardial infarction. Lancet 1980; 2: 1324—27.

53. IMPACT Research Group: International Mexiletine and Placebo Antiarrhythmic Coronary Trial (IMPACT): II. Results from 24-hour electrocardiograms. IMPACT Research Group. Eur Heart J 1986; 7: 749—59.

54. IMPACT Research Group: International mexiletine and placebo antiarrhythmic coronary trial: I. Report on arrhythmia and other findings. Impact Research Group. J Am Coll Cardiol 1984; 4: 1148—63.

55. Hagemeijer F, Glaser B, van Durme JP, Bogaert M: Design of a study to evaluate drug therapy of serious ventricular rhythm disturbances after an acute myocardial infarction. Eur J Cardiol 1977; 6: 299—310.

56. Gottlieb SH, Achuff SC, Mellits D, Gerstenblith G, Baughman KL, Becker L, Chandra NC, Henley S, Humphries J O'N, Heck C, Kennedy MM, Weisfeldt ML, Reid PR: Prophylactic antiarrhythmic therapy of high-risk survivors of myocardial infarction: lower mortality at 1 month but not at 1 year. Circulation 1987; 75: 792—9.

57. The CAPS Investigators: The Cardiac Arrhythmia Pilot Study. Am J Cardiol 1986; 57: 91—95.

58. The CAPS Investigators: Recruitment and baseline description of patients in the Cardiac Arrhythmia Pilot Study. Am J Cardiol 1988; 61: 704—13.

59. The CAPS Investigators: Effects of Encainide, Flecainide, Imipramine, and Moricizine on Ventricular Arrhythmias during the Year after Acute Myocardial Infarction: CAPS Am J Cardiol 1988; 61: 501—9.

60. Bigger JT Jr: Methodology for clinical trials with antiarrhythmic drugs to prevent cardiac death: US experience. Cardiology 1987; 74 (suppl 2): 40—56.

6. Value of beta-blockers in the treatment of ventricular arrhythmias

NINA REHNQVIST

Drugs with beta adrenergic blocking action are classified into Class II of the Vaughan Williams Classification. According to this, their general effect is on phase 4 on the mono action potential. The value of beta-blockers in treating arrhythmias would with this concept be mainly arrhythmias due to increased automaticity. However, the most common underlying mechanism for ventricular arrhythmias is the reentry phenomenon where phase 4 depolarisation has no meaningful contribution. In contrast to this, certain beta-blocking drugs are so far the only drugs able to generally improve prognosis when given to patients prone to sudden death. The studies where this has been documented are particularly in the postinfarction patients but also in acute ischemic heart disease a positive effect on survival has been observed. The mechanism behind this is probably that the reentry plenomenon in these patients is dependent on noradrenaline [1]. Among the beta-blockers there is also the drug sotalol which in addition to Class II action carries Class III effects. During long-term therapy metoprolol also has been shown to have this effect [2].

Effects on single ventricular ectopic complexes

Based on the early studies in the CCU premature ventricular complexes (PVCs) have been considered to be markers of an unfavourable prognosis in heart disease [3]. Therefore many studies have dealt with the suppression of single monoform or multiform PVCs without taking the prognostic aspects into consideration.

Both selective and nonselective beta-blockers with and without intrinsic sympathetic activity (ISA) have been shown to suppress PVCs associated with increased sympathetic tone such as exercise induced PVCs both in patients with and without ischemic heart disease [4—6]. We have compared sotalol with procainamide in patients with frequent PVCs. Sotalol was superior in suppressing the number of PVCs in the study population and especially effective in patients with ischemic heart disease (IHD) [7].

In postinfarction patients the natural course regarding asymptomatic

A. Bayés de Luna et al. (eds.): *Sudden Cardiac Death*, 63–69.
© 1991 Kluwer Academic Publishers, Dordrecht.

ventricular arrhythmias is worsening both in numbers of PVCs and in their severity. This development is counteracted by prophylactic beta-blockade by metoprolol, propranolol or timolol [8—10]. There is also an immediate antiarrhythmic effect after 3 days of metoprolol therapy [4]. We have compared the effect on ventricular arrhythmias in an angina pectoris population where the mean number of PVCs was reduced after one month of treatment both with the calcium-antagonist verapamil and metoprolol, whereas ST-depressions seemed to be more influenced by metoprolol than verapamil.

PVCs due to digitalis intoxication seem to be dependent on sympathetic tone since an excellent effect is observed when propranolol has been given although restraint is advocated since asystole may result [11, 12]. Single PVCs may also be troublesome in patients with the mitral valve prolapse. In this entity autonomous imbalance seems to be one contributing factor to the genesis of palpitations and therapeutic effects have been good without severe side effects and above all without a high incidence of worsening of the arrhythmia which may be encountered by traditional antiarrhythmic drugs [13]. A properly conducted comparative study has however not been performed in this condition. Furthermore the indications for treating the ECG in these patients seldom are very convincing [14].

Apart from the comparison of sotalol and procainamide various beta-blockers have been compared to various antiarrhythmic drugs. The antiarrhythmic efficacy in general tends to be somewhat lower in uncompromised patients with PVCs of various origins compared to Class I drugs. However, arrhythmogenic effects also seem to be higher in the general arrhythmia populations for Class I drugs compared to at least metoprolol which may be the only drug for which the confidence interval to arrhythmogenic effect does overlap 1.0 that is the arrhythmogenic effect is not proven (Table 1) [15]. However, naturally great caution is to be observed when treating patients with harmless disturbances on the ECG with any of these potentially dangerous drugs.

Table 1.

	Arrhythmia suppression%	Arrhythmogenic effects%		CO Change
		−CHF	+CHF	
Class IA	75	3	5—20	−20
IB	60	2	5—10	−15
IC	80	6	10—15	−15
II	50	5	1—10	+25
III	70	1	5—15	−10

Estimation of the degree of suppression in numbers of premature ventricular contractions PVCs and arrhythmogenic effects with and without congestive heart failure CHF. The change in cardiac output CO refers to patients with ischemic heart disease.

Repetitive forms/ventricular tachycardia

The repetitive forms of ventricular arrhythmias and especially ventricular tachycardia (VT) have been shown to be associated with a poor prognosis in various heart diseases such as hypertrophic cardiomyopathy, congestive cardiomyopathy, ischemic heart disease, long QT-interval, mitral valve prolapse and also left heart failure of undefined origin [16]. It seems as though the occurrence of asymptomatic repetetive ventricular arrhythmias is a marker of a more severe heart disease. The depression of the arrhythmia is possibly also a market that prognosis has been influenced [17, 18]. Both beta-1-selective drugs and nonselective beta-blockers with and without Class III action have been shown to reduce both the occurrence of VT and the induction of VT during electrophysiologic stimulation in patients with congestive heart failure and undefined left ventricular failure, ischemic heart disease, the long QT-interval and mitral valve prolapse whereas patients with hypertrophic cardiomyopathy did not respond equally well (Table 2) [6, 11, 19, 20]. In the electrophysiology study laboratory Nademanee studied i.v. sotalol in 37 patients with refractory VT/VF. I.v. sotalol prevented 46% of induced attacks. During long term follow up in 11 patients both the number of PVCs and VTs were significantly reduced and the number of beats in the VTs was reduced by 95% [21].

The arrhythmia responsible for reccurrent sudden death has naturally more often been registered as VT than VF. The reason for this is probably due to the patient selection. However, also in patients with reccurrent VT beta-blockers have been able to improve prognosis when the underlying disease is mitral valve prolapse or the long QT syndrome [22–25].

Postoperative arrhythmias

The postoperative phase of particularly cardiac surgery is associated with both supra ventricular and ventricular arrhythmias responding better to beta-blockade than conventional antiarrhythmic drugs [26, 27]. Furthermore, many patients referred for cardiac surgery have been treated with beta-

Table 2. Effect on arrhythmia

	Class I	II	III	ACE
HCM	+	0	+	0
DCM	+	+	+	+
IHD	+	+	+	0

Comparison on various classes of antiarrhythmic drugs and ACE-inhibitors in hypertrophic cardiomyopathy HCM, dilated cardiomyopathy DCM and ischemic heart disease IHD.

66   *N. Rehnqvist*

blockers for angina pectoris, hypertension or as postinfarction prophylaxis. In these patients the incidence of arrhythmia is greatly reduced if the beta-blockade is not withdrawn [28].

Ischemic heart disease and ventricular fibrillation (VF)

The condition most often responsible for sudden death is ischemic heart disease. Most of these patients do not suffer from a new myocardial infarction, rather a new ischemic event is responsible. All efforts to reduce arrhythmias in this aspect with antiarrhythmic drugs have so far failed if caution has not been taken to identify an antiarrhythmic response. Generalized prophylactic treatment with beta-blockade however has been shown to improve prognosis both in the acute phase and chronic phase [29] (Table 3). In the acute phase the underlying mechanism may not be the arrhythmia suppression since only the early metoprolol study showed a reduced incidence of ventricular fibrillation [30]. In the ISIS II study and the MIAMI study ventricular fibrillation did not seem to be influenced rather the prophylactic effect was considered to be due to reduced myocardial work and maybe reduced incidence of rupture [31, 32]. However in other studies where beta-blockade has been withdrawn during the acute myocardial infarction the incidence of ventricular fibrillation has increased [33]. Interestingly enough the marker PVCs are reduced both in the early phase and later when metoprolol is given in the acute myocardial infarction [34]. Whether acute beta-blockade acts as an antiarrhythmic drug or not may not be generalized to all beta-blocking drugs. Pharmacokinetics may differ and lipid solubility may be one prerequisite for an antiarrhythmic action in the acute phase of ischemic heart disease.

During chronic treatment both the incidence and numbers of single PVCs are reduced as has been mentioned before. The most important point however is that sudden death is reduced by 30% by generalized postinfarction prophylactic treatment with the lipophilic beta-blocking drugs propranolol, timolol and metoprolol [35]. That sudden death in these instances most

Table 3. Effect on mortality

	Class IA	IB	IC	II	III	IV
HCM	0	0	0	0	0	0
DCM	0	0	0	+	(+)	0
IHD	−	−	−	+++	0	0
LQTs	−	−	−	+++	0	0

Comparison of effects on mortality by the various classes of antiarrhythmic drugs in hypertrophic cardiomyopathy HCM, dilated cardiomyopathy DCM, ischemic heart disease IHD and the long QT syndrome LQTs.

often are instantaneous deaths indicates that an antiarrhythmic effect is in fact present. These super acute arrhythmias are associated with disturbances in the autonomic tone and even though in the very early phase of acute myocardial infarction vagal tone may be of higher importance than sympathetic tone the balance is influenced by beta-blockade. In my opinion there is little doubt that in the event of a new ischemic event, prophylactic beta-blockade with the above mentioned drugs reduces the risk for ventricular fibrillation. Whether these drugs also influence the triggers is not yet clarified.

Withdrawal

When beta-blockade is withdrawn sudden death may occur in patients with ischemic heart disease. In our study when beta-blockade was withdrawn in a controlled fashion over 2 weeks, arrhythmias were greatly increased during the withdrawal phase and incidents of VT occurred [35]. This also substantiates or underlines the suggestion that there is an antiarrhythmic effect.

Combination with other drugs

When conventional antiarrhythmic drugs fail they may be combined with beta-blockers. This has successfully been done in several studies. The drugs used have been quinidine, procainamide, mexiletine, disopyramide and tocainide and for each of these, studies can be found in which an additive effect has been observed. However the obvious risk of an arrhythmogenic effect is to be observed. However the doses can be kept lower than with one single drug and side-effects may in some cases diminish [12, 36, 37, 38].

Summary

Ventricular arrhythmia in patients with heart disease indicates a poor prognosis. The only drugs in which an improvement of prognosis on general prescription basis has been observed is for the beta-blockers. However, also for beta-blockers an antiarrhythmic response may indicate that the drug has been particularly effective, as has been shown by Class I antiarrhythmic drugs.

References

1. Wit AL, Bigger JT Jr: Electrophysiology of ventricular arrhythmias accompanying myocardial ischemia and infarction. Postgraduate Med J 1977; 53 (Suppl 1): 98—112.
2. Ahnve S: QT interval prolongation in acute myocardial infarction. Eur Heart J 1985; 6 (Suppl D): 85—95.

3. Lown B, Fakho AM, Hood WB *et al*: Coronary care unit. JAMA 1967; 199: 188.
4. Olsson G, Rehnqvist N, Lundman T, Melcher A: Metoprolol treatment after acute myocardial infarction. Acta Med Scand 1981; 210: 59—65.
5. Coumel P, Rosengarten MD, Leclercq JF, Attuel P: Role of sympathetic nervous system in non-ischemic ventricular arrhythmias. Br Heart J 1982; 47: 137—47.
6. Pratt CM, Lichstein E: Ventricular antiarrhythmic effects of beta-adrenergic blocking drugs: a review of mechanism and clinical studies. J Clin Pharmacol 1982; 22: 335—47.
7. Lidell C, Rehnqvist N, Sjogren A, Yli-Uotila RJ, Ronnevik PK: Comparative efficacy of oral sotalol and procainamide in patients with chronic ventricular arrhythmias: a multicenter study. Am Heart J 1985; 109(5): 970—5.
8. Von der Lippe G, Lund-Johansen P, Kjekshus J: Effect of timolol infarction. Acta Med Scand 1981; Suppl 651: 253—8.
9. Lichstein E, Morganroth J, Harrist R, Hubble E: Effect of propranolol on ventricular arrhythmias. The BHAT experience. Circulation 1983; 67 (Suppl I): I 5—I 10.
10. Olsson G, Rehnqvist N: Ventricular arrhythmias during the first year after acute myocardial infarction: influence of long-term treatment with metoprolol. Circulation 1984; 69 (6): 1129—34.
11. Gilson DG, Sowton E: The use of beta-adrenergic receptor blocking drugs in dysrhythmias. Prog Cardiovasc Dis 1969; XII (1): 16—39.
12. Singh BN, Jewitt DE: Beta-adrenoreceptor blocking drugs in cardiac arrhythmias. Cardiovasc Drugs 1977; 2: 119—59.
13. Muhiddin K, Nathan AW, Hellestrand KJ, Banim SO, Camm AJ: Ventricular tachycardia associated with flecainide. Lancet 1982; 2: 1219—20.
14. Campbell RWF, Murray A, Julian DG: Ventricular arrhythmias in first 12 hours of acute myocardial infarction. Br Heart J 1981; 46: 351—7.
15. Velebit V, Podrid, Lown B, Cohen BH, Graboys TB: Aggravation and provocation of ventricular arrhythmias by antiarrhythmic drugs. Circulation 1982; 65 (5): 886—94.
16. Rehnqvist N: Arrhythmias and their treatment in heart failure patients. Am J Cardiol 1989. In press.
17. Grayboys TB, Podrid PJ, DeSilva R: Long-term survival of patients with malignant ventricular arrhythmias treated with anti-arrhythmic drugs. Am J Cardiol 1982; 50: 437—43.
18. Olsson G, Rehnqvist N: Evaluation of anti-arrhythmic effect of metoprolol treatment after acute myocardial infarction: relationship between treatment responses and survival during a 3 year follow-up. Eur Heart J 1986; 7: 312—9.
19. De Soyza K, Kane JJ, Murphy ML, Laddu AR, Doherty JE, Bisset JK: The long-term suppression of ventricular arrhythmia by oral acebutolol in patients with coronary artery disease. Am Heart J 1980; 100 (5): 631—8.
20. McKenna WJ, Chetty S, Oakley CM, Goodwin JF: Arrhythmia in hypertrophic cardiomyopathy: Exercise and 48 hour ambulatory electrocardiographic assessment with and without beta adrenergic blocking therapy. Am J Cardiol 1980; 45: 1: 1—5.
21. Nademanee K, Feld G, Hendrickson J, Singh BN: Electrophysiologic and antiarrhythmic effects of sotalol in patients with life-threatening ventricular tachyarrhythmias. Circulation 1985; 72 (§): 378—64.
22. Schwartz PJ, Periti M, Malliani A: The long QT syndrome. Am Heart J 1975; 89 (3): 378—90.
23. Ritchie JL, Hammermeister KE, Kennedy JW: Refractory ventricular tachycardia and fibrillation in a patient with the prolapsing mitral leaflet syndrome: successful control with overdrive pacing. Am J Cardiol 1976; 37: 314—6.
24. Winkle RA, Lopes MG, Popp RL, Hancock EW: Life-threatening arrhythmias in the mitral valve prolapse syndrome. Am J Med 1976; 60: 961—7.
25. Milne JR, Camm AJ, Ward DE, Spurrell RAJ: Effect of intravenous propranolol on QT interval. A new method of assessment. Br Heart J 1980; 43: 1—6.

26. Aneglini P, Feldman MI, Lufschanowski R, Leachman RD: Cardiac arrhythmias during and after heart surgery: diagnosis and management. Prog Cardiovasc Dis 1974; XVI (5): 469—95.
27. Cambell TJ, Gavaghan TP, Morgan JJ: Intravenous sotalol for the treatment of atrial fibrillation and flutter after cardiopulmonary bypass. Comparison with disopyramide and digoxin in a randomised trial. Br Heart J 1985; 54: 86—90.
28. Ponten J, Biber B, Henriksson B-A, Hjalmarson A, Jonsteg C, Lundberg D: Beta-reception blockade and neurolept anaesthesia. Withdrawal vs. continuation of long-term therapy in gall-bladder and carotid artery surgery. Acta Anaesth Scand 1982; 26: 576—88.
29. May GS, Eberlein KA, Furberg CD, Passami ER, DeMets DL: Secondary prevention after myocardial infarction: A review of long-term trials. Prog Cardiovasc Dis 1982; 24: 331—51.
30. Rydén L, Ariniego R, Arnman K, Herlitz J, Hjalmarson Å, Holmberg S, Reyes C, Smedgard P, Svedberg K, Vedin A, Waagstein F, Waldenström A, Wilhelmsson C, Wedel H, Yamamoto M: A double-blind trial of metoprolol in acute myocardial infarction. Effect on ventricular tachyarrhythmias. N Engl J Med 1983; 308: 614—8.
31. Hajlmarson Å: Metoprolol in acute myocardial infarction. MIAMI. Am J Cariol 1985; 56: 1G—46G.
32. ISIS study group: Randomized trial of intravenous atenolol among 16027 cases of suspected acute myocardial infarction: ISIS −1. Lancet 1986; 57—66.
33. Norris RM, Brown MA, Clarke ED, Barnaby PF, Georg GG, Logan RL, Sharpe DN: Prevention of ventricular fibrillation during acute myocardial infarction by intravenous propranolol. Lancet 1984; 2: 883—6.
34. Rehbqvist N, Olsson G, Erhardt L, Ekman A-M: Metoprolol in acute myocardial infarction reduces ventricular arrhythmias both in the early stage and after the acute event. Int. J Cardiol 1987 15: 301—8.
35. Yusuf S, Petó R, Lewis J, Collins R, Sleight P: Betablockade during and after myocardial infarction: An overview of the randomized trials. Prog Cardiovasc Dis 1985.
36. Champman JH, Schrank JP, Crampton RS: Idiopathic ventricular tachycardia. Am J Med 1975; 59: 470—80.
37. Leahey EB, Heissenbuttel RH, Giardina E-G V, Bigger JT: Combined mexiletine and propranolol treatment refractory ventricular tachycardia. Br Med J 1980; 281: 357.
38. Ikram H: Haemodynamic and electrophysiologic interactions between antiarrhythmic drugs and beta-blockers with special reference to tocainide. Am Heart J 1980; 100 (6, Part 2): 1076—80.

7. Psychological stress and sudden cardiac death

S. GARCÍA-SÁNCHEZ, J. GUINDO and A. BAYÉS DE LUNA

Several research lines over recent years (Table 1) are strongly beginning to demonstrate that the influence of psychological stress on sudden death is more folk wisdom than folklore [1], and should be taken more seriously. Several excellent reviews on this topic have in fact been published [2—10].

Studies in animals

In recent years, the works of Lown and Verrier et al. [11—14], Skinner et al. [15] and Parker et al. [16] have defined the role of behavioral stress in precipitating ventricular arrhythmias in animal models, concluding that higher nervous activity triggered by psychologic factors can significantly affect cardiac electrophysiologic properties and may result in lowering the threshold for ventricular fibrillation, the underlying basis for sudden cardiac death [4].

In these experiences, both aversive conditioning with mild electric shock and induction of an angerlike state in dogs by denial of access to food decreased the vulnerable period threshold to ventricular fibrillation (VF) by 40%—50% [9]. The finding that VF was induced more easily during an experimentally induced coronary occlusion-release sequence in dogs when exposed to an aversive sling environment [14] is compatible with the observation that a non aversive environment protected pigs against reperfusion induced VF [15, 16].

Richter [17] observed that the situation of physical restraint in rats, of being hopelessly trapped, led to severe fear and rage reaction and, finally, to giving up, slowing heart rate and sudden death. This model of uncontrollability and inhibition has also been observed in other diseases, such as gastric ulcer [18].

Cortical and subcortical electrical stimulation in dogs has been related to life-threatening arrhythmias [3], and nervous cryoblockade from the frontal cortex to the brainsteam has delayed or prevented VF during stress in pigs [16, 19], as observed following left stellectomy [20].

A. Bayés de Luna et al. (eds.): *Sudden Cardiac Death*, 71–81.
© 1991 Kluwer Academic Publishers, Dordrecht.

Table 1. Example of several research lines on stress and sudden cardiac death

	Research line	Ventricular arrhythmias	Coronary vasomotor tone	Platelet function
Animals studies	Behavioral stress CNS stimulation Pharmacological interventions during stress and	[11—18] [3, 16, 19] [21—24]	[13, 25]	[26]

Humans studies	Ventricular arrhythmias during emotional stress testing [33, 40]
	Long QT syndrome [3, 34—38]
	Psychosocial factors and sudden cardiac death in post-myocardial infarction patients:
	    retrospective [1, 31—33, 41—44]
	    prospective [45—48, 55]
	Patients resuscitated following ventricular fibrillation [4]
	Behavioral interventions in patients at risk of SCD [49, 51, 54]			

CNS: central nervous system

Pharmacological studies [21] have shown that beta-blockers and also diazepam protected against malignant ventricular arrhythmias associated with acute coronary artery occlusion in dogs exposed to light, sudden noise and electrical shock stress. DeSilva *et al.* [22] have observed that pretreatment with morphine accentuated vagal tone and completely prevented a decrease in the vulnerable period threshold during stressful environmental conditions.

Administration of tryptophane (a serotonine precursor) and monoamino oxidase inhibitor (IMAO) decreases vulnerability to VF [23], probably due to the effect of serotonine in CNS decreasing sympathetic flow to the heart [24].

While nonspecific emotional arousal or defense reactions increase coronary blood flow as in physical exercise, denial of access of food and consequent anger are associated with a progressive increase in coronary vascular resistance. Verrier *el al.* [25] have observed that this increase persists for 10 to 15 min after the anger episode, when heart rate and arterial pressure have returned to control levels, suggesting emotionally triggered primary coronary vasoconstriction.

Pathologic examination of rats exposed to heat, electrical shock, intense light, sound or audio presentation of noisy ratcat fights showed coronary occlusion due to platelet thrombi and fibrin deposits [26].

Studies in humans

Anecdotal evidence has accumulated over many years regarding sudden death in humans exposed to certain psychosocial conflicts, and prospective studies on this topic have been performed in recent years (Tables 2, 3).

Anthropological reports of death after voodoo practices, collected by Cannon in 1942 [27], are related to the much more recent descriptions of 'entrapment without exit' [4] or animal 'helplessness' [28]. In fact, when a person believes he is under the effect of voodoo, the community withdraw social support, and he sees death as the only way out of his unbearable loneliness. Once he accepts the inevitability of death the community come back, encouraging him to accept this form of exit [29].

From newspapers and colleagues' reports, Engel [1] collected 170 examples of emotional life settings in which sudden death was described to occur; for example, following the impact of death of someone close, under threat of loss of a close person, during mourning or on an anniversary, on loss of status or self-esteem, personal danger or threat of injury, after the danger is over, or even during reunion, triumph or a happy ending. What these emotional situations have in common is that they are impossible to ignore and evoke overwhelming excitation combined with lack of control.

Weisman and Hackett [30] described a *predilection* to death among

Table 2. Example of psychosocial determinants of sudden cardiac death

Low education-socioeconomic status	— no college education [48]; less than 8 years of schooling in the presence of complex ventricular premature beats [46]
Type A behavior pattern	— only for SCD 1 hour after the onset of acute symptoms [47]
Less social support	— not married [50, 58], women with fewer children [58]
Psychiatric history	— depression [58, 59], schizophrenia [58]
Educational incongruity	— women with more years education than husbands [58]
Life changes	— widowing [42, 43], retirement [44], more life events [41]
Hopelessness	— in animal studies: giving up after uncontrollable stress, slow heart rate and death [18]
Entrapment without exit	— Voodoo-like practices [27], biographic circumstances [4]
Sisyphus pattern	— individual strivess incessantly with no chance for satisfaction or success [10]
Predilection to death	— convinced that death is not only inevitable but desirable [30]

Table 3. Prospective studies on psychosocial determinants of sudden cardiac death in post-myocardial infarction patients

Authors (Year/Ref.)	N	Follow-up	Factor	Risk SCD
Weinblatt *et al.* 1978 [46]	1,739	3 yr.	Less 8 years schooling	× 3.3
Marmot *et al.* 1978 [48]	17,530	7.5 yr.	Low work qualification	× 3.6
Ruberman *et al.* 1984 [47]	2,320	3 yr.	Social isolation/low education	× 5
Brackett *et al.* 1988 [55]	1,012	4.5 yr.	Type A behavior	× 1.5
			Low socioeconomic status	× 3.1

critical surgical patients who regarded their impending deaths without anxiety or depression and were convinced that death was not only inevitable but desirable.

Sudden cardiac death may also occur during stressful situations such as sexual intercourse [31] or the first day of medical school [32] even in subjects without CAD.

Lown [33] has described the case of a patient with psychiatric problems and normal coronary arteries experiencing VF twice and numerous PVB, which were provoked by psychophysiologic stress testing (interviews) and reduced by beta-adrenergic blockade, phenytonin and digitalis.

In relation with the descriptions of death on an anniversary or recall of past negative emotional events [1], Figure 1 shows the case of a woman who presented a bidirectional ventricular tachycardia during exposure to a choice-reaction time stress test of uncontrollable basis, and who repeated the presentation of frequent isolated premature ventricular contractions, couplets and runs of ventricular tachycardia several hours later while mentally remembering and describing the previous stress situation to a friend. The clear involvement of such life-threatening ventricular arrhythmias in a conditioning reflex process is noteworthy. This arrhythmia was not observed in two previous conventional 24 hours Holter monitorings, therefore pointing out the usefulness of this kind of *emotional stress testing* [69].

The normal response to arithmetical mental stress is shortening QT even in absense of a simultaneous increase in ventricular rate, as has been shown in patients with permanent pacemaker [34, 35]. In long QT syndrome, sounds, pain, anger, or fright [3, 36—38] can trigger syncopal attacks.

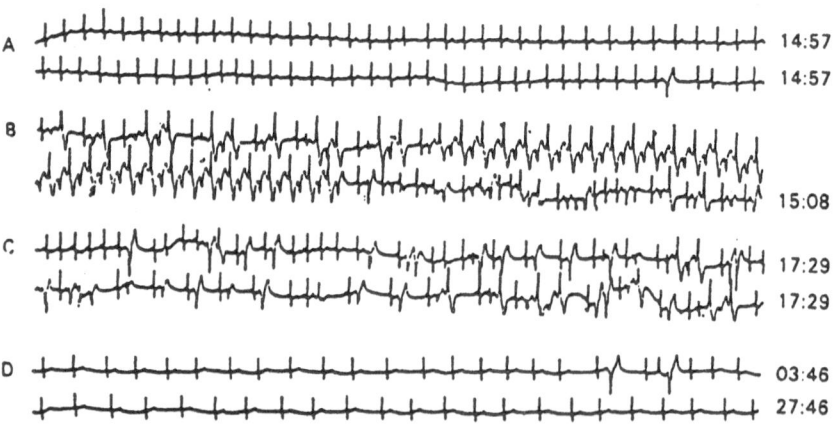

Figure 1. (A) Continuous Holter monitoring recording showing sinus rhythm at rest with some isolated PVBs. (B) Bidirectional VT during psychological stress testing (uncontrollable choice-reaction time task), which obliged to stop the test. (C) Reapparence of frecuent PVBs and couplets on recalling of past emotional event when explaining to friends. (D) Sinus ryhthm during sleep, with some isolated PVBs.

Neurosurgical procedures in the young without coronary artery disease induce long QT and decrease T waves [39]. Wolf [10] has described a *Sysiphus pattern* characterized by incessant striving without satisfaction after success very similar to Type A behavior pattern. In a serie of these men who were also emotionally depressed he observed prolongations of QT interval.

Lown [4] has formulated a tridimensional model to explain the psychophysiologic aspects of sudden cardiac death based on a retrospective study of 117 patients succesfully resuscitated after ventricular fibrillation and evaluated by a interdisciplinary group. The three dimensions are:

1. The presence of electrical instability of the myocardium, usually due to ischemic heart disease, whether symptomatic or not;
2. The presence of a psychological state of entrapment without possible exit intense enough to pervade and burden daily life;
3. A proximate psychologic trigger for the ventricular arrhythmia, which was present in patients with less demonstrable heart disease, consisting in the majority of cases of anger- related conflicts occuring less than one hour before the onset of the arrhythmia.

In a group of 20 patients with complex premature ventricular contractions we have observed [40] that a special biographic situation of 'entrapment without exit' (no way out in work, personal or familiar areas) happens much more frequently in patients without structural heart disease (6 of 12 cases) than in arrhythmic patients with heart disease (1 of 8 cases). The same patients score more depressive on the Minnesota Multiphasic Personality Inventory (MMPI) and Beck questionnaires.

By interviewing spouses or next of kin of individuals dying suddenly from myocardial infarction, Rahe *et al.* [41] found that in the 2 years prior to sudden death there was a 143% increase in the SRE scale (schedule of recent events) of 42 items. Furthermore, bereavement, specially among males [42, 43], and also retirement [44], has been associated with sudden cardiac death.

In a prospective study in post-MI patients, Follick [45] observed a direct relationship between self-reported distress levels (measured by the SCL-90 inventory) and occurrence of premature ventricular contractions. There are also several prospective studies relating increased risk of SCD with low education [46, 47], social isolation [47] and low work qualifications [48].

In a longitudinal study [49], the simple telephonic monitorization of psychological wellbeing in a sample of 453 post myocardial infarction patients was associated with a 47% decrease in mortality in comparison with a control group (4.4% vs. 8.9%). Another example of the importance of social support as a buffer of stress consequences is being married, which has been associated with decreased mortality in post-MI patients [50]. The main objective of self-help groups is to develop this social support.

Powell *et al.* [51] have found that reduction of type A behavior [52] decreases reinfarction but not mortality. In any case, the hostility component of this pattern of behavior is more related to mortality [53] than time urgency or other components.

It has been observed [54] that transfer from a coronary care unit to a general ward has been associated with emotional disturbances, increase in catecholamine excretion, reinfarction and serious ventricular arrhythmias, and specific psychological preparation is associated with fewer cardiac or emotional complications.

The latest demonstration of a direct relationship between psychosocial stress and SCD in a large prospective study has been made by Bracket and Powell [55]. Using data from the Recurrent Coronary Prevention Project (a 4.5 year prospective clinical trial of 1,012 postinfarction patients in San Francisco started in 1978) these authors found that SCD, defined as death occurring within 1 hour of the onset of acute symptoms, had predominantly psychosocial predictors, such as type A behavior (hostility and time urgency) [52], absence of a college education and low socioeconomic status, apart from anterior myocardial infarction. Nevertheless, nonsudden cardiac death and nonfatal reccurrences were predominantly predicated by biologic factors such as severity of angina or abstinence from alcohol. Besides, this study concludes that the risk of sudden death in a postinfarct patient can be reduced by reduction in the degree of type A behavior. Benson et al. [56] have shown that the relaxation response can reduce ventricular arrhythmias through autonomic nervous system influences, which could explain this results.

Nevertheless, Regland and Brand [57] have shown recently that persistence of type A behavior after a MI could predict less mortality after acute episode.

Talbot et al. [58] reported that women who died suddenly were less often married, had fewer children, had greater educational incongruity with their spouses and presented more psychiatric disorders than controls.

Physiopathologic implications

Combination of long standing depression and acute emotional disturbances, which has been proposed as psychophysiological basis of sudden death [4, 59], could provoke neurovegetative responses involving both the fight-flight (sympathetic adrenal-medullary system) and conservation-withdrawal responses (pituitary-adrenal-cortical system) [60, 61]. Corticoids increase the vassopresive action and myocardial degeneration experimentally induced by catecholamines [26]. Furthermore, sympathetic adrenal-medullar activity can facilitate electrolytic changes such as hypokalemia [62] previously induced by adrenal-cortical activation in depressive states [60], precipitating ventricular arrhythmias [63] (Table 4).

In fact, tricyclic antidepressants do not have the cardiac toxicity at therapeutical doses previously supposed [64], and can even have an antiarrhythmic effect, as has been observed in the CAPS study with imipramine [65]. For this antiarrhythmic effect of imipramine the patient need not be depressed, and its mechanism of action can be central or peripheric [66].

Table 4. Psychophysiological mechanism involved in sudden cardiac death

Psychological level:	Chronic depression	+	Acute emotional triggering (anger, fear . . .)
Physiological level:		↓	
Adrenal:	cortical	+	medular
Hormonal:	cortisol	+	catecholamines
Electrolytic:	↓ K⁺	+	↓ K⁺
ANS:	vagal	+	sympathetic (alpha)
ECG:	Long QT	+	short QT

↓

Vulnerable myocardium

↓

Sudden cardiac death

That acute anxiety could be involved in triggering sudden death is supported by the observations of Bayes de Luna *et al.* [67] who describe sinus tachycardization prior to sudden death from ventricular tachycardia.

Why education protects against sudden death is still unknown. Apart from better therapeutic and preventive compliance and access to better health services, education perhaps facilitates resources for coping with psychosocial stress. Association of low education with hostility, ambition, and time urgency (type A behavior pattern [52]) could suppose higher stress to gain social status that could lead to overfunction and disruption of integrating nervous system of cardiovacular function.

In effect, in a group of asymptomatic healthy subjects, we have found by multiple regression analysis considering several individual differences (age, sex, education, type A behavior, psychiatric disturbances by General Health Questionnaire, and basal blood pressure), that the function of more type A behavior pattern (Framingham scale) and less years of schooling is the only equation entering a predictive model of cardiovascular hyperreactivity. This equation is associated to greater increase in diastolic blood pressure (and not heart rate or systolic blood pressure) during exposure to a laboratory test consisting of a choice-reaction time stress of uncontrollable basis [68]. This diastolic blood pressure increase could be associated to a higher alphaadrenergic tone [69], which could be implied in coronary constriction, ischemia and sudden cardiac death.

Preventive implications

All this evidence on psychosocial determinants of sudden cardiac death indicates that some preventive measures in high risk patients should be taken:

1. Depression, not only anxiety, must be correctly diagnosed and treated, with tricyclics if necessary.
2. Social support must be movilized. Group programs can be useful in post-MI patients.

3. Hostility and anger components of Type A behavior pattern should be dealt with by specific intervention (personal counseling, group meetings on life values and relaxation training).
4. Education on coronary risk factors and stress management should be specifically increased in patients with less schooling.
5. Betablockers can be specially helpful in long-QT syndrome, in patients with increasing ventricular arrhythmias under emotional stress testing, and in hostile type A behavior pattern subjects.
6. Efforts to reduce psychological stress in coronary patients are important from the point of view of effective sudden death, decreasing not only for theoretical reasons.

References

1. Engel GL: Sudden and rapid death during psychological stress. Folklore or Folk Wisdom?. Ann Intern Med 1971; 74: 771—782.
2. Dismdale JE: Emotional causes of sudden death. Am J Psychiatry 1977; 134: 1361—1366.
3. Malliani A, Schwartz PJ, Zanchetti A: Neural mechanisms in life-threatening arrhythmias. Am Heart J 1980; 705—715.
4. Lown B, DeSilva RA, Reich P, Murawski BJ: Psychophysiologic factors in Sudden Cardiac death. Am J Psychiatry 1980; 137: 1325—1336.
5. Franck G, Rossi L, Piffer R, Matturri L: Psychosocial and neuropathologic precursors of arrhythmogenic sudden cardiac death: A synthetic reappraisal. New Tends Arrhythm 1985; 1: 125—143.
6. Dimsdale JE, Ruberman W, Carlenton Ra, DeQuattro V, Eaker E, Eliot RS, Furberg CD, Irvin CW, Lown B, Shapiro AP, Shumaker SA: Task force 1: Sudden cardiac death. Stress and cardiac arrhythmias. Circulation 1987; 76 (suppl I): 198—201.
7. Kuller LH, Talbott EO, Robinson C: Environmenntal and psychosocial determinants of sudden death. Circulation 1987; 76 (suppl I): 177—185.
8. Lown B, Sudden cardiac death: biobehavioral perspective. Circulation 1987; 76 (suppl I): 186—196.
9. Verrier RL: Mechanisms of behaviorally induced arrhythmias. Circulation 1987; 76 (suppl I): 48—56.
10. Wolf S: Behavioral aspects of cardiac arrhythmia and sudden death. Circulation 1987; 76 (suppl I): 174—176.
11. Lown B, Verrier RL, Corbalan R: Psychologic stress and threshold for repetitive ventricular response. Science 1973; 182: 834—838.
12. Lown B, Verrier RL, Neural activity and ventricular fibrillation. N Engl Med J 1976; 294: 1165—1170.
13. Verrier RL, Lomabridi F, Lown B: Restraint of myocardial blood flow during behavioral stress. Circulation 1982; 66 (suppl II): 258—262.
14. Verrier RL, Lown B: Influence of psychologic stress on susceptibility to spontaneous ventricular fibrillation during acute myocardial ischemia and reperfusion. Clin Res 1979; 27: 570—576.
15. Skinner JE, Lie JT, Entmen ML: Modification of ventricular fibrillation latency following coronary artery occlusion in the conscious pig: the effects of psychological stress and beta-adrenergic blockade. Circulation 1975; 51: 656—662.
16. Parker GW, Michael LH, Entman KL: An animal model to examine the response to

environmental stress as a factor in sudden cardiac death. Am J Cardiol 1987; 60: 9J—14J.

17. Richter C: On the phenomenon of sudden death in animals and man. Psychosom Med 1957; 19: 190—198.

18. Weiss JM, Pohorecky LA, Salman S, Gruenthal M: Attenuation of gastric lesions by psychological aspects of aggression in rate. J Comp Physiol Psychol 1976; 90: 252—259.

19. Skinner JE, Reed JC: Blockade of frontocortical-brain stem pathway prevents ventricular fibrillation of ischemic heart. Am J Physiol 1981; 240: 156—162.

20. Verrier RL, Lown B: Effects of left stellectomy on enhanced cardiac vulnerability induced by psychologic stress. Circulation 1977; 55/56 (suppl III): 80—84.

21. Rosenfeld J, Rosen MR, Hoffman BF: Pharmacologic and behavioural effects on arrhythmias that immediately follow abrupt coronary occlusion: a canine model of sudden coronary death. Am J Cardiol 1978; 41: 1075.

22. DeSilva RA, Verrier RL, Lown B: The effects of psychological stress and vagal stimulation with morphine on vulnerability to ventricular fibrillation (VF) in the conscious dog. Am Heart J 1978; 95: 197—201.

23. Rabinowitz SH, Lown B: Central neurochemical factors related to serotonin metabolism and cardiac ventricular vulnerability for repetitive electrical activity. Am J Cardiol 1978; 41: 516—522.

24. Antonaccio MJ, Robinson RD: Cardiovascular effects of 5-hydroxy-tryptophan in anesthetized dogs. J Pharm Pharmacol 1973; 25: 495—497.

25. Verrier RL, Hagestad EL, Lown B: Delayed myocardial ischemia induced by anger. Circulation 1987; 75: 249—253.

26. Raab W: Emotional and sensory stress factors in myocardial pathology. Am Heart J 1966; 72: 538—540.

27. Cannon W: Voodoo death. American Anthropologist 1942; 44: 169—181.

28. Seligman MEP: Helplessness: One depression, department, development and death. Freeman. San Francisco, 1975.

29. Cohen SI: La muerte vudú, la respuesta al stress, depresión y SIDA. Psicopatologia 1987; 8: 1—15.

30. Weissman A, Hackett T: Predilection to death. Psychosom Med 1961; 23: 232—256.

31. Vlay SC: Morte d'amour with subsequent electrophysiologic studies. Am J Cardiol 1988; 61: 1364.

32. Vlay SC: Ventricular tachycardia/fibrillation on the first day of medical school. Am J Cardiol 1986; 57: 483.

33. Lown B, Temte JV, Reich P, Gaughan CH, Regestein Q, Hai H: Basis for recurring ventricular fibrillation in the absense of coronary heart disease and its management. New Engl J Med 1976; 294: 623—629.

34. Hedman A, Norlander R: Changes in QT and Q-aT intervals induced by mental and physical stress with fixed rate and atrial triggered ventricular inhibited cardiac pacing. PACE 1988; 11: 1426—1431.

35. Hedman A, Hjemdahl P, Norlander R: Mental stress test in the evaluation of the QT sensing TX pacemaker. PACE 1987; 10: 687—692.

36. Sigurd B, Suenson M, Wennevold A, Sandoe E: Los syndromes de QT largo. In: Bayes A, Cosín J eds. Diagnóstico y tratamiento de las arritmias cardiacas. Doyma. Barcelona 1978; pp 624—630.

37. Vincet GM, Abildskov JA, Burguess MJ: QT interval syndromes. Progr Cardiovasc Dis 1974; 16: 523—525.

38. Schwartz PJ: Experimental reproduction of the long QT syndromes. Am J Cardiol 1978; 41: 374—378.

39. Finkelstein S, Nigagliani A: Electrocardiographic alterations after neurosurgical procedures. Am heart J 1961/ 62: 772—778.

40. García-Sánchez S, Bayés de Luna A, Guindo J, García-Moll M: Complejos ventriculares prematuros y factores psicológicos. Rev Esp cardiol 1985; 38 (suppl II): 48.

41. Rahe RH, Bennet L: Recent life changes, myocardial infarction and abrupt coronary death. Arch Intern Med 1974; 133: 221—228.
42. Helsing KJ, Szklo M, Comstock GW: Factors associated with mortality after widowhood. Am J Public Health 1981; 71: 802—810.
43. Parkes CM, Benjamin G, Fitzgerald RG: Broken heart: a statistical study of increased mortality among widowers. Br med J 1969; 1: 740—743.
44. Casscelles W, Hennnekens CH, Evans D, Rosener et al.: Retirement and coronary mortality. Lancet 1980; 1: 1288—1289.
45. Follick MJ, Gorkin L, Capone RJ, Smith TW, Ahern DK, Stablein D, Niaura R, Visco J: Psychological stress as a predictor of ventricular arrhythmias in a post-myocardial infarction population. Am Heart J 1988; 116: 32—36.
46. Weinblatt E, Ruberman W, Golderg JD, Frank ChW, Shapiro S, Chaudary BS: Relation of education to sudden death after myocardial infarction. New Engl J Med 1978; 299: 60—65.
47. Ruberman W, Weinblatt E, Glodberg JD, Chauhary BS: Psychosocial influences on mortality after myocardial infarction. N Eng J Med 1984; 311: 552—559.
48. Marmot MG, Rose G, Shipley M, Hamilton PJS: Employment grade and coronary heart disease in British civil servants. J Epidemiol Community Health 1978; 32: 244—249.
49. Frasure-Smith N, Prince R: The ischemic Heart Disease Lide Stress Monitoring Program: impact on mortality. Psychosom Med 1985; 41: 431—445.
50. Chandra V, Szklo M, Goldberg R, Tonascia J: The impact of marital status of survival after an acute myocardial infarction: a population-based study. Am J Epidemiol 1983; 117: 320—325.
51. Powell LH, Friedman M, Thoresen CE, Gill JJ, Ulmer DK: Can the Type A behavior pattern be altered after myocardial infarction? A second year report from the Recurrent Coronary Prevention Project. Psychosom Med 1984; 46: 293—314.
52. Friedman M, Rosenman RH: Association of specific overt behavior pattern with blood and cardiovascular findings. JAMA 1959; 96: 1286—1296.
53. Williams RB: Redifining the Type A hipotesis: emergence of the hostility complex. Am J Cardiol 1987; 60: 27J—32J.
54. Klein RF, Kliner VA: Transfer from a coronary care unit. Some adverse responses. Arch Intern Med 1978; 122: 104—108.
55. Brackett Ch D, Powell L: Psychosocial and Physiological predictors of sudden cardiac death after healing of acute myocardial infarction. Am J Cardiol 1988; 61: 979—983.
56. Benson H, Alexander S, Feldman ChL: Decreased premature ventricular contractions through use of the relaxation response in patients with stable ischemic heart-disease. Lancet 1975; 380—382.
57. Ragland DR, Brand RJ: Type A behavior and mortality from coronary heart disease N Engl Med 1988; 318: 65—69.
58. Talbott E, Kuller LH, Detre K, Perper J: Biologic and psychosocial risk factors of sudden death from coronary disease in white women. Am J Cardiol 1977; 39: 856—864.
59. Greene WA, Goldstein S, Moss AJ: Psychosocial aspects of sudden death. Arch Intern Med 1972; 129: 725—731.
60. Henry JP, Stephens PM: Stress, health and the social environment. Springer-Verlag. New York 1977.
61. Selye H: The evolution of the stress concept. Am J Cardiol 1970; 26: 289.
62. Struthers AD, Reid JL, McLean K, Rodger JC: Adrenaline, hypokalemia and cardiac arrhythmias: the effect of beta adrenoceptor antagonists. Clin Sci 1982; 62: 11.
63. Thomas R, Hicks S: Myocardial infarction: ventricular arrhythmias associated with hypokalemia. Clin Sci 1981; 60: 32.
64. Jefferson JW: A review of the cardiovascular effects and toxicity of tricyclic antidepressants. Psychosom Med 1975; 37: 160—179.
65. The Cardiac Arrhythmia Pilot Study (CAPS) Investigators: Recruitment and baseline

description of patients in the Cardiac Arrhythmia Pilot Study. AM J Cardiol 1988; 61: 704—713.

66. Giardina EGV, Bigger JT: Antiarrhythmic effect of imipramine hydrochloride in patients with ventricular premature complexes without psychological depression. Am J Cardiol 1982; 50: 172—179.
67. Bayés de Luna A, Coumel Ph, Leclercq JF: Ambulatory sudden death: mechanisms of production of fatal arrhythmia on the basis of data from 157 cases. AM Heart J 1989; 117: 154.
68. Carcía-Sánchez S: Prueba de Esfuerzo Emocional: Estudio de la psicofisiología cardiovascular en diferentes grupos de sujetos. Doctoral Thesis. Barcelona, 1989.
69. Newlin DB, Levenson RW: Cardiovascular responses of individuals with type A behavior pattern and parental coronary heart disease. J Psychosom Res 1982; 26: 393—402.

8. Acute and chronic components of ischaemia in acute ischaemic syndromes

ATTILIO MASERI

It is now established that thrombosis plays a major role in acute ischaemic syndromes. Thrombosis develops for causes still incompletely understood, on an atherosclerotic background of very variable severity, and leads to a chain of events which often, but not invariably, results in permanent organ damage or death.

When considered in broad terms as a single disease entity, ischaemic heart disease appears to have a very variable, unpredictable onset and course, often punctuated by occasional, usually unheralded, catastrophic events caused by acute ischaemic stimuli.

It is commonly assumed that, by and large, the disease has a long preclinical course and a certain 'threshold' above which ischaemic heart disease becomes more frequent. However, this assumption requires qualification, as it would be useful to establish whether the disconcerting variability of course and outcome results just from random chance on a sub-clinical, gradually progressive evolution, or whether it also reflects an important heterogeneity of prevailing mechanisms.

The consideration of pathogenetic components of ischaemic syndromes should lay the basis for any future attempt to identify clinical subsets with better defined prognosis.

In order to understand the relative contribution of various pathogenetic mechanisms to ischaemic syndromes, it may be useful to identify the individual pathogenetic components. Indeed major distinct components can be identified in the pathogenesis of acute ischaemic syndromes:

— The atherosclerotic background, which develops slowly over a period of years, presumably as a result of a variety of injuries to the vessel wall and of variable blood-vessel wall interactions.
— Acute ischaemic stimuli which occur occasionally and usually unpredictably in the presence of a very variable atherosclerotic background. Their very rare occurrence must be the result of very rare events or of the coincidental occurrence at the same time of multiple, relatively rare, unfavourable events and cannot be explained by alterations which are fairly common or occur frequently [1].

A. Bayés de Luna et al. (eds.): *Sudden Cardiac Death*, 83–86.

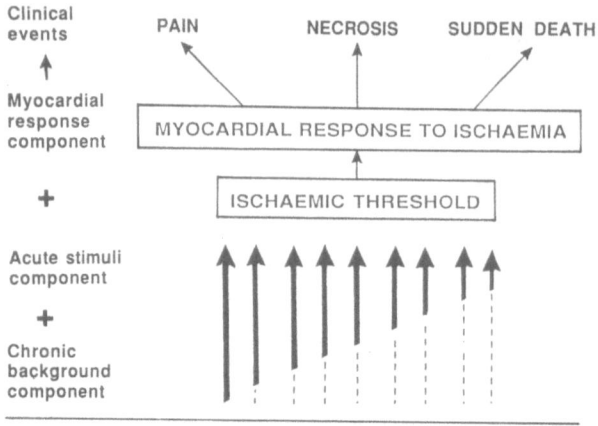

Figure 1.

— The variable response of the heart to ischaemia, particularly in terms of supply of blood via collateral vessels and development of fatal arrhythmias (Figure 1).

In this presentation I will outline the components related to ischaemic stimuli.

The acute ischaemic stimuli

The discrepancies between severity of coronary 'atherosclerosis' and signs of myocardial ischaemia in age- and sex-matched case controls and in population studies are too commonly reported and too obvious to be dismissed as an artefact resulting from inaccurate assessment either of coronary anatomy or of the signs and symptoms of myocardial ischaemia. Therefore, ischaemic stimuli must represent a major, though often elusive, link between the very variable pre-existing 'atherosclerotic' background and acute myocardial ischaemic events.

Acute myocardial ischaemia can result from two types of stimuli:

a) excessive increase of myocardial oxygen consumption in the presence of limitation of coronary blood flow — *secondary to increased myocardial demand*. In this case the coronary circulation plays a predominantly passive secondary role as the acute ischaemic stimulus is in the myocardium. Myocardial ischaemia is simply the consequence of alterations, usually chronic and stable, already established in the coronary circulation;

b) sudden reduction of regional coronary oxygen supply which depends on active transient processes taking place in the coronary circulation. These processes can be due to a variety of causes and all lead to a *primary, sudden reduction of coronary supply*.

A given stimulus can be the only cause of ischaemia for some patients, but often different stimuli occur in the same patient at different times or in combination at the same time.

Ischaemic stimuli caused by a primary acute impairment of coronary flow are much more likely to cause catastrophic coronary events. In particular, the most dangerous acute ischaemic stimuli are coronary thrombosis and spasm because they can cause sudden coronary artery occlusion and massive ischaemia. Coronary thrombosis was traditionally considered as synonymous with infarction, however, nowadays it is recognised as a very dynamic process which plays a major role, possibly in combination with some form of coronary constriction, not only in myocardial infarction and in sudden ischaemic cardiac death but also in those patients with recent onset and worsening of angina requiring aggressive management. Small fresh mural fibrinplatelet thrombi can also be found at the site, or within fissured "atherosclerotic" plaques, in about 10% of a random sample of individuals who died of non-cardiac causes, and in 20% of those with a history of hypertension, diabetes, hypercholesterolaemia. Conversely, in a few instances no fissure can be found at the site of coronary thrombosis. The existence of coronary artery spasm could be demonstrated in patients with variant angina because in these patients it occurs often and it can be reproduced by provocative tests. Spasm can occur both at the site of angiographically normal arteries and at the site of plaques reducing the lumen up to 90%. The susceptibility to develop spasm in response to ergonovine challenge [2] was found to be much higher in unstable angina (38% of the cases) and in recent infarction (20%) than in old infarction (6%), stable angina (4%) or atypical chest pain (2%). However, the role of coronary spasm in occasional acute ischaemic syndromes other than variant angina is difficult to ascertain because spasm is an ischaemic stimulus even more sudden and elusive than thrombus.

In patients with acute infarction angiography showed that, after thrombo-lytic therapy, the severity of the residual stenosis in the infarct-related coronary artery is only mild in about 20% of patients with first myocardial infarction, consistent with their sudden presentation with ischaemic heart disease [3] and the pre-existing stenosis at the site of thrombosis could have been even milder if thrombolysis was not complete. The comparison of the severity of stenoses in infarct-related artery after thrombolytic therapy with that found in the absence of thrombolytic therapy is revealing [4]. In the absence of thrombolytic therapy a much small number of vessels recanalize spontaneously and the stenosis of the infarct-related artery is mild in about 10% of the cases, but on the whole obstruction or very severe stenosis of the infarct-related artery remains after infarction in the absence of thrombolytic therapy. Therefore, ischaemic stimuli leading to the formation of coronary thrombus, but not necessarily to infarction, often do not occur at the site of pre-existing flow-limiting stenoses, and can lead to sudden progression of coronary artery 'atherosclerotic' obstruction, when the thrombus is incompletely lysed. Myocardial infarction with angiographically 'normal' coronary arteries, without critical stenosis or with single vessel disease is more frequent in young patients without previous ischaemic heart disease. Thus, some of the older patients with a previous history of ischaemic heart disease who come to medical attention with severe multi-vessel disease might also have had repeated episodes of occasional thrombus with or without infarction in the past and thus the severity of a coronary artery obstruction could be the result of old ischaemic stimuli rather than only its cause.

Acute ischaemic syndromes happen only occasionally in the life of a patient. Therefore their cause cannot be explained by any of the fairly frequent causes [1]. The precise understanding of the causes of sudden coronary occlusion remains a major challenge.

Reference

1.   Maseri A, Chierchia S, Davies, GJ: Pathophysiology of coronary occlusion in acute infarction. Circulation 1986; 73: 233.
2.   Bertrand ME, La Blanche JM, Tilmant PY, Thieuleux FA, Delfarge MR, Carre G, Asseman P, Berzin B, Libersa C, Laurent JM: Frequency of provoked coronary arterial spasm in 1089 consecutive patients undergoing coronary arteriography. Circulation 1982; 65: 1299.
3.   Hackett D, Davies G, Maseri A: Pre-existing coronary stenoses in patients with first myocardial infarction are not necessarily severe. Eur Heart J 1988; 9: 1317.
4.   Bertrand M, Lefebvre J, Laisne C, Rousseau M, Carre A, Lekieffre J: Coronary arteriography in acute transmural myocardial infarction. Am Heart J 1979; 97: 61.

9. Markers and trigger mechanisms of sudden cardiac death
Exercise and sports activity

F. FURLANELLO, R. BETTINI, G. VERGARA, A. BERTOLDI,
M. DEL GRECO, G. B. DURANTE and L. FRISANCO

Background

Exertion-related cardiac arrest and sudden death may happen both in cardiac patients and in subjects without evident heart disease. This latter group includes young athletes who are also competitive and at a high level of sports activity with asymptomatic cardiopathy [1, 2, 3, 4, 5, 6, 7, 8]. Exertion and sports activity-related cardiac arrest is typically a primary arrhythmic event [9] due to electrical destabilization of underlying heart disease or to primary arrhythmic disorders. Several reports have indicated that there is a small correlation between vigorous exercise and cardiac arrest (CA) — sudden cardiac arrhythmic death (SCAD) in the general population. This correlation ranges from 9 to 17% of all sudden death [10, 11, 12] and is about 11% of patients resuscitated from out-of hospital cardiac arrest due to ventricular fibrillation [9]. However, in young athletes, a cardiac arrest/ SCAD is normally sports activity-related [1, 8]. In fact, serious arrhythmic patterns are possible in athletes during or immediately after athletic activity (post-exertion vulnerable period). These manifestations may cause critical symptoms and/or haemodynamic repercussions which include presyncope, syncope, hyperkinetic or hypokinetic cardiac arrest, aborted sudden death which, if not resuscitated, may lead to sudden death [2].

Exertion-related cardiac arrest/SCAD appears to be confined to patients with structural heart disease or primary electrical disorders. Beyond the age of 35 years 90% of the victims have atherosclerotic coronary heart disease [13, 14, 15].

Indeed in young active athletes many types of so called 'silent arrhythmogenic cardopathy' are possible [1, 2, 4, 5, 8, 16]. This latter condition is characterised by morphostructural or only electrical anomalies of such minor significance from a haemodynamic standpoint that high-level athletic results may be obtained. However, there is the possibility of electrical destabilisation, primarily during or after the athletic activity.

The most important information about silent arrhythmogenic cardiopathy of the young athletes is based both on the pathological examination of the

A. Bayés de Luna et al. (eds.): *Sudden Cardiac Death*, 87–98.
© 1991 Kluwer Academic Publishers, Dordrecht.

athletes who died suddenly [5, 16], and on the arrhythmologic studies of the subjects with aborted sudden death or malignant arrhythmic manifestations which were sports activity related [1, 2, 4, 17]. At present the background of the silent arrhythmogenic cardiopathy of the athletes may be confined to the following heart diseases or primary electrical disorders:

1) coronary heart diesase which was mainly atherosclerosis but which also included congenital anomalies of origin or of course;
2) cardiomyopathy, particularly hypertrophic cardiomyopathy, arrhythmogenic right ventricular dysplasia and dilated cardiomyopathy;
3) myocarditis (active, healing, healed);
4) mitral valve prolapse;
5) conduction system disturbances;
6) WPW syndrome;
7) long QT syndrome.

The identification of the silent cardiopathy in the competitive athletes has led to the development of some preparticipation screening studies [18] and to the formulation of cardio-arrhythmological study protocols. These protocols may be applied, in a sport Arrhythmologic Centre, to the individual athlete with arrhythmias in order to identify the subject at risk of sudden death [1, 2, 3, 4, 17].

The aim of this work is to answer the following questions:

a) can sports activity by considered a *trigger* of electrical destabilization in competitive asymptomatic athletes with silent arrhythmogenic cardiopathy?
b) is it possible to reproduce in a cardiological laboratory the most severe symptoms which are sports-activity related and/or to single out the *markers* of the risk?

The present study concerns a wide experience from 1974 to 1988 which is based on a cardioarrhythmological study protocol for the athlete and which has previously been decribed [1, 2, 4]. In this paper we only report on the most important symptoms and/or arrhythmic manifestations which are sports activity-related and are based on five different subgroups of our athlete population.

Athlete population

This study concerns 410 athletes, 352 males, 58 females, mean age about 23 years (Table 1) who were referred to our Arrhythmologic Centre for serious documented or suspected arrhythmias from 1974 to 1988. In this young population only athletes who had been previously declared fit for sports activity are included. They practiced all kinds of sport [2, 4] even as competitive athletes and at a high level until the appearance of arrhythmic manifestations and/or symptoms for which they were referred to our Centre.

Table 1. Athlete population

---

410 athletes — 352 M, 58 F. Mean age 23 years

Subgroups:

214   WPW
52   Mitral valve prolapse (MVP)
32   Arrhythmogenic right ventricular disease (ARVD)
5   Sudden death
9   Aborted sudden death

---

1) *Aborted sudden death athletes.* 9/410 athletes (mean age 25.9 years) were referred to our Centre after cardiac arrest, 6 during effort and 3 after effort (Table 2 and 3) with subsequent cardiac resuscitation; these cases are typical examples of aborted sudden death.

The clinical arrhythmia was ventricular fibrillation (VF) in 8, which probably followed ventricular tachycardia (VT) in 3 cases and preexcited atrial fibrillation in 4 cases. In one case with clinical arrhythmias which were not documented during arrest, symptomatic prolonged AV block was evidenced during paroxysmal atrial fibrillation. Four athletes had structural heart disease (1 dilated cardiomyopathy, 1 ARVD, 1 minor hypertrophic cardiomyopathy and 1 MVP); 4 had WPW (2 of which instable). The arrhythmologic study with EES allowed us to observe sustained VT in 2 athletes (the one with ARVD and the one with initial dilated cardiomyopathy) and multiform VT in one (with minor hypertrophic cardiomyopathy), as well as preexcited atrial fibrillation (shortest R-R < 190 ms) in the 4 WPW athletes. It was not possible to induce any arrhythmias in the clinical VF athlete with MVP.

Table 2. Aborted sudden death 5 athletes referred to our Centre after cardiac resuscitation

Years	Sport	Exercise	Clinical arrhythmia		Induced arrhythmia	Cardiopathy
1) 22-M	Foot-ball	After	V.F.		Not	MVP
2) 36-M	Swimming	After	?		Prolonged AV block during paroxysmal a.f.	
3) 27-M	Foot-ball	After	V.T.	V.F.	Sustained VT (EES)	ARVD
4) 33-M	Foot-ball	During	V.T.	V.F.	Sustained VT (EES)	Initial dilated cardiomyopathy
5) 33-M	Foot-ball	During	V.T.	V.F.	Multiform VT	Minor hypertrophic cardiomyopathy

Table 3. WPW athletes with cardiac arrest (mean age = 21.7 years)

	WPW	Exercise	Spontaneous acute episode	Induced by TES or EES	
4 cardiac arrest DC shock	Instable	Druing	1) referred V.F.	1) a.f. preexcited with shortest R-R 195 ms	EES
	Stable	During	2) a.f. preexcited with shortest 160—170 ms V.F.	2) a.f. preexcited with shortest R-R 160 ms	EES
	Stable	During	3) a.f. preexcited with shortest R-R 160 ms	3) a.f. preexcited with shortest R-R 190 ms	TES
	Instable	During	4) V.F.	4) a.f. preexcited with shortest R-R 170 ms	TES

2) *WPW athletes.* Of 214 athletes with WPW, 10 were studied after a syncope with spontaneous termination (Table 4) and 4 were studied after a cardiac arrest with DC shock and cardiopulmunary resuscitation (Table 3).

Both syncope (5/6) and cardiac arrest (4/4) were sports activity-related. These athletes had an electrogenetic mechanism that could be reproduced by Electrophysiological Endocavitary Studies (EES) or Transesophageal Electrophysiological Study (TES).

Table 4. WPW athletes with syncope

	WPW	Exercise	Spontaneous acute episode	Induced by TES or EES	
6 syncope with spontaneous termination	Stable	During	No ECG	1) a.f. preexcited shortest R-R 200 ms	TES
	Stable hypertrophic cardiomyopathy	At rest	No ECG	2) preexcited R/T at 220/min cardiac arrest	TES
	Stable	During	Preexcited R/T at 210/min	3) not induced	EES
	Unstable	During	No ECG	4) preexcited a.f. R-R 190 ms	EES
	Unstable	After	Preexcited a.f. R-R 190 ms	5) preexcited a.f. R-R 190 ms	TES
	Stable	During	Preexcited a.f. R-R 180 ms	6) preexcited a.f. R-R 200 ms	EES

This mechanism is mainly due to preexcited atrial fibrillation with shortest R-R < 200 ms (< 190 ms in athletes with cardiac arrest).

3) *Sudden death.* 5/410 athletes (mean age 30.6 years) (Table 5) who were all previously fit for athletic activity, had sudden death, 4 during follow up after arrhythmologic studies; 1 of whom was previously asymptomatic (as a first symptom). Sudden death was sports activity related in 4/5 (Table 6). In the fifth athlete who was on medical-surgical-AICD treatment for ARVD with refractory polymorphous sustained VT with proarrhythmic phenomena, the SD happened 1 month after cardiosurgical cryoablations and AICD

Table 5. Arrhythmias in athletes: Sudden death

---

1. 18 year old basket ball player.
    Palpitations after effort — negative arrhythmological study.
    Sudden death one year later during warm-up before basket ball match.
    Pathological examination: coronary artery obstructive disease.
2. 23 year old 'tug-of-war' player.
    Paroxysmal atrial flutter fibrillation, MVP.
    Sudden death in a discotheque 6 months later.
    Pathological examination: not performed.
3. 47 year old-cyclist.
    Aborted SD during sports activity.
    Refractory polymorphous sustained VT with proarrhythmic phenomena.
    Very slight echo-ventriculographic alterations.
    Multiple cardiosurgical cryoablations, AICD implantation.
    Remarkable bi-ventricular (mainly right) fibroadiposis.
    SD 1 month after while walking: post-defibrillation asystole.
4. A 37 year old athlete, national trainer for cross country skiing.
    Asymptomatic: very good athletic performances.
    Cardiac arrest from VF after taking part in the Marcialonga in which he gave a very good performance and was among the first to arrive at finishing point.
    Anatomo-pathological evidence of acute massive MI.
5. A 28 year old professional footballer
    NsVT multiform type
    ARVD diffused form with LV involvement
    Declared not fit
    SD 'on field' 4 years later while training a football team

---

Table 6. Sudden death athletes (5/410)

---

4 During follow-up:

3 sports activity related despite being declared not fit	1 on medical-surgical-AICD treatment previously aborted SD during competition

1 Asymptomatic (as a first symptom)

---

implantation, for post-defibrillation asystole. This patient had previous aborted sudden death during competition (cyclistic amateur trial).

In 3 athletes, even though they had been declared not fit, SD happened during follow-up and was exercise-related. As regards the substrate (Table 7) 2 had ischemic heart disease, 2 had ARVD and 1 had 'complicated' MVP. Sports activity can be considered a trigger because 4/5 SD and 1/5 previous aborted SD were exercise related. Good athletic performance was a typical situation for a silent cardiopathy of the athletes in this population.

4) *Arrhythmogenic Right Ventricular Dysplasia (ARVD).* In 32 athletes with ARVD, mean age 23.4 years, 59.4% of the most serious arrhythmias and symptoms (including syncope, sustained VT, cardiac arrest) were sports activity-related (Table 8). However there was not a high correlation (41.2%) between clinical severe arrhythmic manifestations which were exercise related and arrhythmias induced or worsened by ergometric test (ET) or which were recorded by Holter monitoring (HM). Moreover 19/32 ARVD athletes had clinical sustained VT, which were sports activity related in 95% (19/20) and accompanied by severe symptoms (5 syncopes, 9 presyncopes, 1 cardiac arrest). The reproducibility in laboratory of these sustained VT (Table 9) was 3.1% by HM and 6.8% by ET, higher by EES with specificity 100% (but with sensitivity of only 60% and accuracy of 68%). Two athletes died during follow up (see section 1).

5) *Mitral Valve Prolapse (MVP) athletes.* 52 of 410 athletes admitted to our Centre for documented or suspected arrhythmias had MVP. Sports activity-related symptoms were less than 50% (32.7% during, 5.8% after exercise)

Table 7. Sudden death athletes (5/410)

Substrate:	Trigger:
2 ischemic heart disease	4/5 SD and 1/5 previously aborted SD sports activity related in
2 ARVD	subjects with good athletic performance.
1 complicated MVP	

Table 8. ARVD athletes. Mean age 23.4 years. Most serious arrhythmias. 19/32 (59.4%) sports activity related

Non sustained VT	8/32
Sustained VT	19/32
Cardiac arrest (VT → FV)	1/32
Presyncope	9/32
Syncope	5/32
SD (during follow-up)	2/32
(1 while training a football team)	

Table 9. 32 ARVD athletes. 19/32 clinical sustained VT. 19/20 (95%) during sports activity. Documented in laboratory.

Holter monitoring	1/32	(3.1%)
Bicycle ergometric test	2/29	(6.8%)
Induced (EES), all with clinical VT	12/25	(48%)

Sensitivity: 60%; Specificity: 100%; Accuracy: 68%

but included cardiac arrest and presyncope (Table 10). One ex-athlete died during follow up during exercise (Table 11). By ergometric tests only 36% of MVP athletes increased or worsened the basal arrhythmias but the most serious forms (non sustained VT, sustained VT) were included.

MVP is a very common arrhythmic syndrome in athletes and is frequently benign (22/52 athletes are still active in sports). Sports activity-related exercise arrhythmias are not very frequent but the most serious forms can appear during effort.

Table 10. 52 MVP athletes symptoms and sport activity.

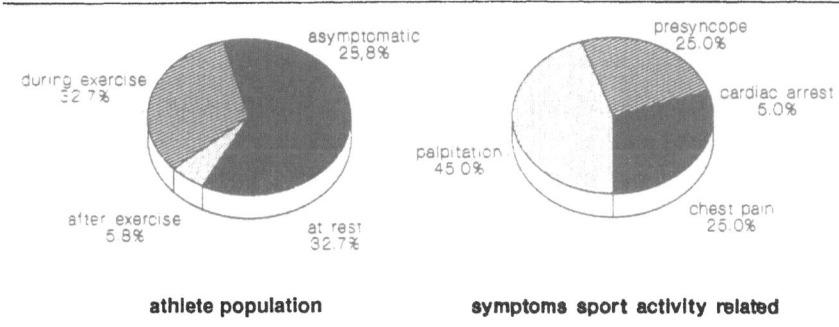

athlete population   **symptoms sport activity related**

Table 11. 52 MVP athletes follow up.

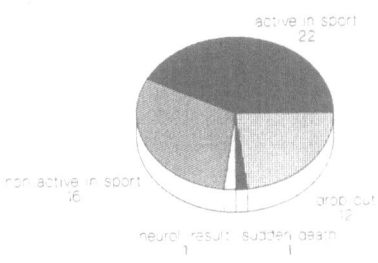

Comments

Vigorous effort including sports activity can be a *trigger* of electrical destabilization and can lead to Sudden Cardiac Arrhythmic Death (SCAD) in susceptible patients with myocardial vulnerability due to underlying disease or to primary arrhythmogenic cardiopathy (WPW, prolonged QT, pathology of the conduction system). SCAD can be avoided in patients with even severe damage of myocardium during supervised exercise tests [9, 19] and rehabilitation programmes [20, 21].

Cardiac arrest and SCAD are not frequent (about 10—15% of all S.D.) in the previously asymptomatic general population, who performs vigorous effort and sports activity, but are possible and unpredictable in susceptible subjects, especially when they are occasionally involved in physical exercise.

Both retrospective and prospective studies on the incidence of exertion-related cardiac arrest and SCAD in persons without evident heart disease are epidemiologically incomplete, especially since they include subjects of different ages (i.e. from 25 to 75 years [22]) and with different degrees of exercise activity. As an indication, one CA occurred in 375,000 people hours of exercise [23], one SD per 396,000 hours of jogging [24]. In our personal experience of the popular famous 50—70 Km competition of cross-country skiing (The Marcialonga) with thousands of skiers participating [1] there have been 2 deaths (one during and one after) in 17 years. It means 1 death in 42,334.5 participants, 1 for every 2,963,415 Km of skiing. There are some, though not conclusive, reports on the estimate additional risk of cardiac arrest/SD during physical exertion in relation to other time [25]. For instance, SD related to jogging was 10 fold greater than the SD due to non vigorous activity [26]; the incidence of CA was 5 to 56 times greater during high intensity exercise. The relative risk of SD during strenuous exercise as compared with other times increased by a factor 56 [22] in men with relatively low levels of normal activity. There is general agreement that in the asymptomatic population over the age of 35 obstructive coronary artery disease secondary to atherosclerosis is the leading cause of CA/SCAD which is exercise and sports activity-related. As a final comment on the problem of SCAD in the general and not very young population, we can say that strenuous physical exertion and sports activity may trigger cardiac arrest in some apparently normal but susceptible subjects with underlying disease which is mainly coronary atherosclerosis, and that the events are frequently unpredictable.

Sports activity related cardiac arrest-sudden cardiac arrhythmic death in athletes

The problem is quite different from that in the general population for different reasons including age, training, competitions, medical supervision, compulsory fitness and type of underlying arrhythmogenic silent cardiopathy.

Given the aims of this work, our patient population can be considered as a valid sample of athletes with severe symptoms and arrhythmic manifestations which are sports activity-related (including aborted SD, CA and SCAD) because all types of sports are represented and because the athletes are young (mean age about 23 years) and all were previously declared fit.

For the discussion we considered 5 different subground, aborted SD and sudden death, WPW, ARVD and MVP athletes. These groups are quite representative of all possible conditions reponsible for sports activity-related electrical destabilization.

The first question regards sports activity as a trigger of cardiac arrest/SCAD in young athletes. There is conclusive documentation that SCAD in the majority of cases is closely correlated to sports activity and normally happens during or immediately after (vulnerable period post-exercise) effort. In our athlete population major clinical arrhythmic symptoms such as presyncope, syncope, severe non sustained VT (including multiform type) sustained VT, preexcited atrial fibrillation, VF, aborted SD, Sudden Death, were present in almost all subjects during effort or immediately after. In three ex-athletes, declared not fit, Sudden Death happened during follow up, while exercising, even though sports activity had been forbidden to them. Thus the improvement in the arrhythmological studies of the athletes at risk for arrhythmogenic silent cardiopathy may create a new clinical problem, for the long term prevention of SCAD in identified subjects who have been warned of risk. Consequently, the follow up of these selected ex-athletes has to be careful and should include the therapeutic control of potentially severe arrhythmic manifestations.

The second question regards the reproducibility in laboratory of the most serious symptoms and arrhythmic manifestations that happen spontaneously and are sports activity-related in athletes. In addition, in the presence of a silent arrhythmogenic cardiopathy several different conditions are necessary for the triggering of severe arrhythmic manifestations during sports activity. The electrical destabilisation that may take place during or after the athletic activity needs a particular variation of the neurovegetative tone in subjects with a pre-existing arrhythmogenic substratum and with activation of possible present or latent trigger arrhythmias. Moreover, psychobiological components, such as emotion, fatigue, and/or specific type of sport play and additional important role in the realisation of lethal arrhythmias during sports activity (see ARVD) as was observed in the 'normal' population in individual cases [27, 28]. Sometimes it is not easy to reproduce these conditions in a laboratory study, particularly when the electrogenetic mechanism of the spontaneous arrhythmias is not reinducible or when the ventricular irritability is too erratic.

That is not the case of the WPW athletes in whom it is easy to reproduce the clinical symptoms and the most severe arrhythmias (preexcited AF, VF) by electrophysiological transesophageal atrial pacing and during ergometric test [29, 30].

The substrate of sports activity related cardiac arrest/SCAD is a silent cardiopathy with good athletic performance. If the patophysiologic mechanism of SD is an independent contribution of two factors, i.e. ventricular arrhythmias and myocardial vulnerability [31], in competitive asymptomatic athletes the substrate is only a potential arrhythmogenic situation which permits good performance. In contrast to cardiac patients with extensive myocardial disease and underlying vulnerability, the silent cardiopathy of the athletes requires a strong provocation (trigger) to precipitate life-threatening arrhythmias; the trigger is both physiologic (sports activity) and due to a sympathetic-vagal drive including psycobiological components.

The need for strong trigger to destabilize an underlying good ventricular function justifies the fact that the cardiac arrest in competitive athletes is a rare event which is sometimes difficult to reproduce but easier to control than in cardiac patients.

When it is not possible to reproduce the spontaneous sports activity related arrhythmic events, as we observed in some athletes with sustained symptomatic VT and ARVD, it is necessary to identify, by careful arrhythmic study, a useful markers of the individual risk. For instance, in our experience we can indicate as markers of risk for ARVD athletes [3]:

a) T waves inversion the anterior precordial leads (V1 V2 V3 V4);
b) presence of RBBB;
c) syncope and/or sustained VT during sports activity;
d) clinical and/or induced sustained VT, including pleomorphic type reliable marker of left ventricle involvement [31, 32];
e) multiform VT.

For MVP athletes, we can consider the following as markers of risk [4]:

a) family history of sudden death;
b) 'complicated' mitral valve prolapse;
c) presyncope, syncope, severe nsVT, sustained VT;
d) severe arrhythmias due to effort and/or sports activity related;
e) prolonged QT interval.

In severe arrhythmic sports activity-related manifestation, the first arrhythmic symptoms may be the most serious ones as we observed in all five subgroup of the patient population, including WPW, aborted sudden death, SD athletes. In general, there are premonitory exercise related symptoms which should be carefully evaluated, though they are sometimes vague and non specific. Some athletes may ignore prodromal symptoms such as a common tendency to sudden cardiac death in the general population [33].

Conclusions

Sports activity (during and immediately after) can be considered as a trigger of electrical destabilization with major arrhythmic manifestations (syncope, VT/VF) Aborted Sudden Death, Cardiac Arrhythmic Sudden Death in susceptible athletes who may be even asymptomatic, competitive and at a high level. The substrate is represented by a typical silent arrhythmogenic cardiopathy with good athletic performance.

In the athlete population first and/or premonitory symptoms and arrhythmic sports activity related manifestations are being carefully studied to identify the risk for Sudden Cardiac Arrhythmic Death by reliable markers, particularly when it is not easy to reproduce the major spontaneous clinical events in a laboratory study.

In identified athletes at risk with silent arrhythmogenic cardiopathy and who have been declared not fit, the continuation of forbidden sports activity may represent a new clinical problem for the prevention of sudden cardiac arrhythmic death. The follow up of these selected and warned ex-athletes should be careful.

Reference

1. Furlanello F, Bettini R, Cozzi F, Del Favero A, Disertori M, Vergara G, Durante GB, Guarnerio M, Inama G, Thiene GL: Ventricular arrhythmias and sudden death in athletes. Ann NY Acad Sci 1984; 253—279.
2. Furlanello F, Vecchiet L, Bettini R, Cozzi F, Vergara G, Antolini R, Resina A: Arrhythmias in athletes. In: Cosin J. Bayés de Luna AJ, Garcia Civera R, Cabadés A (eds),: Cardiac Arrhythmias. Diagnosis and Treatment, Pergamon Press 1988; 457—467.
3. Furlanello F, Bettini R, Bertoldi A, Vergara G, Visonà L, Durante GB, Inama G, Frisanco L, Antolini R, Zanuttini D: Arrhythmias patterns in arrhythmogenic right ventricular dysplasia athletes. Eur Heart J 1989; 10, 16—18.
4. Furlanello F, Bettini R, Bertoldi A, Visonà L, Vergara G, Cozzi F, Del Greco M, Braito G, Durante GB, Inama G, Antolini R: Malignant Arrhythmias in Athletes. A clinicopathological overview. New trend Arrhyt 1989; in press.
5. Thiene G, Gambino A, Corrado D, Nava A: The pathological spectrum underlying sudden death in athletes. New trend Arrhyt, 1, 1985; 3: 323—330.
6. Thiene G, Nava A, Corrado D, Rossi L, Pennelli N: Right Ventricular Cardiomyopathy and Sudden Death in Young People. N Engl J Med 1988; 318, 3: 129—133.
7. Northcote RJ, Flannigan C, Ballantyne D: Sudden death and Vigorous exercise — a study of 60 deaths associated with squash. Br Heart J 1986; 55: 198.
8. Maron BJ, Epstein SE, Roberts WC: Causes of Sudden Death in Competitive Athletes. JACC 1986; 7, 1: 204—214.
9. Cobb LA, Weaver WD: Exercise: A Risk for Sudden Death in Patients With Coronary Heart Disease. JACC 1986; 7. 1: 215—219.
10. Liberthson RR, Nagel EL, Hirschman JC, Nussenfielf JD, Blackbourne BD, Davis JD: Pathophysiologic observation in prehospital ventricular fibrillation and sudden cardiac death. Circulation 1974; 49: 790—798.
11. Kala R, Romo N, Siltanen P, Halonen PI: Physical activity in sudden cardiac death. Adv Cardiol 1978; 25: 27—34.
12. Vuori I, Makarainen M, Jaaskelainen A: Sudden death and physical activity. Cardiology 1978; 63: 287—304.
13. Coplan NL, Gleim GW, Nicholas JA: Exercise and sudden cardiac death. Am Heart J 1988; 115, 1: 207—212.

14. Waller BF: Exercise-related sudden death in young (age ≤ 30 years) and old (age > 30 years) conditioned subjects. In: Wenger NK (ed), Exercise and the heart. Philadelphia: FA Davis Co. 1985; 9—74.
15. Bayés de Luna, J Guindo Soldevila: Sudden Cardiac Death. Editorial MCR, Barcelona 1989.
16. Rossi L, Thiene G: Arrhythmologic pathology of sudden cardiac death. Milano. Casa Editrice Ambrosiana, 1983.
17. Furlanello F, Bettini R, Bertoldi A, Visonà L, Vergara G, Antolini R, Resina A, Vecchiet L: Holter monitoring in sports medicine. JAM 1989; 1, 3, in press.
18. Epstein SE, Maron BJ: Sudden Death and the Competitive Athlete: Perspectives on Preparticipation Screening Studies. JACC 1986; 7, 1: 220—230.
19. Weaver WD, Cobb LA, Hallstrom AP: Characteristics of Survivors of Exertion — and Nonexertion — Related Cardiac Arrest: Value of Subsequent Exercise Testing. Am Heart J 1982; 50: 671—676.
20. Tavazzi L, Ignone G: Rehabilitation: effect on exercise arrhythmias. Eur. Heart J. 8 (Suppl. D) 1987; 83—90.
21. Van Camp SP: Risk of Sudden Death With Exercise. JACC 1986; 8, 4: 991—992.
22. Siscovick DS, Weiss NS, Fletcher RH, Lasky T: The incidence of primary cardiac arrest during vigorous exercise. N Engl J Med 1984; 311: 874—877.
23. Gibbons LW, Cooper KH, Meyer BM, Ellison RC: The acute cardiac risk of strenuous exercise. JAMA 1980; 244: 1799—1801.
24. Thompson PD, Funk EJ, Carleton RA, Sturner WQ: Incidence of Death During Jogging in Rhode Island From 1975 Through 1980. JAMA 1982; 247, 18: 2535—2538.
25. Kannel WB, Belanger A, D'Agostino R, Israel I: Physical activity and physical demand on the job and risk of cardiovascular disease and death: The Framingham Study. Am Heart J, 1986; 112, 4: 820—825.
26. Yater WM, Traum AH, Brown WG, Fitzgerald RP, Geisler MA, Wilcox BB: Coronary artery disease in men 18 to 39 years of age. Report of 866 cases, 450 with necropsy examinations. Am Heart J, 1948; 36: 334—372.
27. Lown B: Sudden cardiac death: biobehavioral perspective. Circulation 1987; 76 (Suppl. I): 1—186—196.
28. Kuller LH, Talbott EO, Robinson C: Environmental and psychosocial determinants of sudden death. Circulation 1987; 76 (Suppl.I): 1—177—185.
29. Furlanello F, Vergara G, Bettini R, Disertori M, Inama G, Guarnerio M, Visonà L: Progress in the study of Wolff-Parkinson-White syndrome of the athletes. The transesophageal atrial pacing during bycicle exercise. J Sports Card 1984; 1: 101.
30. Vergara G, Furlanello F, Disertori M, Inama G, Guarnerio M, Bettini R, Cozzi F: Induction of supraventricular tachyarrhythmia at rest and during exercise with transesophageal atrial pacing in the electrophysiological evaluation of asymptomatic athletes with Wolff-Parkinson-White syndrome. Eur Heart J 1988; 9: 1119—1125.
31. Keefe DL, Schwartz J, Somberg JC: The substrate and the trigger: The role of myocardial vulnerability in sudden cardiac death. Am Heart J 1987; 113, 1: 218—225.
32. Vergara G, Bettini R, Inama G, Guarnerio M, Durante GB, Frisanco L, Furlanello F: La malattia aritmogena del ventricolo destro. Cardiologia 88, Ediz. Librex 1988; 638—645.
33. Thompson PD, Stern MP, Williams P, Duncan K, Hskell WL, Wood PD: Death During Jogging or Running. JAMA 1979; 242, 12: 1265—1267.

10. Lessons from recordings of sudden death by Holter monitoring

JEAN-FRANÇOIS LECLERCQ and PHILIPPE COUMEL

Prevention of sudden death (SD) remains one of the major therapeutic challenges in cardiology in 1989. It is then crucial to know as precisely as possible the mechanisms of SD, particularly in coronary patients. We decided to study the modalities of SD occuring during Holter monitoring. Some series are available in the literature, each including a more or less limited number of cases [1—6]. The cooperative study of the French Working Group on Arrhythmias collected a reasonable number of SD recordings [7], and we recently added 10 cases to this series. The aims of the present study were: to precise the mechanisms responsible for SD, and to look for the determinants of these mechanisms of SD.

Material and methods

Out of a total of 97 tapes including SD, we excluded patients with a recent myocardial infarction (less than 3 weeks) or NYHA functional class-IV heart failure, in order to restrict our subject to sudden unexpected death. Death was considered sudden if occuring within 30 min after the first symptom. Patients successfully resuscitated by external DC shocks were included. Seventy nine cases met these criteria and were considered for analysis.

All tapes were analysed manually, including full disclosure on a optic-fiber system. Computerized processing was performed using the ATREC-II system [8].

The analysis of each tape included the following items:
— Hourly mean heart rate in the 3 hours before SD
— Mean heart rate during the 3 minutes before the onset of the ventricular tachyarrhythmia leading to SD.
— Presence of atrial arrhythmias.
— ST segment changes before SD.
— Existence of a pause (defined as a RR interval exceeding 125 p. 100 of the average cycle duration over the 5 preceding beats) just preceding the onset of the ventricular tachyarrhythmia.

A. Bayés de Luna et al. (eds.): *Sudden Cardiac Death*, 99–111.
© 1991 Kluwer Academic Publishers, Dordrecht.

— Coupling interval (CI) of the extrasystole initiating the ventricular tachy-arrhythmias, compared to the shortest CI of other extrasystoles.
— Prematurity index, defined as the ratio of CI and the immediately preceding RR cycle.
— Morphology of the extrasystole initiating the ventricular tachyarrhythmia, by comparison with the preceding extrasystoles.
— Rate and morphology of the ventricular tachycardia at its onset, and immediately before its transformation into ventricular fibrillation.

Statistical analysis was performed using Student's paired t test when applicable, analysis of variance or chi square test. Numbers indicate the mean values ± standard deviation.

Results

The 79 patients were divided in 3 groups, according to the nature of the terminal event:
1) asystoles;
2) torsades de pointe;
3) ventricular fibrillation (VF).

Group I (asystoles)

This group includes 17 patients (21.5%), 11 males and 6 females, with a mean age of 73.5 ± 2.4 years. Fourteen had a coronary artery disease, 2 an aortic stenosis, and 1 an atrial septal defect. In 13/17 cases, asystole was due to a progressive slowing of the atrial rate accompanied by a QRS widening, traducing an electromechanical dissociation (Figure 1), and not to a primary SA or AV block. In the 4 other cases, SD was due to AV block (3 cases) or SA block (1 case). Two of the 3 AV blocks were iatrogenic (flecainide and verapamil).

The causal role of a myocardial ischemia appears predominant, as judged by the ST segment modifications in the minutes preceding the asystole: 12/17 (70.5%) SD (11 EM dissociations and 1 AV block) were clearly preceded by ST segment changes. In fact, only one patient (the SA block) died from a primary conduction disorder, without ischaemia or iatrogenic factor, and without underlying heart disease.

Group II (torsades de pointe)

This group includes 13 patients (16.5%), 7 females and 6 males, with a mean age of 63.1 ± 14.4 years. The diagnosis was based on strict classical criteria:

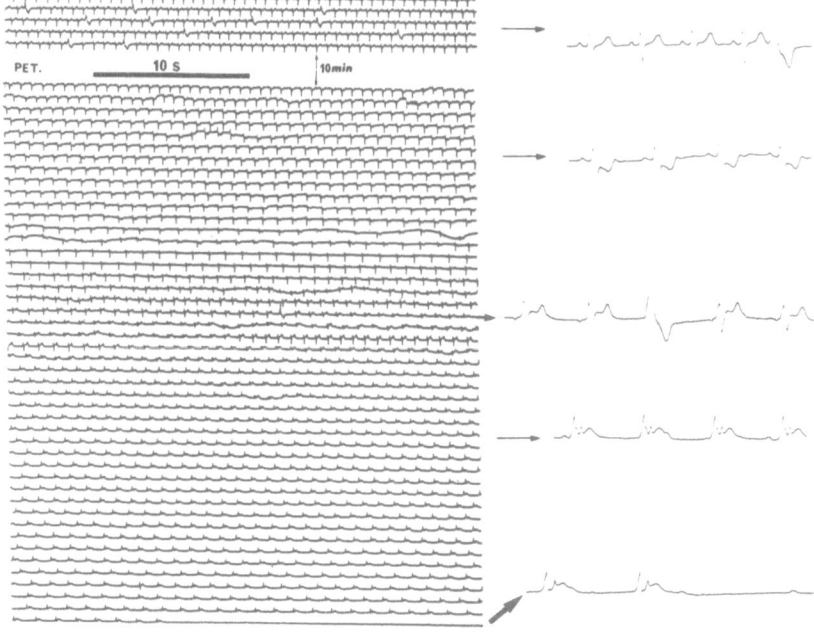

Figure 1. Sudden death by asystole due to an ischaemic electromechanical dissociation in a coronary patient. ST segment depression persisted for more than 6 minutes, then a ST segment elevation for 10 minutes. After that occured a progressive widening of QRS complexes with AV dissociation.

QT interval prolongation, long coupling interval of the initiating beat, and a typical pattern of the ventricular arrhythmia. Three patients died out of the hospital, and 10 SD occured in the hospital (7 were successfully resuscitated). Only 5/13 had an underlying heart disease: 2 were coronary patients, and 3 had a valvular disease.

The contributing etiological factors were:
— Class I-A antiarrhythmic drugs in 8/13
— Potassium depletion (diuretics) in 7/13
— Amiodarone therapy in 3/13.

The two main determinants found in the Holter tape before the initial torsades de pointes were:
1) a progressive bradycardia from 77.5 ± 2.5 to 60.6 ± 2.7 b/min for the mean hourly heart rate of the 3rd and the last hour before SD (n = 13, $p < 0.001$ by paired t test);
2) a long-short cycle sequence related to a post-extrasystolic pause (13/13).

The importance of the bradycardia and of the pause is in keeping with the timing of the event: 8/13 occured between 8 pm and 8 am.

Group III (VF)

This group includes 49 patients (62%), 39 males and 10 females. The mean age was 65.7 ± 11.9 years. Twenty-one SD occurred out of the hospital and 28 in the hospital (only 8 could be resuscitated). Almost all patients were known as coronary patients with healed myocardial infarction, except 1 with an aortic stenosis, and 1 with a congenital long QT syndrome. Two had no detectable heart disease. Eighteen patients (37%) were treated by antiarrhythmic drugs for previous atrial or ventricular arrhythmias.

The terminal event: VF
Only 12 patients died from primary VF, and the majority of VF (37/49) followed a sustained VT that was polymorphic in 13 cases and monomorphic in 24. The transformation of VT into VF was related to three factors: the VT duration and rate, and the widening of the QRS of ventricular origin.

The VT duration before transformation into VF was 42 ± 67 sec for the polymorphic VT and 180 ± 197 sec for the monomorphic VT ($p < 0.05$ by ANOVA). In the 19 patients with previous runs of VT, the duration of the VT leading to VF was longer than the longest run of VT recorded before: 442 ± 571 vs. 42 ± 93 beats ($p < 0.01$ by paired t test).

The transformation of VT into VF was preceded by an acceleration of the VT rate, from 220.6 ± 55 beats min-1 at the onset to 241.5 ± 69 immediately before VF (n = 37, $p < 0.001$ by paired t test).

A progressive widening of QRS was present in 8 cases. Three of them occured early after introduction of flecainide, a class-IC drug that most probably played a favouring role by depressing the intraventricular conduction.

The precipitating factors of VT and VF: the initiating premature beat
Three characteristics of the initiation of VT or VF could be analysed and compared with the preceding events: the coupling interval of the initiating extrasystole, the RR cycle immediately preceding it, and the morphology of the ventricular extrasystole.

The morphology of the initiating beat was particularly scrutinized in 35 patients with more than 100 extrasystoles in the 3 hours preceding SD. In 13 cases, the initiating extrasystole was never seen before, thus appearing 'de novo'. This fact was relatively more frequent in primary VF (6/12 cases) than in VT. In 20 cases, similar extrasystoles were indeed present before SD, usually with a longer coupling interval. In 2 patients, the defect of sensing of an implanted VVI pacemaker was the cause of SD, with a spike falling early after a non sensed extrasystole.

The mean coupling interval (CI) initiating VT or VF was 378.7 ± 87 ms for the whole group, with slightly different values according to the type of the arrhythmia: 341.7 ± 46.5 ms for the 12 primary VF, 370.8 ± 60.8 ms for the 13 polymorphic VT, and 392.5 ± 98 ms for the 24 monomorphic VT (p = NS). In 9 of the 24 patients with sustained monomorphic VT (37.5%)

the VT was not directly initiated by a single extrasystole, but by a run of VT of different morphology, or polymorphic.

A long RR cycle was present in 22 of the 49 cases (45%): 7/12 primary VF, 6/13 polymorphic VT, 9/24 monomorphic VT (p = NS). In 21 cases the pause formed the last or the penultimate cycle preceding the tachyarrhythmia, and was usually due to a post-extrasystolic compensatory pause. In one case, this long RR cycle occured during the sustained VT immediately before its acceleration into VF. Figure 2 shows an example of VF occuring after a post-extrasystolic pause.

The CI initiating VT or VF was not different in cases with (379 ± 71 ms, n = 22) or without (378 ± 101 ms, n = 27) a cardiac pause. However, when this last CI was compared with the shortest CI of the preceding extrasystoles that did not induce VT or VF in the same patient a dramatic shortening (421.4 ± 92.3 to 377.6 ± 94.5, p < 0.01 by paired t test), was evidenced in the group without any pause, whereas no significant difference was seen in the 22 patients with a pause (405.5 ± 88.2 to 378.6 ± 70.6, p = NS). The prematurity index was of course lower in patients with a pause than in those without, but also in primary VF compared to poly- and monomorphic VT: 0.415 ± 0.23 vs. 0.58 ± 0.19, p < 0.05). Figure 3 shows an example of the crucial role of both the short CI and the pause, provoking an extrasystole with a low prematurity index triggering a primary VF.

The favouring factors in the hour preceding VF
In the hour preceding SD by VF, other determinants were analyzed: the basic heart rate, the ventricular repolarization and the ventricular extrasystoles.

We observed a significant heart rate increase (sinus rhythm, or rate of ventricular response for patients in chronic atrial fibrillation) during the last hour preceding SD. In the 46 patients in whom it could be evaluated, after exclusion of the 2 cases of pacemaker-induced arrhythmia and of 1 case with

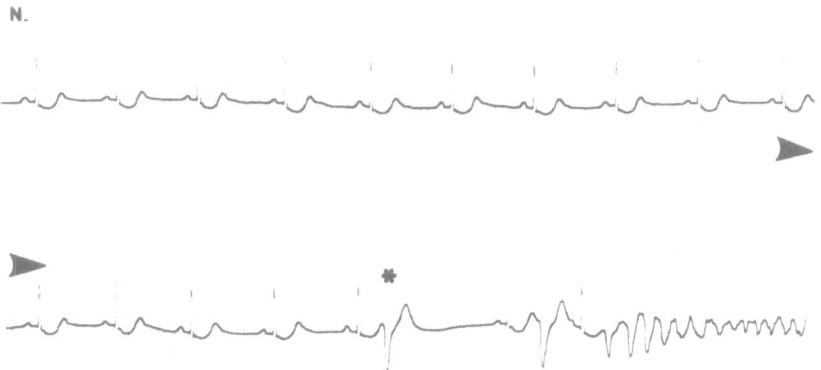

Figure 2. Sudden death by primary VF. The first extrasystole (star) induced a compensatory pause and the successive one is interpolated, permitting a short coupling interval of a third one, and VF ensues.

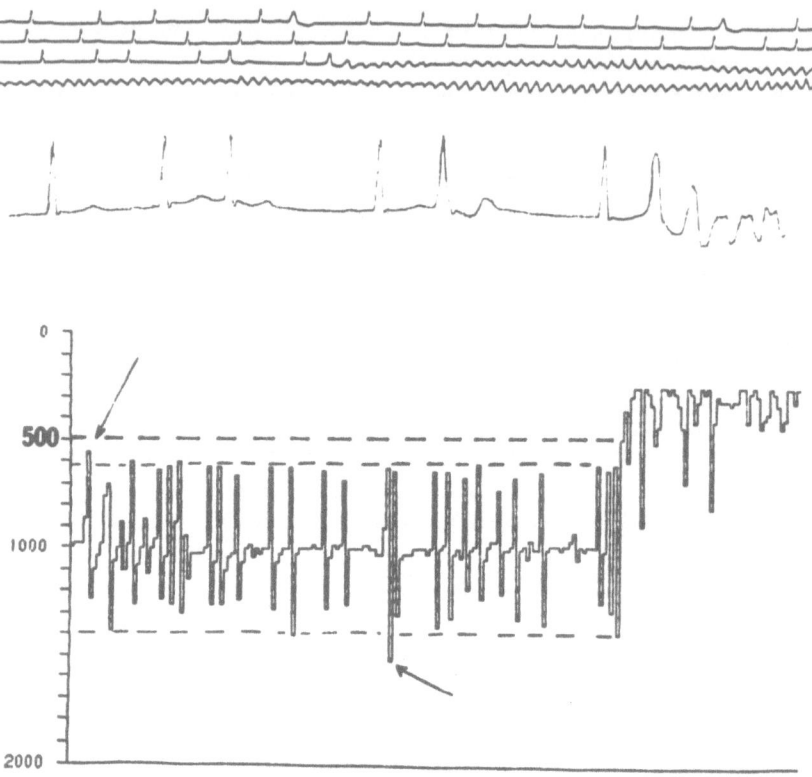

Figure 3. Sudden death by primary VF induced by an extrasystrole with short coupling interval, and following a long pause. Beat-to-beat analysis of the last 5 minutes of Holter recording (bottom) showed that this combination of events was not encountered before SD: one short CI (first arrow) was not preceded by a pause, and a long pause (2nd arrow) was not followed by a short CI.

less than 1 hour of ECG, the heart rate increased from 82.8 ± 20 to 92.0 ± 26.7 beats min-1 (p < 0.001 by paired t test), by comparison of the values during the hour and the 3 minutes preceding SD. A clear difference was found between primary VF and VT leading to VF, the latter occuring in the setting of a much higher heart rate: 72.4 ± 10.4, n = 11, vs. 93.2 ± 25.2 beats min-1, n = 35 (p < 0.05). However, the heart rate acceleration in the last hour concerns only the cases without a preceding pause (from 85.0 ± 22.8 to 99.1 ± 31.1, p < 0.001), and not the cases with a pause (from 79.85 ± 15.5 to 80.8 ± 16.3, p = NS). As a result, if the 3 last minutes are considered isolately, a great difference appears according to the presence or the absence of a pause, the latter including a higher heart rate (p < 0.05). These differences are schematically displayed in figure 4.

Atrial arrhythmias were often observed during the last hour before SD due to VF: 7 patients were in chronic atrial fibrillation, 5 had a paroxysmal

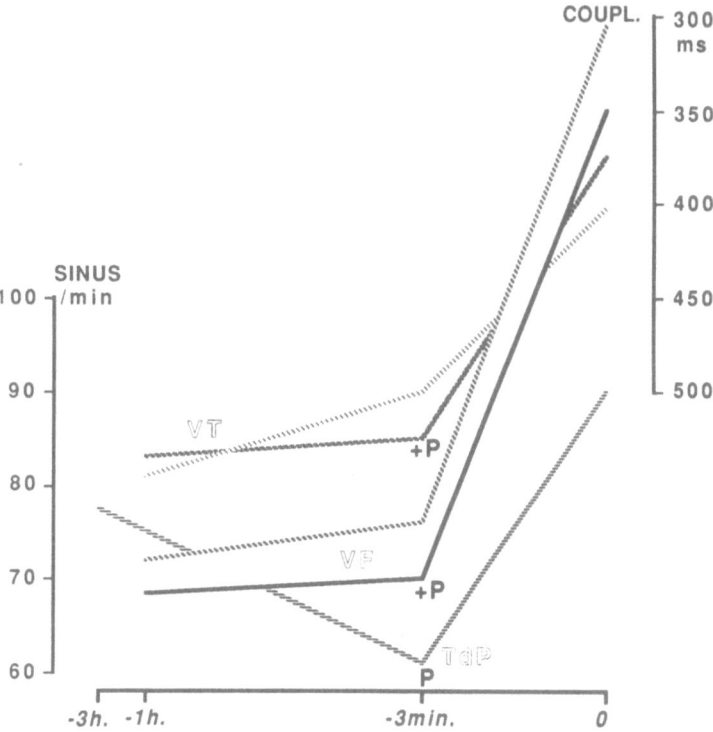

Figure 4. Schematic representation of heart rate and CI values before SD by ventricular tachyarrhythmias. In TdP, a decrease of heart rate occurs in the 3 preceding hours, and the initiating CI is long. In primary VF, the heart rate is lower than in VF secondary to VT, and the initiating CI is shorter. In both cases of primary and secondary VF, the heart rate immediately before SD is higher in VT/VF not preceded by a pause (P), and the sinus rate increase during the preceding 3 minutes is more pronounced.

sustained atrial tachyarrhythmia starting less than 1 hour before SD, and in 3 the sustained VT was started by an atrial premature beat. Thus in 15/49 patients (31%), atrial arrhythmias apparently played a role in the genesis of the ventricular tachyarrhythmia, or had the same determinants. Not surprisingly, a majority of these patients were older than 65 years (12/15). Figure 5 shows three examples of the determinant role of atrial premature beats in the genesis of SD.

In contrast to the heart rate changes, an increase in the extrasystolic rate was rare: out of 49 patients, 11 (22%) had no ventricular extrasystoles in the 3 hours before SD, and only 11 of the other 38 had an increase of more than 50% in the last hour compared to the preceding two hours.

ST segment changes in the 2 leads of Holter monitoring were very unusual in these coronary patients, seen only in 5 cases (10%) in the minutes preceding SD. Of these 5 cases, 2 had primary VF, 2 a polymorphic VT, and

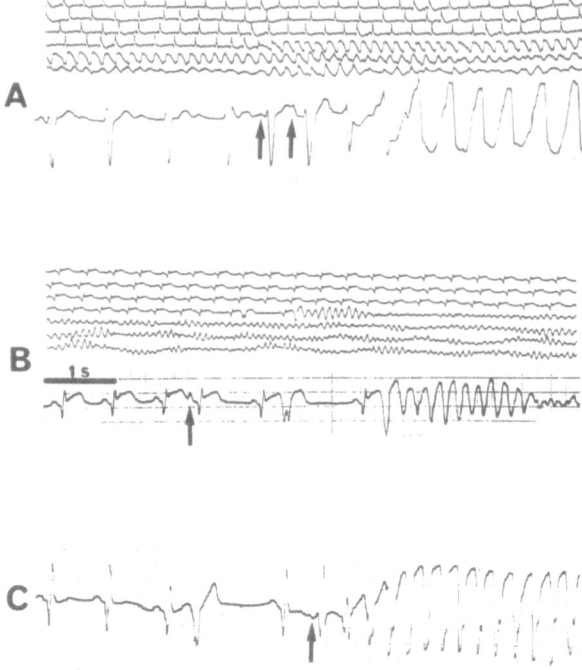

Figure 5. Three examples of SD in which atrial premature beats play a determinant role. In A, an atrial couplet triggered directly the VT. In B, the atrial premature beat induced a succession of post-extrasystolic pauses leading to VF. In C, it is the reverse situation: the atrial extrasystole occured after a postextrasystolic pause and triggered the VT.

one a monomorphic VT. An increasing heart rate was also present in 4 of these patients, and a long RR cycle in 3.

Discussion

The major findings of this analysis of 79 cases of recorded SD were the existence of 3 different terminal events: asystoles in 17 patients, torsades de pointe of iatrogenic origin in 13, and ventricular fibrillation in 49. Asystoles were primarily due to an ischaemic process in the vast majority of cases and not to a primary conduction disturbance. The role of torsades de pointe in the genesis of SD should be clearly individualized. The 2 major determinants, bradycardia and long-short RR sequence, contribute to prolong and to make inhomogeneous the ventricular refractory period [9, 10, 11]. In the literature devoted to SD, the distinction between usual VF and torsades de pointe is not always clear [12, 13]. This distinction appears of crucial importance as the determinants of either form of lethal arrhythmia, hence the therapeutic implications are different.

In the present study, the most frequent mechanism of SD, particularly in coronary patients, is formed by VF, as in some preceding series [1, 4, 5, 6]. The role of cardiac asystole in the genesis of SD appears restricted to electromechanical dissociation and related to an ischaemic process [7]. By contrast, VT or VF directly related to an electrocardiographically evident ischaemia seems relatively rare in these coronary patients: as judged on the 2 leads of the Holter recording, the majority of asystoles, but few VT/VF are preceeded by ST segment changes in the 3 main series of the literature [3, 5, 7]. Although it is not possible to exclude a localized ischemia, SD appears usually due to a primary electrophysiological phenomenon, a VF, or more frequently a sustained VT which leads to VF. This mechanism, underlined in some series [2, 6], is well correlated with the high incidence of SD in coronary patients with paroxysmal VTs [14]. In a recent study (15) comparing coronary patients presenting aborted SD with those presenting sustained VT not leading to SD, the major differences were a higher incidence of polymorphic VT, and a higher rate of the monomorphic VT. The other recognized predisposing factor to SD is the left ventricular dysfunction [16, 17]. The relationship between these 2 factors may be that the more the left ventricle is impaired, the less the patient can tolerate a fast VT. It has been demonstrated that both rate and hemodynamic consequences of the VT induced by provocative studies are well correlated with the increase in catecholamines blood level [18], reflecting an adaptative sympathetic stimulation.

The 2 main determinants of VT/VF are the sympathetic tone and the long RR cycles. An increase in the sympathetic drive favors all the potential mechanisms of ventricular arrhythmias. Its main clinical marker, an increasing heart rate, has been already signaled before SD [3]. There is a balance between these two factors, and SD occuring after a pause is preceeded by a less marked heart rate acceleration than SD without pause.

Long RR cycles induce an instantaneous increase in sympathetic nervous discharges [19, 20], in addition to the prolongation of the ventricular refractory period. An increase in the inhomogeneity of refractoriness between ventricle and His-Purkinje system [11], may favour an electrical instability. Abrupt changes of cycle duration in patients with a low rate may be responsible for extrasystoles with a low prematurity index leading to primary VF.

It is possible that a latent localized ischaemia is one of the physiological supports of the changes in the vagosympathetic balance evidenced by the heart rate acceleration before SD. However, its role remains clinically limited, since ECG signs of patent ischemia are rare in the Holter recordings.

Repolarisation changes, reflected by the QT interval, is often difficult to appreciate in Holter recordings. There is some series in the literature indicating a trend to a QT increase before SD [21], but this point remains to establish.

The prevention of SD remains yet difficult and controversial. In this regard recorded SD suggests several possible therapeutic implications:

Prevention of SD due to asystoles is not possible by rythmological means. It is a more general problem of prevention of the genesis and progression of the coronary artery disease.

Antiarrhythmic drugs are primarily implicated in 'torsades de pointe'. Some VF are also favored by drugs that depress intraventricular conduction. On the other hand, antiarrhythmic drugs prolong CI and VT cycle length which constitute immediate determinants of VF [3, 22, 23] and may be useful for the control of paroxysmal atrial arrhythmias, which are also a determinant of VT/VF. Such a balance of potentially beneficial and deleterious actions of antiarrhythmic drugs probably explains the absence of statistical 'effects of these drugs in various trials. A tailored therapy, adapted to individual cases is theoretically suitable, yet difficult to manage practically.

The role of long RR cycles, especially the post-extrasystolic pause is important: all torsades de pointes and fifty per cent of VT/VF are concerned. The preventive effect of pacing is well known for the torsades, and could be expected for some VT/VF. On the other hand, any pacemaker dysfunction is potentially dangerous and an accurate sensing of all morphologic types of ventricular extrasystoles is never certain [22].

Finally, considering that an increased heart rate, reflecting a change in the vago-sympathetic drive, is almost never absent and often critical in the genesis of VF, the role of beta-blocking agents appears fundamental. It is important to realize that the apparent limited increase in the heart rate (mean: 9.2 beats min-1/hour) should not be taken as an argument for the limited role of the sympathetic drive. On the contrary, it may reflect a greater sensitivity of the arrhythmogenic substrate to this factor. The hypothesis of such an 'adrenergic paradox' necessarily implies a less marked (hence less evident) sinus acceleration before the event [24]. The results of prospective trials with beta-blockers after myocardial infarction, concluding to their preventive effect against SD [25, 26, 27] could then be explained. The fact that an ECG detectable myocardial ischaemia is rare before SD is consistent with the absence of beneficial effect of other anti-anginal drugs in terms of reduction of the mortality rate in the post-myocardial infarction trials [28, 29, 30]. It is then probable that the anti-anginal effect of beta-blockers does not play a major role in their SD preventive effect.

Summary

Seventy-nine Holter recordings of sudden unexpected death were analysed by full disclosure and computerized processing. Seventeen were due to asystoles, principally in coronary patients (14/17), and preceded by a clearly visible myocardial ischaemia, evidenced by ST segment changes. Thirteen sudden deaths were due to torsades de pointe in non-coronary subjects (11/13), related to quinidine-like drugs and/or hypokaliemia: they were always initiated by a long RR cycle due to a post-extrasystolic pause, and announced by a progressive decrease of mean heart rate (from 77.5 ± 2.5 to 60.6 ± 2.7 b/min, p < 0.001), in the 3 preceding hours. The other cases were due to ventricular fibrillation (VF) occurring in coronary patients (45/49), by acceleration of ventricular tachycardia (VT), monomorphic in 24 cases, polymorphic in 13, the ventricular rate increasing from 220.6 ± 55 to 241.5 ± 69 b/min, rather than by primary VF (12 cases). A cardiac pause (RR cycle exceding 125% of the mean 5 preceding cycles) was present in 22/49 cases immediately before the onset of VT/VF. The coupling interval of the extrasystole initiating VT/VF was shorter than the shortest value encountered before: 377.6 ± 94.5 ms vs. 421.4 ± 92.3. The prematurity index (coupling interval/preceding RR cycle ratio) was lower in primary VF, ST changes were unusual (5 cases), whereas heart rate increased from 82.8 ± 20 to 92.0 ± 26.7 b/min (p < 0.001). This acceleration was in fact present only in cases without pause before onset of VT/VF: from 85.0 ± 22.8 to 99.1 ± 31.1 (n = 27, p < 0.001) whereas no change exists in cases with preceding pause: from 79.8 ± 15.5 to 80.8 ± 16.3 (n = 22, p = NS). As a result, VT/VF without a preceding pause occurs in the setting of a higher heart rate, most probably reflecting a higher sympathetic drive. Prevention of these two main determinants by pacing and betablocking therapy should be more efficient than the use of antianginal or antiarrhythmic drugs.

References

1. Nikolic G, Bishop RL, Singh J: Sudden death recorded during Holter Monitoring. Circulation 1982; 66: 218—25.
2. Panidis IP, Morganroth J: Sudden death in hospitalized patients: cardiac rhythm disturbances detected by ambulatory electrocardiographic Monitoring. J Am Coll Cardiol 1983; 2: 798—805.
3. Pratt CM, Francis MJ, Luck JC, Wyndham CR, Miller RR, Quinones MA: Analysis of ambulatory electrocardiograms in 15 patients during spontaneous ventricular fibrillation with special reference to preceding arrhythmic events. J Am Coll Cardiol 1983; 2: 789—97.
4. Kempf FC, Josephson ME: Cardiac arrest recorded on ambulatory electrocardiograms. Am J Cardiol 1984; 53: 1577—82.
5. Roelandt J, Klootwijk P, Lubsen J, Janse MJ: Sudden death during longterm ambulatory monitoring. Europ Heart J 1984; 5: 7—20.
6. Milner PG, Platia EV, Reid PR, Griffith LSC: Ambulatory electrocardiographic recordings at the time of fatal cardiac arrest. Am J Cardiol 1985; 56: 588—92.
7. Leclercq JF, Coumel P, Maisonblanche P, Cauchemez B, Zimmermann M, Chouty F, Slama R: Mise en évidence des mécanismes déterminants de la mort subite. Enquête coopérative portant sur 69 cas enregistrés par la méthode de Holter. Arch Mal Coeur 1986; 79: 1024—33.
8. Coumel P, Leclercq JF, Maisonblanche P, Attuel P, Cauchemez B: Computerized analysis of dynamic electrocardiograms: a tool for comprehensive electrophysiology. A description of the ATREC II system. Clin Progress 1985; 3: 181—201.
9. Browne KF, Prystowsky E, Heger JJ, Chilson DA, Zipes DP: Prolongation of the QT interval in man during sleep. Am J Cardiol 1983; 52: 55—9.

10. Kay GN, Plumb VJ, Arciniegas JG, Henthorn RW, Waldo AL: Torsades de pointe: the long-short initiating sequence and other clinical features. Observations in 32 patients. J Am Coll Cardiol 1983; 2: 806—17.

11. Lehmann MH, Denker S, Mahmud R, Akhtar M: Postextrasystolic alterations in refractoriness of the His- Purkinje system and ventricular myocardium in man. Circulation 1984; 69: 1096—1102.

12. Denes P, Gabster A, Huang SK: Clinical, electrocardiographic and follow-up observations in patients having ventricular fibrillation during Holter monitoring. Role of quinidine therapy. Am J Cardiol 1981; 48: 9—16.

13. Lewis BH, Antman EM, Graboys TB: Detailed analysis of 24 hour ambulatory electrocardiographic recordings during ventricular fibrillation or torsades de pointe. J Am Coll Cardiol 1983; 2: 426—36.

14. Swerdlow CD, Winkle RA, Mason JW: Determinants of survival in patients with ventricular tachyarrhythmias. N Engl J Med 1983; 308: 1436—42.

15. Stevenson WG, Brugada P, Waldecker B, Zehender M, Wellens HJJ: Clinical, angiographic and electrophysiologic findings in patients with aborted sudden death as compared with patients with sustained ventricular tachycardia after myocardial infarction. Circulation 1985; 71; 1146—52.

16. Marchlinski FE, Buxton AE, Waxman HL, Josephson ME: Identifying patients at risk of sudden death after myocardial infarction: value of the response to programmed stimulation, degree of ventricular ectopic activity and severity of left ventricular dysfunction. Am J Cardiol 1983; 52: 1190—6.

17. Mukharji J, Rude RE, Poole K, Gustafson N, Thomas LJ et al: Risk factors for sudden death after acute myocardial infarction. Two-years follow-up. Am J Cardiol 1984; 54: 31—65.

18. Morady F, Halter JB, Dicarlo LA, Baerman JM, De Buitler M: The interplay between endogenous catecholamines and induced ventricular tachycardia during electrophysiologic testing. Am Heart J 1987; 113: 227—33.

19. Herre MJ, Thames M: Responses of sympathetic nerves to programmed ventricular stimulation. J Am Coll Cardiol 1987; 9: 147—54.

20. Welch WJ, Smith ML, Rea RF, Bauernfeind RA, Eckberg DL: Enhancement of sympathetic nerve activity by single premature ventricular beats in Humans. J Am Coll Cardiol 1989; 13: 69—75.

21. Bayes De Luna A, Coumel P, Leclercq JF: Ambulatory sudden cardiac death: mechanisms of production of fatal arrhythmia on the basis of data from 157 cases. Am Heart J 1989; 117: 151—9.

22. Leclercq JF, Maisonblanche P, Cauchemez B, Coumel P: Respective role of sympathetic tone and of cardiac pauses in the genesis of 62 cases of ventricular fibrillation recorded during Holter monitoring. Europ Heart J 1988; 9: 1276—83.

23. Swerdlow B, Axelrod, Kilman B, Perry D, Merk R: Ambulatory ventricular tachycardia: characteristics of the initiating beat. Am Heart J 1983; 106: 1326—31.

24. Coumel P: The management of clinical arrhythmias. An overview on invasive versus non-invasive electrophysiology. Europ Heart J 1987; 8: 92—9.

25. The Norvegian Multicenter Study Group: Timolol-induced reduction in mortality and reinfarction in patients surviving acute myocardial infarction. N Engl J Med 1981; 304: 801—7.

26. Beta-blocker Heart Attack Trial Research Group: A randomized trial of propranolol in patients with acute myocardial infarction. I. Mortality results. J Am Med Ass 1982; 247: 1707—14.

27. Chadda K, Goldstein S, Byington R, Curb JD: Effect of Propranolol after acute myocardial infarction in patients with congestive heart failure. Circulation 1986; 73: 503—10.

28. The Danish Study Group of Verapamil in Myocardial Infarction: Verapamil in acute myocardial infarction. Europ Heart J 1984; 5: 516—28.

29. Moss AJ and the Multicenter Diltiazem Post-Infarction Research Group: Long-term effect of Diltiazem on mortality and reinfarction after myocardial infarction. The MDPIT study. J Am Coll Cardiol 1988; 11: Suppl. A, 27A (abstract).
30. The Israeli Sprint Study group: Secondary prevention reinfarction Israeli Nifedipine trial (SPRINT). A randomized intervention trial of Nifedipine in patients with acute myocardial infarction. Europ Heart J 1988; 9: 354—64.

11. Profile of the candidate for sudden cardiac death

Introduction

Sudden cardiac death is a problem of epidemic proportions. A majority of instances are caused by lethal arrhythmias, ventricular fibrillation being the most common. Sudden cardiac death and acute myocardial infarction are near synonymous in the mind of the general public but coronary artery disease is by no means the only responsible pathophysiology. Valvular heart disease, particularly aortic stenosis, is associated with sudden cardiac death and there is a small but important incidence in patients with mitral valve prolapse. Sudden cardiac death occurs in a variety of cardiomyopathies including hypertrophic cardiomyopathy and dilated cardiomyopathy associated with heart failure. In all these situations, progress is being made towards profiling the high-risk candidates for sudden cardiac death.

Sudden cardiac death also occurs in apparently normal people. For them, sudden death is their first, and last, manifestation of cardiac disease. These individuals present a major and near insuperable challenge to prospective identification.

Techniques to identify high-risk candidates for sudden death

Although an arrhythmia is the final mechanism for the majority of instances of sudden cardiac death, electrophysiological markers are not well developed. Prognostically significant ventricular ectopic beats which may trigger ventricular fibrillation can be detected by standard electrocardiography or dynamic electrocardiography. The electrophysiological substrate for VF is less accessible but QT prolongation, signal averaged late potentials and programmed stimulation responses may be markers of arrhythmogenic potential.

Clinical history, features of examination, chest X-rays, echocardiography, ST analysis on exercise stress testing, nuclear scintigraphy, angiography, enzyme profiles, etc, can identify high-risk candidates for sudden death.

A. Bayés de Luna et al. (eds.): *Sudden Cardiac Death*, 113–120.
© 1991 Kluwer Academic Publishers, Dordrecht.

These features characterise the basic cardiovascular disease and help stage its severity.

High risk profiles and specific conditions

Survivors of out-of-hospital ventricular fibrillation. VF recurrence in survivors of out-of-hospital cardiac arrest is a major concern. A surprising finding of community rescue services has been that many patients who were resuscitated from and survived out-of-hospital cardiac arrest had not suffered an acute myocardial infarction. At first this was considered to carry a good prognosis but in fact it was these individuals who suffered the highest recurrence rates. Patients who infarcted had destroyed their arrhythmogenic mechanism whilst those with only ischaemia could reactivate it again in the future. All survivors of out-of-hospital ventricular fibrillation who have not suffered a myocardial infarction should be investigated, seeking significant coronary lesions for surgical or angioplasty procedures [1].

Acute phase myocardial infarction. Sudden death, the major complication of acute phase myocardial infarction, is most usually due to ventricular fibrillation. The risk of primary ventricular fibrillation (no shock and/or heart failure) is highest in the first minutes at a time when ischaemic cells have not yet begun the process of necrosis. With maturation of the infarct and the loss of electrical activity in the jeopardised cells, the risk of ventricular fibrillation gradually falls to become rare after 6—8 hours. The individual at risk of primary ventricular fibrillation, cannot be identified reliably. Ventricular ectopic beat patterns which were considered to pressage primary ventricular fibrillation are neither sensitive nor specific for this complication [2]. Low serum potassium levels are associated with a risk of developing primary ventricular fibrillation but the relationship is insufficiently reliable to be of clinical use.

Consequences of primary VF. Primary ventricular fibrillation is not always successfully reverted to sinus rhythm. Whether those who die were potentially salvageable or whether their intractable ventricular fibrillation represents an irretrievable progression of their initial ischaemic event is unknown. Concern about failed resuscitation from primary ventricular fibrillation has raised interest in the prophylaxis of this arrhythmia [3]. Lidocaine offers efficacy, reducing the early VF rate fivefold, but at the risk of a significant increase in asystole [4].

Individuals successfully resuscitated from primary ventricular fibrillation during acute infarction have been shown to resume normal activities and to have good prospects for long-term survival [5]. This would be consistent with the hypothesis that primary ventricular fibrillation reflects transient unstable electrical conditions during the early hours of infarction and is unrelated to infarct size, coronary anatomy or left ventricular function. It has been suggested, however, that when primary ventricular fibrillation complicates anterior infarction, the long-term prognosis may be as poor as a 32% one-year mortality [6]. Other studies have not confirmed this situation [7]. For the present it would seem that any adverse prognostic significance of ventricular fibrillation in acute phase infarction must be modest.

Secondary ventricular fibrillation. The extremely bad prognosis for secondary VF (VF complicating AMI in the presence of shock and/or failure) has long been recognised. Reliable resuscitation and survival figures are scarce but a 70% mortality from the initial event and a further 70% one-year mortality for the resuscitated survivors is a reasonable estimate. In our department, examination of the prognosis for all types of ventricular fibrillation, confirmed the initial high mortality of this type of VF but indicated that for hospital survivors, the long-term prognosis was better than expected [7]. Nonetheless, these patients must still be considered high-risk candidates for subsequent sudden death.

Predicting late VF. Infarct survivors at greatest risk of late VF (more than 48 h after first infarct in the absence of evidence of fresh ischaemia) are those who have suffered anteroseptal infarction complicated by right bundle branch block and axis shifts [8]. When survivors of these infarct patterns were followed in a prospective study, the late VF risk was confirmed but perhaps surprisingly was confined to the first six weeks after infarction [9].

The risk of reperfusional ventricular fibrillation. In experimental infarction, early thrombolytic therapy is associated with reperfusional arrhythmias including ventricular fibrillation. It was feared that in man, this arrhythmic complication of intra-coronary clot dissolution would prove a contraindication to acute thrombolysis.

In practice, reperfusion arrhythmias proved rare, suggesting either species variation or that clinical reperfusion occurs too late. Certainly at highest risk are those successfully reperfused within two hours from the onset of symptoms. The late prognostic impact of reperfusional ventricular fibrillation has not been assessed. Its occurrence might signify substantial myocardial salvage and therefore be of good rather than of adverse prognostic significance, assuming that the patient is speedily resuscitated.

The risks post thrombolysis. Concerns that patients who had undergone successful thrombolysis would be at high risk of further occlusive events with the threat of ventricular fibrillation have proved largely unfounded. Anti-coagulation should be continued for a sufficient period of time to allow repair of the ulcerated or fissured plaque and to permit remodelling. Exercise stress testing will help define individuals in whom high-grade stenoses persist and who may benefit from further investigation.

Survivors of acute myocardial infarction. Survivors of acute myocardial infarction are identified as having coronary atheroma with the prospect of further, possibly fatal events. In reality the post-infarct population comprises a large low-risk group and a much smaller group with a significant risk of either sudden arrhythmic death or fatal reinfarction. These high-risk patients are characterised more by their coronary anatomy, left ventricular function and evidence of ischaemia than by features which might reflect an electrical propensity of the ventricle to fibrillate.

High-risk non-electrophysiological features associated with sudden death include: left main coronary artery disease, extensive three-vessel coronary artery disease, impaired left ventricular function, size of myocardial infarction, increased cardiothoracic ratio, clinical features of cardiac failure, a poor effort test and continuing angina particularly if unstable.

Electrical indicators of a poor prognosis include high-frequency ventricular ectopic beats, sustained monomorphic ventricular tachycardia, left bundle branch block, bundle branch block and axis shift complicating anteroseptal infarction, QT prolongation, signal averaged late potentials and electrophysiologically provoked repetitive responses.

It might be anticipated that the non-electrophysiological features would correlate with sudden ischaemic or sudden functional (contractile) death and the electrophysiological features with VF. The natural history is not so clear-cut. New ischaemic events may prove fatal through a mechanism of ventricular fibrillation and some electrophysiological features (LBBB, frequent VEBs,) are related to infarct size and need not necessarily pressage VF death.

Late potential detection and positive electrophysiological repetitive responses probably identify the same pathology [10]: an infarct which has healed in a mottled pattern to create re-entrant pathways for VT and/or VF. There is growing interest in the prospect that signal averaging might be a useful non-invasive screening tool to identify patients in whom more detailed investigations would be appropriate. Disappointingly, the signal averaged QRS shows no reliable alteration when clinically successful antiarrhythmic drug therapy is prescribed for the patient.

Modifying prognosis for high-risk patient groups depends upon the nature of the threat. Dynamic ischaemia related to coronary artery disease is prognostically benefited by surgery, by angioplasty or perhaps even by drug therapy. Functional impairment perhaps will be improved by ACE inhibitor therapy. Improving prognosis against an electrophysiological risk is possible using electrophysiologically guided antiarrhythmic therapy, implantable cardioverter defibrillators or surgery. Although high-frequency ventricular ectopic beats identify high-risk individuals, management of these patients is more complex. Ectopic beat suppression by conventional antiarrhythmic drugs has not proved beneficial [11] whilst therapy with beta- adrenoreceptor blocking therapies has reduced mortality without necessarily affecting ventricular ectopic beat patterns [12]. Both these aspects are now being challenged. Criticisms of early studies employing conventional antiarrhythmic drugs have prompted new investigations of the role of conventional membrane depressant antiarrhythmic agents in acute infarction [13]. Furthermore, it has been suggested that the prognostic benefit of beta-blockers may accrue only to those patients in whom ventricular ectopic beats are beneficially influenced by prescription of that therapy [14]. Further work on these two aspects is awaited. The results have important implications for clinical management.

Angina. Unstable angina, Prinzmetal variant angina and decubitus angina are associated with a high risk of sudden death. The risk of sudden death in patients with stable angina is higher than for the normal population but is very much lower than for these special categories of angina. Nonetheless, stress testing, dynamic electrocardiography, echocardiography and nuclear scintigraphy can identify a group of patients with stable angina who are at high risk. These tests identify patients with critical degrees or sites of atheroma who should be offered early coronary angiography with a view to surgery or angioplasty.

The congenital long QT syndromes. The overall risk of death in patients with the congenital long QT syndrome is not known accurately but appears substantial. High-risk individuals are identified by their history of syncope, by their manifest ventricular arrhythmias and by the severity of their repolarization changes. The Valsalva manoeuvre has been suggested as usefully exaggerating QT prolongation to identify those at risk [15]. Observational results of an International Registry for this condition have been persuasive in directing therapy [16]. Management strategies have not been tested by standard scientific methods but the rarity of the condition, the biologic variability of its presentation and the psychosocial problems of the afflicted families, are a major impediment to standard controlled and blinded studies. For the present, it appears reasonable to accept that beta-adrenoreceptor blockers and/or left stellate ganglionectomy improve prognosis for high-risk individuals with these syndromes.

Patients on antiarrhythmic drugs. Antiarrhythmic drugs can aggravate existing arrhythmias or cause new arrhythmias. Florid events are relatively easily recognised but more subtle problems may escape attention. Concerns have been voiced that an important proportion of sudden deaths may reflect not failure of antiarrhythmic drugs but active toxicity. For example, antiarrhythmic drugs have been incriminated in out-of-hospital cardiac arrests [17] and digoxin-treated elderly survivors of acute myocardial infarction fare less well than their non-digoxin taking counterparts [18]. These situations are perhaps numerically modest but it is likely that awareness of potentially dangerous arrhythmogenic situations will grow with time. It is prudent to consider that all patients taking drugs which modify cardiac electrophysiology are at some increased risk of sudden death. Fortunately for most that risk is negligible but even then it must be carefully weighed against the anticipated benefits of therapy.

Hypertrophic cardiomyopathy. Hypertrophic cardiomyopathy may pursue a benign course but in most studies an important and persistent sudden death risk extends from infancy to childhood. The highest risk individuals are those with manifest ventricular arrhythmias on 24-hour ECGs and with a family history of sudden death [19]. In selected high-risk patients, amiodarone, despite its adverse effects, offers a significantly improved prognosis [20].

Mitral valve prolapse. Sudden death in mitral valve prolapse is rare. ST and T wave changes on the surface ECG, QT prolongation and manifest ventricular arrhythmias may identify the high-risk patient [21], but neither the sensitivity nor specificity of these features is known.

Aortic stenosis. Sudden death in aortic stenosis correlates with the pressure difference across the aortic valve; emergency management is appropriate for those with a 100 mmHg or more transvalvular pressure difference. Haemodynamic considerations may have obscured that not all aortic stenotic sudden death is mechanical. Patients may die in ventricular fibrillation and ventricular ectopic beats found in aortic stenotic patients have been identified as a risk factor [22].

Heart failure. Heart failure mortality does not necessarily reflect slow inexorable mechanical decline. Sudden, presumptively arrhythmic death, is not uncommon, the risk correlating loosely with the presence of ventricular arrhythmias on 24-hour ECG recordings [23]. Hopes that an observed antiarrhythmic action of captopril might indicate that ACE inhibitors could reduce sudden death rates in heart failure were not confirmed by the Consensus Study in which enalapril significantly reduced mortality but through an effect on mechanical rather than sudden death [24].

Apparently normal individuals. Sudden cardiac death prediction in normal individuals is not practical at the present time. A family history of precocious cardiac death and a background of multiple risk factors for atheroma might indicate a high-risk individual but the specificity and sensitivity offered by these features is unacceptably poor. High frequency ventricular ectopic beats on a conventional surface electrocardiogram have been advanced as a predictor of subsequent mortality [25], but other studies have failed to confirm this relationship [26], and for the present such ectopic beat patterns should be considered as of no practical significance.

Conclusions

Sudden arrhythmic death is the final common result of many types of cardiac disease. Profiling high-risk candidates is an attractive proposition but will have relevance only if specificity and sensitivity are high. No single investigation will offer this information. Although the heart is a relatively unsophisticated organ capable of only a few failure modes, the complex pathophysiology which produces disease mandates that any profile will be the result of a wide range of investigations. Predicting preventable sudden arrhythmic death is an even greater clinical challenge; knowledge and technology must advance much further if it is to be realised.

References

1. Weaver WD, Cobb LA, Hallstrom AP, Fahrenbruch C, Copass MK, Ray R: Factors influencing survival after out-of-hospital cardiac arrest. J Am Coll Cardiol 1986; 7: 752—7.
2. Campbell RWF, Murray A, Julian DG: Ventricular arrhythmias in first 12 hours of acute myocardial infarction. Natural history study. Br Heart J 1981; 46: 351—7.
3. Kertes P, Hunt D:Prophylaxis of primary ventricular fibrillation in acute myocardial infarction. The case against lidocaine. Br Heart J 1984; 52: 241—7.
4. Koster RW, Dunning AJ: Intramuscular lidocaine for prevention of lethal arrhythmias in the prehospitalisation phase of acute myocardial infarction. N Engl J Med 1985; 313: 1105—10.
5. Dunn HM, McComb JM, Mackenzie G, Adgey AAJ: Survival to leave hospital from ventricular fibrillation. Am Heart J 1986; 112: 745—51.
6. Schwartz PJ, Zaza A, Grazi S *et al*: Effects of ventricular fibrillation complicating acute myocardial infarction on long term prognosis. Influence of site of infarction. Am J Cardiol 1985; 57: 384—9.
7. Dougeni-Christacou V, Dougenis D, Tai YT, McComb J, Campbell RWF: Hospital mortality of ventricular tachycardia and fibrillation. Br Heart J 1989; 61: 125.
8. Lie KI, Liem KL, Schuilenberg RM, David GK, Durrer D: Early identification of patients developing late in-hospital ventricular fibrillation after discharge from the coronary care unit. A 5.5 year retrospective study of 1897 patients. Am J Cardiol 1978; 41: 674—7.
9. Hauer RNW, Lie KI, Liem KL, Durrer D: Long term prognosis in patients with bundle branch block complicating acute anteroseptal infarction. Am J Cardiol 1982; 449: 1581—5.
10. Denniss AR, Richards DA, Cody DV *et al*: Prognostic significance of ventricular tachycardia and fibrillation induced at programmed stimulation and delayed potentials detected on the signal-averaged electrocardiograms of survivors of acute myocardial infarction. Circulation 1986; 74: 731—45.
11. May GS, Eberlein KA, Furberg CD, Passamani ER, DeMets DL: Secondary prevention after myocardial infarction. A review of long term trials. Prog Cardiovasc Dis 1982; 24: 331—52.
12. Furberg CD, Hawkins CM, Lischstein E: Effect of propranolol in post infarction patients with mechanical or electrical complications. Circulation 1984; 49: 761—5.
13. CAPS Investigators: The Cardiac Arrhythmia Pilot Study. Am J Cardiol 1984; 54: 87—90.
14. Olsson G, Rehnqvist N: Evaluation of antiarrhythmic effects of metoprolol treatment

after acute myocardial infarction: relationship between treatment responses and survival during a 3 year follow up. Eur Heart J 1986; 7: 312—9.

15. Mitsutaki A, Takeshita A, Kuroiwa A, Nakamura M: Usefulness of the Valsalva manoeuvre in management of the long QT syndrome. Circulation 1981; 63: 1029—35.

16. Schwartz PJ: The idiopathic long QT syndrome. The need for a prospective registry. Eur Heart J 1983; 4: 529—31.

17. Ruskin JN, McGovern B, Garan H, DiMarco JP, Kelly E: Antiarrhythmic drugs: a possible cause of out-of-hospital cardiac arrest. N Engl J Med 1983; 309: 1302—6.

18. Bigger JT, Fleiss JL, Rolnitzky LM, Merab JP, Ferrick KJ: Effect of digitalis treatment on survival after myocardial infarction. Am J Cardiol 1985; 55: 623—30.

19. McKenna WJ, England D, Doi YL, Deanfield JE, Oakley CM, Goodwin JF: Arrhythmia in hypertrophic cardiomyopathy: I Influence on prognosis. Br Heart J 1981; 46: 168—72.

20. Morady F, Sledge C, Shen E, Sung RJ, Gonzales R, Scheiman MM: Electrophysiological testing in the management of patients with the Wolff-Parkinson-White syndrome and atrial fibrillation. Am J Cardiol 1983; 51: 1623—8.

21. Campbell RWF, Godman MJ, Fiddler GI, Marquis RMM, Julian DG: Ventricular arrhythmias in syndrome of balloon deformity of mitral valve. Definition of possible high risk group. Br Heart J 1976; 38: 1053—7.

22. Chizner MA, Pearle DL, de Leon AC: The natural history of aortic stenosis in adults. Am Heart J 1980; 99: 419—24.

23. Chakko S, Gheorghiade M: Ventricular arrhythmias in severe heart failure: incidence, sigificance and effectiveness of therapy. Am Heart J 1985; 109: 497—504.

24. The CONSENSUS Trial Study Group: Effects of enalapril on mortality in severe congestive heart failure: results of the Co-operative North Scandinavian Enalapril Survival Study (CONSENSUS). N Engl J Med 1987; 316: 1429—35.

25. Cullen K, Stenhouse NS, Wearne KL, Cumpston GN: Electrocardiographic and 13 year cardiovascular mortality in Bussleton study. Br Heart J 1982; 47: 209—12.

26. Kennedy HL, Whitlock JA, Sprague MK, Kennedy LJ, Buckingham TA, Goldberg RJ: Long term follow up of asymptomatic healthy subjects with frequent and complex ventricular ectopy. N Engl J Med 1985; 312: 193—7.

12. Sudden death in patients with intraventricular conduction disorders

HENRI E. KULBERTUS

In 1913, Graybiel and Sprague [1] reported on a group of 395 patients with bundle branch block (BBB) generally associated with coronary artery or hypertensive heart disease. Adequate follow up of 77% of this cohort was available and the authors observed 223 fatal cases with an average survival of 14 months.

Perera *et al.* [2] studied 104 cases of right bundle branch block (RBBB), 95% of whom had heart disease. Of 91 cases with adequate follow up, one third had died over a mean period of 4 years. Their series also contained 60 cases of left bundle branch block (LBBB): 60% were dead at one year.

Among hospitalized patients with LBBB or RBBB, Messer *et al.* [3] observed a mean survival of 3.3 and 3.9 years respectively. Similarly, Campbell [4] followed up 50 patients with BBB of whom 48 had cardiovascular disease; 39 died with a mean survival of two years.

These publications which consider BBB as an ominous sign were all derived from observations of hospital based series. It was soon realized that the prognosis was much better when BBB was detected in individuals without clinical evidence of cardiovascular disease [5—13]. For example, Rotman *et al.* [14] reported their follow up study of 394 subjects with RBBB and 125 with LBBB. Most of these subjects were asymptomatic at the time of the bundle branch block diagnosis. Complete follow up information was available in 94% of the RBBB and 91% of the LBBB patients. The mean follow up was 10.8 ± 4.4 years and 8.8 ± 4.8 years, respectively. Only 14 (4%) RBBB and 9 (8%) LBBB subjects died during this follow up period.

The same contrast between studies reporting either a guarded or a favorable prognosis depending on the population from which the patients were derived still persisted in the seventies.

In 1978, Mc Anulty *et al.* [15] reviewed all 42,000 electrocardiograms recorded at their university from 1969 to 1971. 325 patients had LBBB or RBBB with axis deviation. Survival at 5 years of 164 LBBB patients (40.7 ± 4.1%) was approximately equal to that of 161 patients with RBBB and axis deviation (49.5 ± 4.2%). Patients with coronary artery disease had a particularly poor prognosis (survival at 5 years: 33.7%), especially if they had

A. Bayés de Luna et al. (eds.): *Sudden Cardiac Death*, 121–126.
© 1991 Kluwer Academic Publishers, Dordrecht.

evidence of a previous myocardial infarction (survival at 5 years: 23.5%). Primary conduction disease occurred in 20%; with a survival of 50.6% at 5 years, it was not without risks of its own. The same group [16] prospectively followed up 257 patients with LBBB or RBBB with axis deviation who had undergone His bundle studies. During a follow up of 25 months, 50 patients died, 27 suddenly. Actuarial analysis revealed an annual mortality rate of 19 ± 2.6% and a mortality rate from sudden death of 10.2 ± 2.6%. In their series, in contrast with the results of Narula *et al.* [17], HV interval duration failed to influence the outcome. Some authors indicated that only greatly prolonged HV time may identify a subgroup of patients at high risk of sudden death, especially when heart failure is associated [18, 19].

Dinghra *et al.* [20] in 1978 reported that, among 102 patients with chronic LBBB followed up for 32 to 2,271 days, the cumulative mortality at 4 years was close to 70% and the mortality by sudden death to 60%. According to the same authors (21), among 452 patients with RBBB and axis deviation followed up for a period of 1.066 ± 97 days, the cumulative mortality by sudden death was 20% ± 2.3 at 4 years.

In the mean time, reports dealing with patients culled from a private practice outpatient population [22] or from a screening examination carried out in more than 18,000 London male civil servants [23] yielded the dominant impression that among individuals with intraventricular conduction disorders and no symptomatic history the risk of sudden death is indeed very low.

Prognosis of intraventricular conduction disorders in asymptomatic subjects

The Manitoba Study [24] was designed to evaluate the predictive value of the ECG for sudden death in the absence of preexisting manifestations of heart disease. 3,983 individuals, all former canadian air force pilots, pilots in training or licensed pilots, were followed up for 30 years (1948—1978).

Cases were selected if they fulfilled two criteria: (a) an electrocardiographic abnormality detected during routine examination, and (b) no clinical evidence of ischaemic or valvular disease in either that examination or in the previous one since entry.

Of this group, 70 died suddenly (natural death occurring immediately or within an estimated period of 24 hours after the onset of acute objective or subjective symptoms of ischaemic heart disease). Fifty (71.4%) of the 70 had electrocardiographic abnormalities; these included 22 cases (31.4%) with ST-T wave changes, 11 (15%) with ventricular premature beats, 9 (12.9%) with left ventricular hypertrophy on voltage criteria only, 5 (7.1%) with LBBB and 4 (5.7%) with abnormal left axis deviation (LAD: −45° to −90°). None had RBBB.

Left bundle branch block. In the Manitoba Study, LBBB without evidence of heart disease was noted in 33 cases. Cardiovascular mortality (all by sudden death) was 15.2% (5/33). The age-adjusted sudden death incidence rate was 17.2 per 1000 person-years, i.e. almost 14 times the incidence in men without LBBB. Prognosis in LBBB was dependent on the age of the patient at its detection [25]. For men aged 35 to 44 years, there was no increased risk of sudden death. On the opposite, among men in the age range of 45 to 64 years, the 5 year incidence of sudden death as the first manifestation of coronary artery disease was more than 10 times higher than among men without LBBB. This difference might reflect a difference in etiology. In young people, LBBB might be due to a congenital malformation with no adverse prognosis [26].

Electrocardiographic characteristics of the QRS complex (axis, duration) did not influence prognosis although a trend for wider QRS durations to indicate a lower survival rate was noted [25].

The results of this study indicate that LBBB is a serious finding when it develops in men after the age of 40 years.

Other population studies have indicated that cardiovascular mortality in newly acquired LBBB was significantly increased even after considering in multivariate analysis age, blood pressure, diabetes, coronary heart disease and congestive heart failure [23, 27, 28].

Right bundle branch block. Different population studies with control or comparison groups have demonstrated that complete RBBB with or without axis deviation is not a predictor of sudden cardiac death [29, 30].

Marked left axis deviation. In men aged 40—59 years , LAD is associated with a significantly increased risk of ischaemic heart disease. It is not however a predictor of sudden cardiac death [23, 28, 31—33].

Personal data. Our modest study of 161 subjects with RBBB, 57 with LBBB and 45 with LAD-RBBB, all without evidence of cardiovascular disease, followed up for an average of 40 months and compared with controls matched for age and sex and devoid of cardiovascular disease failed to show any difference in mortality between patients with conduction disorders and controls. The projected 5-years mortality rate of all subjects with BBB was 10%, i.e. exactly the same figure as that obtained among controls. This figure is in keeping with the annual mortality rate within the whole French speaking part of Belgium which, at the age of 65 years (the men age of our population) is 1.75% for women and 4% in men [34—35].

Prognosis of BBB in patients with cardiovascular disease

Due to the lack of accurate data, I shall restrict my remarks to patients with myocardial infarction. It is well known that the presence of BBB in the course of a myocardial infarction worsens the prognosis. Several series have demonstrated this phenomenon which is illustrated by our own results [35] and by pooled results from 12 different studies [36]. One would expect that the risk is more dramatically increased in patients with new versus pre-existing BBB, especially if one considers that myocardial infarction patients who develop a new BBB generally have larger infarcts which carry the risk of cardiogenic shock or heart failure. This hypothesis has been confirmed by some [37, 38], but not by others [39].

In a study published in 1980, Lie *et al.* [40] reported that of 1.008 hospital survivors of a myocardial infarction, 26 died suddenly within one year of the infarct. Five of them had developed a BBB during their stay in the CCU: 4 died within 6 weeks and the last one within 3 months of their acute event.

This is in keeping with data from our own unit [41]. Out of 428 patients admitted to the CCU with a diagnosis of myocardial infarction 45 (10.5%) died between 0—3 months after admission. Another 45 (11.7% of survivors) died between 3 to 33 months. Using a stepwise logistic discrimination technique, the following predictors of early mortality (which in the great majority was due to sudden death) were discovered: LV function score, ventricular fibrillation in the CCU, bundle branch block, history of previous myocardial infarction, age, AV block during hospital stay.

The predictors of late mortality were different and comprised age, anterior site of infarction and relatively small MB-CCK peak of less than 650 units. The latter finding probably reflects the incomplete character of the infarction and indicates that after 3 months, the prognosis is primarily influenced by the amount of remaining jeopardized myocardium. The influence of BBB has disappeared. This observation may account for the surprising finding that in the Coronary Drug Project men with a complete RBBB and a history of remote myocardial infarction had no increased risk [42].

Conclusions

Patients with RBBB and without evidence of cardiovascular disease have no increased risk of dying suddenly. Controversial results have been obtained as regards LBBB which, even if there is no symptomatology, should be regarded as a serious finding, at least in men after the age of 40 years.

In patients with cardiac disease, a BBB indicates a threat of sudden death. New BBB's developping during a myocardial infarction are associated with a very high mortality, especially by sudden death and during the first three months after the infarction. At a later stage, the BBB looses its prognostic significance. The residual amount of jeopardized myocardium then plays a major role.

References

1. Graybiel A, Sprague HB: Bundle branch block: an analysis of 395 cases. Am J Med Sci 1933; 185: 395.
2. Perera G, Leine SA, Erlanger H: Prognosis of right bundle branch block: a study of 104 cases. Brit heart J 1942; 4: 35.
3. Messer AL, Birmingham A, Johnson RP, Schreevinas M, White PD: Prognosis in bundle branch block III. A comparison of right and left bundle branch block with a note on the relative incidence of each. Amer Heart J 1951; 41: 239.
4. Campbell M: The outlook with bundle branch block. Brit Heart J 1969; 31: 575.
5. Schreevinas M, Messer AL, Johnson RP, White PD: Prognosis in bundle branch block I. Factors influencing the survival period in right bundle branch block. Amer Heart J 1950; 40: 891.
6. Wood FC, Jeffers WA, Wolferth CC: Follow up study of 74 patients with a right bundle branch conduction defect. Amer Heart J 1935; 10: 1056.
7. Rodstein M, Gubner R, Mills JP, Lovell JF, Ungerleider HE: A mortality study in bundle branch block. Arch Intern Med 1951; 87: 663.
8. Wolfram J: Bundle branch block without significant heart disease. Amer Heart J 1951; 41: 656.
9. Vazifdas JP, Levine SA: Benign bundle branch block. Arch Intern Med 1952; 89: 568.
10. Lamb LE, Johnson RC: Left bundle branch block is flying personnel. A report of 56 cases. Aerosp Med 1964; 35: 97.
11. Massing GK, Lancaster MC: Clinical significance of acquired complete right bundle branch block in 59 patients without overt cardiac disease. Aerosp Med 1969; 40: 867.
12. Beach TB, Gracey JG, Peter PH: Benign left bundle branch block. Ann intern Med 1969; 70: 269.
13. Smith RF, Jackson DH, Harthorne JW, Sanders CA: Acquired bundle branch block in a healthy population. Amer Heart J 1970; 80: 746.
14. Rotman M, Triebwasser JA: A clinical follow up study of right and left bundle branch block. Circulation 1975; 41: 477.
15. Mc Anulty JH, Kauffman S, Murphy E, Kassebaum DG, Rahimotoola SH: Survival in patients with intraventricular conduction defects. Arch Intern Med 1978; 138:30.
16. Mc Anulty JH, Rahimtoola SH, Murphy EJ, Kauffman S, Ritzmann LW, Kanarek P, De Mots H: A prospective study of sudden in 'high risk' bundle branch block. New Engl J Med 1978; 299: 209.
17. Narula OS, Gann D, Samet Ph: Prognostic value of HV intervals in His bundle electro-cardiography and clinical electrophysiology. Narula OS (ED), Philadelphia, FA Davis Company 1975; p. 437.
18. Scheinman M, Weiss A, Kunke F: His bundle recordings in patients with bundle branch block and transient neurologic symptoms. Circulation 1973; 43: 322.
19. Scheinman M, Peters RW, Moden G, Brennan M, Mies C, O'Young J: Prognostic value of infranodal conduction time in patients with chronic bundle branch block. Circulation 1977; 56: 240.
20. Dinghra RC, Amat-Y-Hem F, Wyndham C, Sridhar SS, Wu D, Denes P, Rosen KM: Significance of left axis deviation in patients with chronic left bundle branch block. Amer J Cardiol 1978; 42: 551.
21. Dinghra RC, Wyndham C, Amat-Y-Hem F, Denes P, Wu D, Sridhar SS, Bustin AG, Rosen KM; Incidence and site of atrioventricular block in patients with chronic bifascicu-lar block. Circulation 1979; 59: 238.
22. Lister JW, Kline RS, Lesser ME: Chronic bilateral bundle branch block. Long term observations in ambulatory patients. Brit Heart J 1977; 39: 203.
23. Rose GA, Baxter PJ, Reid D, Mc Cartney P: Prevalence and prognosis of electrocardiog-raphic findings in middle-aged men. Brit Heart J 1978; 40: 636.

24. Rabkin SW, Mathews FAL, Tate RB: The electrocardiogram in apparently healthy men and the risk of sudden death. Brit Heart J 1982; 47: 546.
25. Rabkin SN, Mathewson FAL, Tate RB: Natural history of left bundle branch block. Brit Heart J 1980; 43: 164.
26. Rabkin SN: Electrocardiographic abnormalities in apparently healthy men and the risk of sudden death. Drugs 1984; Suppl I: 28.
27. Schneider JF, Thomas Jr HE, Kuger BE, McNamara PM, Kannel WB: Newly acquired left bundle branch block. The Framingham Study. Ann Intern Med 1979; 90: 303.
28. Blackburn A, Taylor HL, Key SA: The electrocardiogram in prediction of five year coronary heart disease incidence among men aged forty through fifty-nine. Circulation 1970; 41 & 42; suppl I: 154.
29. Rabkin SW, Mathewson FAL, Tate RB: The natural history of right bundle branch block and frontal plans QRS axis in apparently healthy men. Chest 1981; 80: 191.
30. Schenider RF, Jackson DH, Hawthorne JW, Sanders CA: Acquired bundle branch block in a healthy population. Amer Heart J 1980; 92: 37.
31. Rabkin SW, Mathewson FAL, Tate RB: The relationship of left axis deviation in apparently healthy men to the risk of ischemic heart disease. International Journal of Cardiology 1981; 1: 169.
32. Cullen K, Stenhouse NS, Wearne KL, Cumpston GN: Electrocardiograms and 13 year cardiovascular mortality in Busselton study. Brit Heart J 1982; 47: 209.
33. Tunstall-Pedoe HD: Predictability of sudden death from resting electrocardiograms: effect of previous manifestation of coronary heart disease. Brit Heart J 1978; 40: 630.
34. Kulbertus HE: De Level-Rutten F, Albert A, Dubois M, Petit JM: Electrocardiographic changes occurring with advancing age, In: What's New in Electrocardiography. HJJ Wellens and HE Kulbertus (eds). Martinus Nijhoff Publishers. The Hague (1981), p. 300.
35. Kulbertus HE: Prognostic significance of fascicular blocks in acute myocardial infarction, In: The first 24 Hours in Myocardial Infarction. F. Kainde, O. Pachinger, P. Probst (eds). Verlag Gerhard Witzotrock, Baden-Baden (1977), p. 33.
36. Mullens CB, Atkins JM: Prognosis and management of ventricular conduction blocks in acute myocardial infarction. Mod Concepts Cardiovasc dis 1976; 45: 129.
37. Lie KI, Wellens HJJm, Schnilenburg RM: Bundle branch block and myocardial infarction, In: The Conduction System of the Heart. HJJ Wellens, KI Lie, MJ Janse (eds). Stenfert Kroese, Leiden, 1976.
38. Nimetz AA, Shubrooks SJ Jr, Hutter AM Jr, De Sanctis RW: Significance of chronic versus acute myocardial infarction. Amer Heart J 1975; 90: 439.
39. Gann D, Balachandran PK, El Sherif N, Samet P: Prognostic significance of chronic versus acute bundle branch block in acute myocardial infarction. Chest 1975; 67: 298.
40. Lie KI, Manger Cats V, Durrer D: CCU findings useful for identification of sudden death candidates in the post-hospital phase of myocardial infarction, In: Sudden Death. HE Kulbertus, HJJ Wellens (eds). [Developments in Cardiovascular Medicine, Vol. 4.] Martinus Nijhoff, The Hague (1980), p. 232.
41. Piérard L, Chapelle JP, Albert A, Dubois Ch, Kulbertus HE: Differing characteristics associated with early versus late mortality after acute myocardial infarction (in press).
42. Blackburn H, Tominaga S: Prognostic significance of electrocardiogram after myocardial infarction. Ann Inter Med 1972; 77: 677.

13. Acute drug test

A. BAYÉS DE LUNA, J. GUINDO, S. GARCÍA-SÁNCHEZ,
P. TORNER and R. OTER

Initially introduced by Lown *et al.*. [1—4], these authors demonstrated the efficacy of this test in the treatment of patients with malignant ventricular arrhythmias. The test consists of the administration of acute oral doses of antiarrhythmic drug so as to determine whether the drug can suppress the premature ventricular contractions. If this is the case, it is probable that chronic administration of the antiarrhythmic will be useful. The acute drug test also allows us to know if the drug has an arrhythmogenic effect. *The aims of the acute drug test*, therefore, are:
a) to identify therapy for arrhythmias more scientifically and less empirically;
b) to objectively prove whether the therapeutic efficacy of the drugs administered acutely is maintained with chronic administration;
c) to avoid iatrogenic risks (specially arrhythmogenesis) of antiarrhythmic drugs.

Design of the test

The test was originally divided by Lown *et al.* [1—4] into 4 phases. With a slight modification [5—7], we presently perform the test as follows:

Phase 0. Inclusion criteria comprise patients with any type of ventricular arrhythmia to be treated. This includes patients with previous malignant ventricular arrhythmias (symptomatic ventricular tachycardia or ventricular fibrillation outside acute infarction), patients with potentially malignant ventricular arrhythmias and the rare cases of patients with benign ventricular arrhythmias that we consider must be treated. Prior to inclusion a 48 hour Holter monitoring is performed to determine the exact amount of premature ventricular contractions and the spontaneous variability. Although this spontaneous variability exists these patients are included because we want to be sure that the drug being used is not arrhythmogenic. All antiarrhythmic

A. Bayés de Luna et al. (eds.): *Sudden Cardiac Death*, 127–133.

medication is stopped and data from Holter monitoring, effort testing, echocardiography and/or isotopic ventriculography are collected.

Phase 1. Acute test. After one hour of continuous basal ECG recording which shows the actual number of ventricular arrhythmias, half the maintenance dose of the chosen antiarrhythmic drug is administered in order to prove the reduction of premature ventricular complexes (PVC). Although we do not find PVC during this hour we performed the test in order to be sure that the drug is not arrhythmogenic. Continuous ECG recording during 3—5 hour control, bicycle stress test (until functional limit), mental stress and plasma levels are carried out every hour. In patients with malignant ventricular arrhythmias even if the test is positive, ideally several tests should be performed (one every 24 hours, with an average of 6 tests per patient in Lown's experience). The most effective agent or combination of agents is then selected.

The protocol as designed by Lown *et al.* [1—4] represent a real antiarrhythmogram for the patient, found to be very useful in cases of malignant ventricular arrhythmias. However testing so many drugs is very cumbersome, complicated and impractical, especially in patients with potentially malignant ventricular arrhythmias in which it is difficult to justify such effort when the benefit of antiarrhythmic treatment in such cases is still not well known. For this reason in our modified protocol (Figure 1) in patients with non-malignant ventricular arrhythmias [5—7], if we find a positive response to the first drug, we immediately go to phase 2, with the same drug. Therefore, as we are using a very effective antiarrhythmic agent as a first choice drug we only use one drug in nearly 80% of the patients. Thus, we are not performing a full antiarrhythmogram. Besides, if the test is negative, as the arrhythmia is not malignant we can give the drug until we know the response in phase 2.

Phase 2. Following several days of treatment with the chosen antiarrhythmic drug as a first choice drug and when the steady-state of the drug is established, a 24—48 hours Holter monitoring and an effort test are performed. Concordance between the suppression of premature ventricular

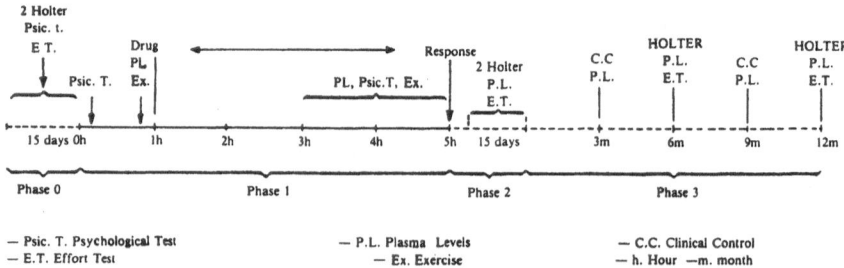

Figure 1. Scheme of our modified protocol of acute drug test. (Adapted from Bayés de Luna *et al.* [5])

contractions in the acute test (phase 1) and phase 2 has been found in 80—85% of cases [1, 6]. If we find that the response to the drug is negative, treatment with another drug is begun.

Phase 3. Clinical follow-up with repeated Holter monitoring. It is interesting to note that in our experience with potentially malignant ventricular arrhythmias, no patient with positive response in phase 2 developped arrhythmogenia in the follow-up [6, 7].

Discussion

Lown's group [1] affirmed that they were able to carry out acute drug tests in over 70% of their patients with malignant ventricular arrhythmias (123/175) as they had frequent spontaneous arrhythmias. Using this methodology in 123 patients with malignant ventricular arrhythmias they demonstrated that annual mortality declined from 41% to 2.3% in individuals in whom grade 4B and 5 ventricular arrhythmias (runs of ventricular tachycardia and R-on-T phenomenon) were supressed (Figure 2). The same group recently published a paper [4] that reaffirmed the effectiveness of antiarrhythmic treatment in the prevention of sudden death. They found that after several years without recurrences withdrawal of treatment was followed by a high incidence of recurrent malignant ventricular arrhythmias and sudden death. Of 24 patients who discontinued treatment for different motives, 12 (50%) suffered recurrence of malignant ventricular arrhythmia (9 with cardiac arrest), and in 11 (46%) the ventricular arrhythmia was of the same degree as before treatment.

It seems surprising that the spectacular results of Lown's group [1] have

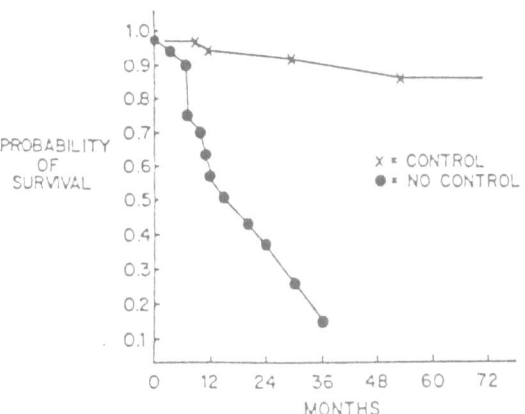

Figure 2. Efficacy of the acute drug test in the treatment of malignant ventricular arrhythmias in Lown's group (from Graboys *et al.* [2]).

received more criticism than praise. It is obvious that the work may be criticized for not having a control group, but we think it is evident that this is not ethically justified in a group of patients at such high risk of mortality. There are other limitations, but nevertheless it seems strange that, contrary to what occurred with the evaluation of antiarrhythmic treatment by intra-cardiac electrophysiological studies with corroboration by numerous groups [8—12] there have been almost no other studies with a reasonable number of patients with malignant ventricular arrhythmias which have duplicated Lown's results. Lown's results [1—4] with acute drug testing in patients with malignant ventricular arrhythmias are similar to those obtained in other groups by selecting the drug by intracardiac electrophysiological studies [12] (Table 1). There are no large series of comparative studies of the acute drug test and programmed electrical stimulation. However, in the recent paper of Mitchell *et al.* [13], programmed electrical stimulation seems to offer better results than the acute drug test, although the series is small. This finding will have to be confirmed in larger series. If the two techniques are found to be similarly effective, we recommend the acute drug test in all patients with frequent arrhythmias in Holter monitoring, and electrophysiologic studies in the other cases. Nevertheless, the acute drug test can even be useful in the group of patients with malignant arrhythmias but without ventricular arrhyth-mias in phase 0 in order to to rule out arrhythmogenesis. In these patients, the treatment could be controlled by monitoring the plasma levels of the antiarrhythmic drugs.

Both the acute drug test and programmed electrical stimulation have some drawbacks [14]. In the first place, in order to be sure of the antiarrhythmic efficacy of the drug, the acute drug test has limitations in patients without frequent ventricular arrhythmias in the Holter recording and great day-to-day variability, although it can be adjusted to rule out arrhythmogenesis. More-over, criteria for efficacy and arrhythmogenesis have been determined intui-tively and it is not known if they are the most adequate. Nevertheless, in some cases the results in phase 1 are not the same in phase 2 and 3. Programmed electrical stimulation as well as being more invasive, is even more expensive and complex than the acute drug test, thus notably limiting its repeated use. This invasiveness also affects the cardiologist who performs

Table 1. Outcome of treatment programs for malignant ventricular arrhythmias. (From Swerdlow *et al.* N Engl J Med 1983; 308: 1436).

	Responder		Nonresponder	
	3 year		3 year	
	N	mortality rate	N	mortality rate
Holter/exercise	98	14%	25	84%
Electrophysiologic studies	103	20%	102	68%

the test, since the provocation of a malignant ventricular arrhythmia and the necessary resuscitation maneuvers produce intense psychic stress. Moreover, there is no uniform stimulation protocol, and the true significance of the arrhythmias induced artificially in the laboratory and whether they correlate with the patient's spontaneous arrhythmias is unknown. Furthermore, it has been demonstrated that certain antiarrhythmic drugs that do not prevent the reinduction of arrhythmias are highly effective in chronic treatment (for example amiodarone and propafenone).

The value of the acute drug test in the choice of drug for patients with potentially malignant ventricular arrhythmias is unknown, although it seems logical, and more after withdrawn flecainide and encainide of CAST due to its proarrhythmic effects, that in patients in whom the efficacy of the drug is not established, we must at least rule out provocation of arrhythmias. Nevertheless we have to consider that proarrhythmia in CAST trial appears not only early (detected by acute drug test) but also late in the follow-up (15), and acute drug test in this case cannot predict the later. Early proarrhythmia has been observed by Velebit *et al.* [16] that can be produced by all antiarrhythmic agents. We think that the best acute drug testing approach in patients with benign or potentially malignant ventricular arrhythmias is the form which we have used, looking for an effective drug and not carrying out the complete screening (Figure 1). Our drug of first choice is propafenone, but we feel that quinidine, procainamide, mexiletine, flecainide and tocainide, etc., may also be useful. The problem with amiodarone is that due to its pharmakocinetic characteristics it requires hospitalization for 8—10 hours and in the case of failure it interferes with the administration of other drugs. However, Coumel *et al.* [17] have demonstrated that amiodarone can be used in an acute drug test.

We consider that the acute drug test can be useful in patients with potentially malignant ventricular arrhythmias, although we need to be able to answer several questions, including:

a) the number of positive cases in phase 1 which continue to be positive in phase 2 and 3;
b) the number of negative cases in phase 1 which are positive in phases 2 and 3;
c) to see whether the arrhythmogenesis seen in phase 1 continues in phase 2;
d) to see if there are cases in which arrhythmogenesis occurs in phase 2 but not in phase 1.

At present we can partly answer (a), (b) and (d). It does not seem ethical to discuss (c) although the criteria for arrhythmogenesis are debatable. We cannot be sure when an increase in the number of premature ventricular contractions is truly dangerous but when confronted with a clear increase of the arrhythmia it is obvious that this medication should not be continued. The true incidence of arrhythmogenesis is probably less than that suggested in publications [16].

Table 2. Results of acute drug test in patients with potentially malignant ventricular arrhythmias using propafenone as a drug of choice.

	Phase I	Phase II
Positive response	27/40 (67.5%)	37/38 (71%)
Negative response	11/40 (27.5%)	11/38 (29%)
Arrhythmogenesis	2/40 (5%)	0/38 (−)

In our experience with our modified protocol and using propafenone [7] as the drug of first choice we think we can answer some of the above problems:

a) the number of cases with a positive response in phase 1 was 67.5% and of these, 71% were also positive in phase 2 (Table 2);

b) there is a good correlation between phase 1 and phase 2 (84%). The percentage of negative cases in phase 1 that become positive in phase 2 or positive cases in phase 1 that become negative in phase 2 is quite low (16%);

c) the arrhythmogenesis of propafenone is low (5%) and it is noteworthy that no patient with positive response in phase 2 developped arrhythmogenia in the follow-up.

The acute drug test therefore appears to be a good method for avoiding the risk of early proarrhythmic effects of antiarrhythmic drugs.

In conclusion, we think that the acute drug test is a valid method to treat patients with ventricular arrhythmias, and also to avoid early proarrhythmia.

References

1. Lown B, Graboys TB: Management of the patient with malignant ventricular arrhythmias. Am J Cardiol 1977; 39: 910.
2. Graboys TB, Lown B, Podrid PJ, De Silva R: Longterm survival of patients with ventricular arrhythmia treated with antiarrhythmic drugs. Am J Cardiol 1982; 50: 437.
3. Graboys TB: Non-invasive assessment of antiarrhythmic drugs. In Bayés de Luna A, Betriu A, Permanyer G: Therapeutics in cardiology. Kluwer Academic Press, Dordrecht 1988, p. 59.
4. Graboys TB, Almeida EC, Lown B: Recurrence of malignant ventricular arrhythmias after antiarrhythmic drug withdrawal. Am J Cardiol 1986; 58: 59.
5. Bayés de Luna A, Guindo J, Torner P, Borja J, Caturla MC, García S, Domínguez JM, Oter R, Jané F: Value of effort testing and acute drug testing in the evaluation of antiarrhythmic treatment. Eur. Heart J 1987; 8 (Suppl A): 77.
6. Guindo J, Bayés de Luna A, Borja J *et al.*: Valoración terapéutica de la propafenona en pacientes con arritmias ventriculares potencialmente malignas mediante la prueba aguda incruenta farmacológica. Rev Lat Cardiol 1986; 7: 507.
7. Guindo J, Bayés de Luna A, Torner P *et al.*: Valor del test agudo incruento en el tratamiento de las arritmias ventriculares potencialmente malignas. Rev Esp cardiol 1987; 40 (Suppl I): 51.

8. Josephson MR, Horowitz LN: Electrophysiologic approach to therapy of recurrent sustained ventricular tachycardia. Am J Cardiol 1979; 43: 631.

9. Mason JW, Winkle RA: Accuracy of the ventricular tachycardia-induction study for predicting long-term efficacy and inefficacy of antiarrhythmic drugs. N Engl J Med 1980; 303: 1073.

10. Horowitz LN, Josephson ME, Kastor JA: Intracardiac electrophysiologic studies as a method for the optimization of drug therapy in chronic ventricular arrhythmia. Prog. Cardiovasc Dis 1980; 23: 81.

11. Ruskin JN, Dimarco JP, Garan H: Out-of-hospital cardiac arrest. Electrophysiologic observations and selection of long-term antiarrhythmic therapy. N Engl J Med 1980; 303: 607.

12. Swerdlow CD, Winkle RA, Mason JW: Determinants of survival in patients with ventricular tachyarrhythmias. N Engl J Med 1983; 308: 1436.

13. Mitchell LB, Duff HJ, Manyari DE, Wyse DG: A randomized clinical trial of the noninasive and invasive approaches to drug therapy of ventricular tachycardia. N Engl J Med 1987; 317: 1681.

14. Podrid PJ: Treatment of ventricular arrhythmia. Applications and limitations of noninvasive vs invasive approaches. Chest 1985; 88: 121.

15. CAST Investigators. Preliminary Report: effect of encainide and flecainide on mortality in a randomised trial of arrhythmia supression after myocardial infarction. N Engl J Med 1989; 321: 406.

16. Velebit V, Podrid P, Lown B: Aggravation and provocation of ventricular arrhythmias by antiarrhythmic drugs. Circulation 1982; 65: 886.

17. Escoubet B, Coumel P, Poirier JM *et al.*: Suppression of arrhythmias within hours after a single oral dose of amiodarone and relation to plasma and myocardial concentations. Am J Cardiol 1985; 55: 696.

14. Malignant ventricular arrhythmias
Serial electrophysiologic testing

JESÚS ALMENDRAL and ANGEL ARENAL

The majority of patients with sustained ventricular tachyarrhythmias are characterized by a scarce number of arrhythmic events but with serious clinical compromise.

The scarce number of spontaneous episodes make therapeutic efficacy difficult to assess: the favorable course of a given patient after the initiation of an antiarrhythmic drug treatment may represent therapeutic efficacy, but that may also happen just by chance.

The usually serious clinical compromise of these arrhythmic events, make the "empiric method" (in which the physician infers the therapeutic efficacy only by the absence of recurrences during the follow-up) undesirable for the selection of antiarrhythmic drugs in this context. It will be preferable to have "guidelines" in this choice.

First Wellens *et al.* [1] and then Josephson *et al.* [2] observed that in patients with recurrent sustained ventricular tachycardias (VT) a morphologically similar tachyarrhythmia could usually be initiated by programmed electrical stimulation. As a consequence, it was hypothesized that, if a drug was efficacious in the prophylaxis of arrhythmic recurrences, it should prevent the initiation of these arrhythmias by programmed electrical stimulation. Otherwise, the arrhythmia would persist inducible. The attempts to support or reject this hypothesis on the basis of a scientific analysis have generated a lot of literature, but the subject still remains controversial. The purpose of the present chapter is to review this information and critically analyze the role of programmed electrical stimulation as a guide in the choice of pharmacologic therapy.

The method: description and general considerations

Table 1 describes the method of serial electrophysiologic testing. It is necessary to perform programmed electrical stimulation on the baseline (without antiarrhythmic therapy) to show that, on the baseline state, the

A. Bayés de Luna et al. (eds.): *Sudden Cardiac Death*, 135–145.
© 1991 Kluwer Academic Publishers, Dordrecht.

Table 1. The method of programmed electrical stimulation to guide the selection of anti-arrhythmic drugs.

1.	Baseline programmed electrical stimulation
2.	Positive response: initiation of a sustained ventricular tachyarrhythmia
3.	Antiarrhythmic drug A
4.	Programmed electrical stimulation on antiarrhythmic therapy
5.	If a positive response: return to 3 with another antiarrhythmic drug (B . . .)
6.	If a negative response (no initiation of tachyarrhythmias): continue with the same antiarrhythmic drug on a chronic basis

arrhythmia is inducible, i.e. it can be initiated by programmed electrical stimulation.

There has been some controversy as to what can be considered a satisfactory drug response. Table 2 includes several criteria proposed to represent a satisfactory pharmacologic response. It has been suggested that a mere narrowing of the tachycardia zone or an increase in the number of extra-stimuli required for the initiation of the tachyarrhythmia are indicators of a good drug response. It has also been suggested that the slowing of the induced tachycardia is a good prognostic sign. In contrast, other authors consider a drug prophylactic only if nonsustained tachycardia, longer than 3 to 6 beats, was also abolished. At the present time, it seems to us that the most adequate criterium is the absence of an inducible sustained tachyar-rhythmia, in response to a complete stimulation protocol, provided that a sustained arrhythmia was induced in the baseline study.

Table 2. Electrophysiologic criteria for efficacy of antiarrhythmic drugs.

Narrowing of tachycardia 'window'
Need for a more "aggressive" stimulation for initiation
Suppression of inducibility of non sustained VT
Slowing of the tachycardia induced
Suppression of inducibility of the clinical arrhythmia

However, two recent studies [3, 4] emphasize the possible clinical efficacy related to responses other than a complete suppression of inducibility, as will be discussed later.

Prior to the review of individual studies, several considerations need to be pointed out because they influence the bulk of the available information (Table 3). The patients whose clinical presentation is cardiac arrest have worse prognosis and distinct electrophysiologic characteristics as compared to those presenting with sustained ventricular tachycardia without cardiac arrest [5]. Likewise, the cardiac diagnosis influences the prognosis [6]. In the majority of studies the end point is described as either sudden death or recurrence of sustained tachycardia; although it is quite clear that they are distinct events, they only tend to be considered separately in the most recent

Table 3. Important considerations in assessing the information related to ventricular tachyar-rhythmias.

1. Clinical presentation: cardiac arrest vs sustained VT
2. Structural heart disease: coronary artery disease, dilated cardiomyopathy, right ventri-cular dysplasia, absence of structural heart disease.
3. End point of the study: sudden death vs recurrence of sustained VT
4. Presence/absence of other therapeutic alternatives: subendocardial resection, implant-able devices, cardiac fulguration.

studies. Finally, the studies are biased to some extent by the introduction of non pharmacologic therapy to a variable degree depending upon the group and the time of the study.

Having raised all these considerations we should try to answer 3 basic questions regarding the method of programmed electrical stimulation: is it applicable? Is it reliable? Is it appropriate?

Inducibility of the clinical arrhythmia

Patients with sustained ventricular tachycardia. Table 4 reflects the percent-ages of inducibility reported by different groups in patients presenting clinically with sustained uniform VT, excluding the first 48 hours of an acute myocardial infarction [7—12]. Considering these series together, in 90% of such patients a uniform, sustained, morphologically similar arrhythmia can be induced by programmed electrical stimulation. The incidence appears to be higher when the stimulation protocol includes a third extrastimuli [13], multiple right ventricular sites [14] an eventually the left ventricle [15]. Although the majority of cases in the reported series had coronary artery disease, patients with VT and no organic heart disease also appear to have a high incidence of inducibility. In patients with cardiomyopathy, the results are more discordant, the inducibility rate ranging from 52 to 100% [10, 16, 17].

Table 4. Inducibility in patients with sustained ventricular tachycardia.

Authors	Number of patients	Inducible	
		No.	%
Fisher *et al.* (1978) [7]	19	18	95
Horowitz *et al.* (1978) [8]	20	20	100
Mason *et al.* (1978) [9]	186	165	89
Naccarelli *et al.* (1982) [10]	39	27	69
Buxton *et al.* (1983) [11]	102	101	99
Schoenfeld *et al.* (1985) [12]	91	81	89

Patients with out-of-hospital arrest. In patients presenting clinically with out-of-hospital cardiac arrest, the initial arrhythmia causing the episode is usually unknown. However, when the arrest is not the initial event of an acute myocardial infarction, in 60 to 90% a fast ventricular arrhythmia, that could have been the cause of the arrest, can be induced by programmed electrical stimulation [18—22] (Table 5). The induced arrhythmia is sustained VT in the majority of cases, ventricular fibrillation in some 15% and VT degenerating to ventricular fibrillation in about 10% [21]. A relationship has been suggested between the initial documented rhythm at the time of the arrest and the chances of inducibility, being the arrhythmias less likely to be induced if the initial rhythm was ventricular fibrillation as opposed to VT [23].

Table 5. Inducibility in patients with cardiac arrest.

Authors	Number of patients	Inducible	
		No.	%
Kehoe et al. (1982) [18]	44	28	64
Benditt et al. (1983) [19]	34	30	88
Morady et al. (1983) [20]	45	34	76
Roy et al. (1983) [21]	119	72	61
Wilber et al. (1988) [22]	166	131	79

Relationship between the response to programmed electrical stimulation and the clinical outcome

The crucial step to the electrophysiologic approach is the correlation between drug response in the laboratory and clinical outcome. Unfortunately, there are almost no controlled studies addressing this issue. However, several non-controlled studies have been reported, involving small number of patients with rather short follow-up, and using mainly Type IA antiarrhythmics. It has to be realized that the results could be partially biased because some of the nonresponders to conventional antiarrhythmics were operated on or received experimental drugs.

Predictive value of suppression of inducibility. Tables 6, 7 and 8 summarize the information concerning patients in whom inducibility of tachyarrhythmias was suppressed by antiarrhythmic agents [3, 10, 18, 22, 24—29]. Despite some variability in percentages overall, the life expectancy free of arrhythmic events is 85 to 90%. It is interesting to note that differences between older and more recent series are not apparent.

Predictive value of persistence of inducibility. Tables 9, 10, and 11 summarize

Table 6. Sustained ventricular tachycardia. Suppression of inducibility: favorable outcome.

Authors	Favorable outcome		
		No.	%
Ruskin *et al.* [25]	17	15	88
Naccarelli *et al.* [10]	9	9	100
Horowitz *et al.* [26]	65	61	94
Kim *et al.* [27]	23	19	83
Total	114	104	91

Table 9. Sustained ventricular tachycardia. Persistence of inducibility: unfavorable outcome.

Authors	Arrhythmic events		
		No.	%
Ruskin *et al.* [25]	5	4	80
Naccarelli *et al.* [10]	15	6	40
Horowitz *et al.* [26]	46	42	91
Total	66	52	79

Table 7. Out of hospital cardiac arrest. Suppression of inducibility: favorable outcome.

Authors	Favorable outcome		
		No.	%
Kehoe *et al.* [18]	5	5	100
Morady *et al.* [20]	9	6	66
Benditt *et al.* [19]	21	20	95
Roy *et al.* [21]	24	17	71
Wilber *et al.* [22]	91	90	88
Total	150	128	85

Table 10. Out of hospital cardiac arrest. Persistence of inducibility: unfavorable outcome.

Authors	Arrhythmic events		
		No.	%
Kehoe *et al.* [18]	9	7	78
Benditt *et al.* [19]	5	2	40
Roy *et al.* [21]	9	3	33
Wilber *et al.* [22]	36	12	33
Total	59	24	41

Table 8. Series including patients with cardiac arrest and sustained ventricular tachycardia. Suppression of inducibility: favorable outcome.

Authors	Favorable outcome		
		No.	%
Mason *et al.* [28]	39	28	72
Swerdlon *et al.* [29]	100	88	88
Mitchell *et al.* [24]	15	14	93
Borggrefe *et al.* [3]	34	32	94
Total	188	162	86

Table 11. Series including patients with cardiac arrest and sustained ventricular tachycardia. Persistence of inducibility: unfavorable outcome.

Authors	Arrhythmic events		
		No.	%
Mason *et al.* [28]	19	6	32
Swerdow *et al.* [29]	103	39	38
Borggrefe *et al.* [3]	54	17	32
Total	176	62	35

data related to patients treated chronically with antiarrhythmic drugs with which inducibility of ventricular tachyarrhythmias persisted [3, 10, 18, 19, 21, 22, 25, 26, 28, 29]. In the analysis of these data, we would like to emphasize:

1. In all the studies the probability of an arrhythmic recurrence is higher among patients in whom ventricular arrhythmias remain inducible than among those in whom inducibility of ventricular arrhythmias have been suppressed (Tables 6, 7, and 8). This means that programmed stimulation allows either the prediction of which antiarrhythmic drugs are more useful than others in each patient, or at least the selection of high and low risk subgroups under a particular drug regimen (a marker of risk).
2. The probability of recurrence tends to be lower in patients presenting clinically with cardiac arrest (Table 10), than in those with sustained VT (Table 9), although the clinical consequences of a recurrence are more serious in the former group.
3. The predictive value of persistence of inducibility for a clinical recurrence is, in general, low, ranging between 30 and 50%.

Sudden death and suppression/persistence of inducibility. Most reported series describe sudden death and sustained VT together as 'arrhythmic events'. Although the latter is an undersirable and serious event, sudden death is obviously more relevant, and needs to be considered separately.

Swerdlow *et al.* [29] reported on 239 patients and 44 sudden deaths. The incidence of sudden death was 12% among 100 patients with a favorable electrophysiologic response, and 31% in 63 patients with an unfavorable response (Figure 1). Moreover, the lack of a favorable electrophysiologic

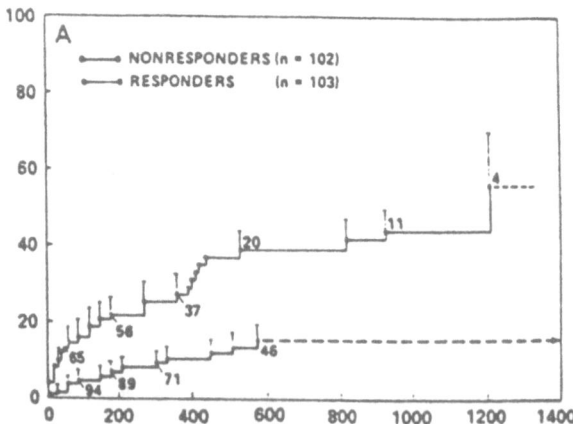

Figure 1. Acturial curve of patients free of sudden death, according to whether they had a good response ("responders") or a poor response ("nonresponders") to programmed electrical stimulation. Reproduced from Swerdlow *et al.* [29].

response and the functional class were the only independent predictors of sudden death [29].

Wilber *et al.* [22] reported on 166 patients with out-of-hospital cardiac arrest. The recurrence rate of cardiac arrest among 91 patients in whom a ventricular tachyarrhythmia was inducible in the baseline study, but it was suppressed with antiarrhythmic agents, was 12% (6 of 11 patients that recurred had discontinued the prescribed treatment). This is in contrast significantly lower than the 36% cardiac arrest recurrence rate among the 36 patients who had inducible ventricular tachyarrhythmias on the baseline state, but that were still inducible on the antiarrhythmic regimen with which they were discharged (Figure 2). In a multivariate analysis, only persistence of inducibility and ejection fraction were independent predictors of risk [22].

Waller *et al.* [4] observed that both sudden death and total mortality were lower in patients in whom inducibility of ventricular arrhythmias was suppressed. These investigators identified a subgroup of patients in whom a sustained VT remained inducible but was significantly slowed by antiarrhythmic drugs. The sustained VT recurrence rate in these patients (39%) was similar to that of the other patients in whom ventricular tachyarrhythmias remained inducible (50%). However, in patients whose VT were slowed down, both total mortality (12%) and sudden death (4%) were similar to those in whom inducibility of VT was suppressed, and significantly lower than in those in whom VT were not slowed down.

Our own series. We have recently reported on a series of patients in whom

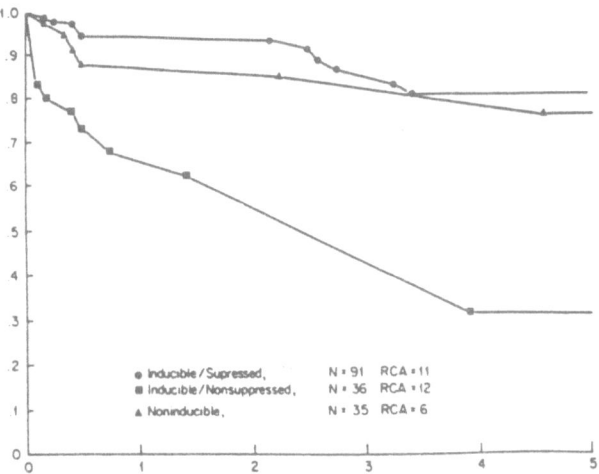

Figure 2. Acturial curve of patients free of cardiac arrest, according to whether ventricular tachyarrhythmia was "inducible" or "non inducible" in the baseline state, and whether inducibility was "suppressed" or not ("nonsuppressed") with antiarrhythmic drugs. RCA: recurrent cardiac arrest X-axis: years. Reproduced from Wilber *et al.* [22].

antiarrhythmic therapy was guided by programmed stimulation [30]. Forty-six patients with sustained or syncopal ventricular tachyarrhythmias (10 with cardiac arrest) underwent programmed ventricular stimulation on the base-line and on antiarrhythmic therapy. Inducibility of ventricular tachyarrhythmias was suppressed with type I drugs in 16/42 (38%), after subendocardial resection in 5/6 (83%) and with amiodarone in 1/15 (7%). After a minimum follow-up of 6 months (mean 19 months) in 45 patients (1 patient lost to follow-up), there have been no deaths or arrhythmic recurrences among 19 patients in whom inducibility of VT was suppressed (Table 12), although 1 patient had syncope after 36 months of follow-up. There have been 4 deaths (3 of them arrhythmic, 14%), and 2 arrhythmic recurrences (1 of them suspected) among the other patients. These 2 groups are not comparable but confirm the favorable outcome of patients in whom inducibility of arrhythmias have been suppressed.

Table 12. Clinical follow-up of 46 patients with sustained ventricular tachyarrhythmias (6—36 month follow-up, mean 19 months).

Inducibility suppressed (n = 19):	Amiodarone (n = 22):
— Deaths: 0	— Deaths: 4 (18%)
— Recurrences: 0	— Arrhythmic deaths: 3 (14%)
— Clinical events: 1 syncope	— Recurrences: 1 documented, 1 suspected
	— Clinical events: 0

New criteria of antiarrhythmic efficacy. Recently, Borggrefe *et al* have reported a new criteria for antiarrhythmic efficacy [3]. These investigators perform an stimulation protocol that includes 4 basic cycle lengths. They identify a subgroup of patients in whom VT remains inducible on anti-arrhythmic agents but it is induced with a basic cycle length faster than that necessary for induction on the baseline study. The prognosis of such patients is favorable, similar to that of those in whom inducibility of VT is suppressed, and significantly better than the remaining patients in whom VT remains inducible with a similar basic cycle length (Figure 3).

Waller *et al.* [4] in a study previously alluded to [4], identified the subgroup of patients with a marked slowing of the induced VT, as having a good life expectancy despite a high VT recurrence rate.

Conclusions

Although today, after more than 20 years of programmed stimulation of the heart, there are still problems with the stimulation protocols, the findings, and their interpretation, we feel that the bulk of the available information can be summarized into a few conclusions:

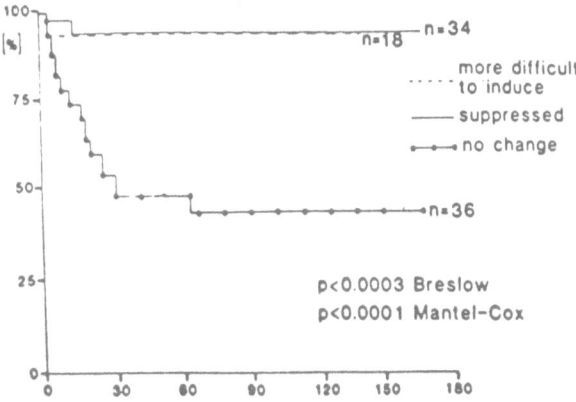

Figure 3. Actuarial curve of patients free of arrhythmic events according to whether inducibility was "suppressed", tachyarrhythmia was "more difficult to induce" or persisted the same ("no change"). X-asis: weeks. Reproduced from Borggrefe *et al.* [3].

1. The method of programmed stimulation as a guide for the selection of antiarrhythmic agents, is applicable to a majority of patients with sustained ventricular tachyarrhythmias (to 90% of patients presenting with sustained VT, and to 70% of those presenting clinically with cardiac arrest).
2. Suppression of inducibility of ventricular arrhythmias (that were inducible on the baseline study) by antiarrhythmic drugs, can be obtained in 30—40% of patients, and accurately predicts a good prognosis regarding both sudden death and arrhythmic recurrences.
3. Although the probability of recurrence and sudden death are, in general, higher when inducibility persists despite therapy, its predictive value of arrhythmic events is relatively low (30—50%).
4. In this context, the recently identified electrophysiologic predictors of efficacy, although requiring further evaluation, are of prime interest.
5. In view of the existence of non pharmacologic therapeutic alternatives highly efficacious although with a higher risk and/or cost (surgical subendocardial resection, implantable cardioverter defibrillator), we feel that the more severe the clinical presentation, the more appropriate the programmed stimulation method and the more recommended its use.

References

1. Wellens HJJ, Durrer DR, Lie KL: Observations on mechanisms of ventricular tachycardia in man. Circulation 1976; 54: 237—244.
2. Josephson ME, Horowitz LN, Farshidi A, Kastor JA: Recurrent sustained ventricular tachycardia. I. Mechanisms. Circulation 1978; 57: 431—440.

3. Borggrefe M, Trampisch H, Breithardt G: Reappraisal of criteria for assessing drug efficacy in patients with venticular tachyarrhythmias: complete versus partial suppression of inducible arrhythmias. J Am Coll Cardiol 1988; 12: 140—149.
4. Waller TJ, Kay HR, Spielman SR, Kutaled SP, Greenspan AM, Horowitz LN: Reduction in sudden death and total mortality by antiarrhythmic therapy evaluated by electrophysiologic drug testing: criteria of efficacy in patients with sustained ventricular tachyarrhythmia. J Am Coll Cardiol 1987; 10: 83—89.
5. Adhar GC, Larson LW, Bardy GH, Greene HL: Sustained ventricular arrhythmias: differences between survivors of cardiac arrest and patients with recurrent sustained ventricular tachycardia. J Am Coll Cardiol 1988; 12: 159—165.
6. Trappe HJ, Brugada P, Talajic M, Della Bella P, Lezaun R, Mulleneers R, Wellens HJJ: Prognosis of patients with ventricular tachycardia and ventricular fibrillation: role of underlying etiology. J Am Coll Cardiol 1988; 12: 166—174.
7. Fisher JD, Cohen ML, Mehra R, Altschuler M, Escher DJN, Furman S: Cardiac Pacing and pacemakers. II. Serial electrophysiologic-pharmacologic testing for control of recurrent tachyarrhythmias. Am Heart J 1977; 93: 658—668.
8. Horowitz LN, Josephson ME, Farshidi A, Spielman SR, Michelson EL, Greenspan AM: Recurrent sustained ventricular tachycardia. 3. Role of the electrophysiologic study in selection of antiarrhythmic regimens. Circulation 1978; 58: 986—997.
9. Mason JW, Winkle RA: Electrode-catheter arrhythmia induction in the selection and assessment of antiarrhythmic drug therapy for recurrent ventricular tachycardia. Circulation 1978; 58: 971—985.
10. Naccarelli GV, Prystowsky EN, Jackman WM, Heger JJ, Rahilly GT, Zipes DP: Role of electrophysiologic testing in managing patients who have ventricular tachycardia unrelated to coronary artery disease. Am J Cardiol 1982; 50: 165—171.
11. Buxton AE, Wawman HL, Josephson ME: Electrical stimulation techniques to predict and assess antiarrhythmic drug efficacy in patients with ventricular arrhythmias. In: Van Durme JP, Bogaert MG, Julaina DG, Kulbertus HK (eds). Chronic antiarrhythmic therapy. Molndal, A.B. Hassle, 1983; 151—163.
12. Schoenfeld MH, McGovern B, Garan H, Kelly E, Grant G, Ruskin JN: Determinants of the outcome of electrophysiologic study in patients with ventricular tachyarrhythmias. J Am Coll Cardiol 1985; 6: 298—306.
13. Buxton AE, Waxman HL, Marchlinski FE, Untereker WJ, Waspe LE, Josephson ME: Role of triple extrastimuli during electrophysiologic study of patients with documented sustained ventricular arrhythmias. Circulation 1984; 69: 532—540.
14. Doherty JV, Kienzle MG, Buxton AE, Marchlinski FE, Waxman HL, Josephson ME: Discordant results of programmed ventricular stimulation at different right ventricular sites in patients with and without spontaneous sustained ventricular tachycardia: a prospective study of 56 patients. Am J Cardiol 1984; 54: 366—342.
15. VandePol CJ, Farshidi A, Spielman SR, Greenspan AM, Horowitz LN, Josephson ME: Incidence and clinical significance of induced ventricular tachycardia. Am J Cardiol 1980; 45: 725—731.
16. Poll DS, Marchlinski FE, Buxton AE, Doherty JU, Waxman HL, Josephson ME: Sustained ventricular tachycardia in patients with idiopathic dilated cardiomyopathy. Circulation 1984; 70: 451—456.
17. Liem LB, Oradia M, Sasson Z, Franz MR, Swerdlow CD: Value of electrophysiologic study in patients with idiopathic dilated cardiomyophathy and sustained ventricular tachyarrhythmias. J Am Coll Cardiol 1987; 9: 107A (Abstract).
18. Kehoe RF, Moran JM, Zheutlin T, Tommasco C, Lesch M: Electrophcysiologic study to direct therapy in survivors of prehospital ventricular fibrillation. Am J Cardiol 1982; 49: 928 (Abstract).
19. Benditt DG, Benson DW, Klein GJ, Pritzker MR, Kriett JM, Anderson RW: Prevention of recurrent sudden cardiac arrest: role of provocative electropharmacologic testing. J Am Coll Cardiol 1983; 2: 418—425.

20. Morady F, Scheinman MM, Hess DS, Sung RJ, Shen E, Shapiro W: Electrophysiologic testing in the management of survivors of out-of-hospital cardiac arrest. Am J Cardiol 1983; 51: 85–89.
21. Roy D, Waxman HL, Kienzle MG, Buxton AE, Marchlinski FE, Josephson ME: Clinical characteristics and long-term follow-up in 119 survivors of cardiac arrest: relationship to inducibility at electrophysiologic testing. Am J Cardiol 1983; 52: 969–974.
22. Wilber DJ, Garan H, Finkelstein D, Kelly E, Newell J, Mcgovern D, Ruskin JN: Out-of-hospital cardiac arrest: Use of electrophysiologic testing in the prediction of long-term N Engl J Med 1988; 318: 19–24.
23. Myerburg RJ, Sung RJ, Conde C, Malon SM, Castellanos A: Intracardiac electrophysiologic studies in patients resuscitated from unexpected cardiac arrest outside the hospital. Am J Cardiol 1977; 39L 275 (Abstract).
24. Mitchell LB, Duff HJ, Manyari DE, Wyse DG: A randomized clinical trial of the non invasive and invasive approaches to drug therapy of ventricular tachycardia. N Engl J Med 1987; 317: 1681–1687.
25. Ruskin JN, Garan H: Chronic electrophysiologic testing in patients with recurrent sustained ventricular tachycardia. Am J Cardiol 1979; 43: 400.
26. Horowitz LN, Spielman SR, Greenspan AM, Josephson ME: Role of programmed stimulation in assessing vulnerability to ventricular arrhythmias. Am Heart J 1982; 103: 604–608.
27. Kim SG, Seiden SW, Felder SD, Waspe LE, Fisher JD: Is programmed stimulation of value in predicting the long-term success of antiarrhythmic therapy for ventricular tachycardias? N Engl J Med 1986; 315: 356–362.
28. Mason JW, Winkle RA: Accuracy of the ventricular tachycardia-induction study for predicting long-term efficacy and inefficiacy of antiarrhythmic drugs. N Engl J Med 1980; 303: 1073–1077.
29. Swerdlow CD, Winkle RA, Mason JW: Determinants of survival in patients with ventricular tachyarrhythmias. N Engl J Med 1983; 308: 1436–1442.
30. Almendral J, Arenal A, San Roman D, Albertos J, Delcán JL: Tratamieto guiado por estimulación eléctrica programada en pacientes con taquiarritmias ventriculares. Rev Esp Cardiol 1988; 41: 38 (Abstract).

15. Non pharmacological treatment of ventricular tachycardia

HANS-JOACHIM TRAPPE, HELMUT KLEIN, GUENTER FRANK, PAUL WENZLAFF and PAUL R. LICHTLEN

Introduction

Sudden death represents the most frequent mode of death in patients with coronary artery disease, particularly during the first year after a myocardial infarction [1, 2].

Although the majority of patients with malignant ventricular arrhythmias suffer from coronary artery disease, there is a group of patients who have recurrent episodes of sustained monomorphic ventricular tachycardia or ventricular fibrillation with either no identifiable heart disease or a structural heart disease due to causes other than coronary artery disease [3—5].

There are several approaches to treat patients with ventricular tachycardia or ventricular fibrillation: medical treatment with antiarrhythmic drugs, endocardial catheter ablation, mapping guided surgery and implantation of electrical devices such as the automatic implantable cardioverter defibrillator (AICD).

The purpose of this presentation is to summarize our experience with patients who have frequent episodes of sustained monomorphic ventricular tachycardia or ventricular fibrillation and to discuss the various non-pharmacological therapeutic approaches in these patients.

Catheter ablation of ventricular tachycardia

Patients

We attempted the ablation of ventricular tachycardia foci in 44 patients (43 men, 1 woman, mean age 49 ± 12 years).

There were 28 patients with coronary artery disease, all of them with an old myocardial infarction: 17 pts had an anterior, 7 patients an inferior and 4 patients had both an anterior and an inferior myocardial infarction (Table 1). In addition, there were 16 pts without coronary disease: In 12 patients right ventricular angiography demonstrated arrhythmogenic right ventricular dys-

A. Bayès de Luna et al. (eds.): *Sudden Cardiac Death*, 147–162.
© 1991 Kluwer Academic Publishers, Dordrecht.

Table 1. Characteristics of patients with non pharmacological treatment of ventricular tachycardia

	Group I (Ablation)	Group II (VT-Surgery)	Group III (AICD)
No of pts	44	108	94
Males	43 (98%)	98 (91%)	85 (90%)
Age (years)	49 ± 11	53 ± 11	56 ± 11
CAD	28 (64%)	97 (90%)	74 (79%)
AMI	17 (61%)	64 (66%)	38 (51%)
IMI	7 (25%)	19 (19%)	24 (32%)
Both	4 (14%)	14 (14%)	12 (17%)
1-VD	21 (76%)	65 (67%)	12 (16%)
2-VD	5 (17%)	20 (20%)	25 (34%)
3-VD	2 (7%)	12 (12%)	37 (50%)
No CAD	16	11 (10%)	20 (21%)
RVD	12 (75%)	6 (54%)	7 (35%)
LVD	3 (19%)	4 (36%)	2 (10%)
COCM	1 (6%)	—	8 (40%)
HOCM	—	—	3 (15%)
OTHER	—	1 (10%)	—
EF (%)	31 ± 9%	36 ± 11	25 ± 11

Abbreviations: pts = patients, CAD = coronary artery disease, AMI = anterior myocardial infarction, IMI = inferior myocardial infarction, RVD = right ventricular dysplasia, LVD = left ventricular dysplasia, COCM = congestive cardiomyopathy, HOCM = hypertrophic cardiomyopathy, EF = left ventricular ejection fraction, VT = ventricular tachycardia.

plasia, in 3 patients a left ventricular dysplastic area was present and one patient suffered from congestive cardiomyopathy (Table 1).

All patients in this study group had recurrent episodes of sustained monomorphic ventricular tachycardia (duration > 30 sec) and in all patients antiarrhythmic drug therapy had failed to suppress sufficiently these ventricular arrhythmias.

The hemodynamic status was studied in all patients prior to the ablation procedure. The mean left ventricular ejection fraction was 31 ± 9% (range 15—17%) (Table 1).

Ablation procedure

Catheter ablation of ventricular tachycardia was performed in all patients under general anesthesia with oral intubation from the beginning. Programmed ventricular stimulation was performed in either the right or the left ventricle in order to induce the clinical documented sustained monomorphic ventricular tachycardia. We then start endocardial mapping during the induced ventricular tachycardia from about 25 different points in the right (10 points) or the left (15 points) ventricle.

The purpose of catheter mapping during the induced ventricular tachycardia was to find the earliest endocardial activation (earlier than the onset of the QRS complex) (Figure 1) or to find the area of slow conduction, defined as an area with mid-diastolic potentials (Figure 2), maximal delay between stimulus and QRS as well as identical QRS morphology during pace mapping. At the earliest endocardial activation or at the area of slow conduction we deliver the first DC shock during ventricular tachycardia. After 15 minutes we repeat programmed ventricular stimulation to test the inducibility of the tachycardia. In patients with inducible ventricular tachycardia we repeat the catheter mapping after the first DC shock and deliver further DC shocks as often as a sustained ventricular tachycardia is inducible or as long as the hemodynamic situation is well tolerated.

Results

Catheter ablation at the earliest endocardial activation. In the first consecutive 32 patients catheter ablation of ventricular tachycardia foci was performed at

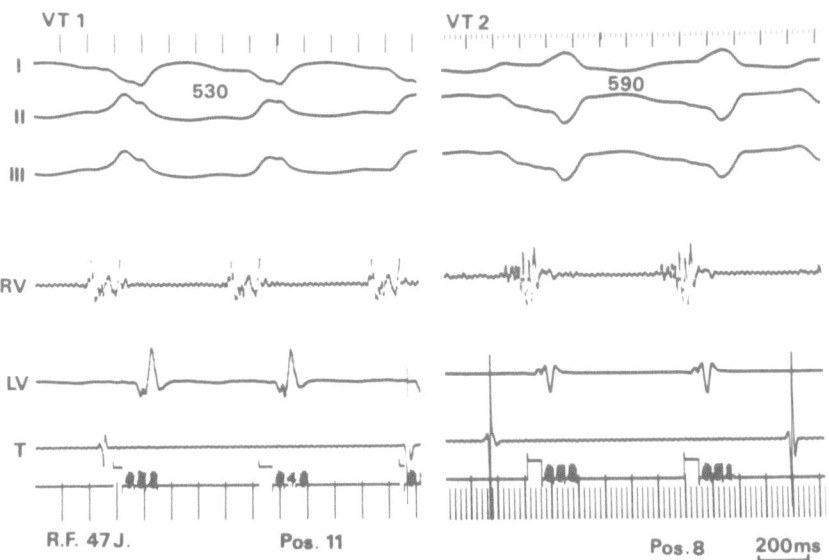

Figure 1. Endocardial catheter mapping during induced ventricular tachycardia (VT) in order to detect the earliest endocardial activation. Note that there are 2 VT morphologies with the earliest endocardial activation at position 11 (VT 1) and position 8 (VT 2) respectively. Tracings from top to bottom: Standard ECG leads I, II, III, a bipolar recording from the right ventricle (RV), from the mapping electrode in the left ventricle (LV). T = interval counting system between LV and RV recordings.

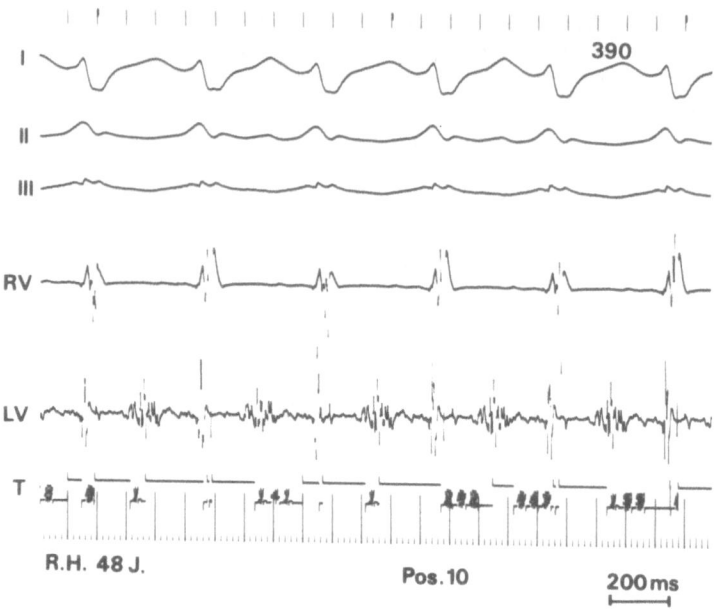

Figure 2. Endocardial catheter mapping during induced ventricular tachycardia in order to detect the area of slow conduction. Note the mid-diastolic potentials at position 10. Tracings from top to bottom: Standard ECG leads I, II, III, a bipolar recording from the right ventricle (RV), from the mapping electrode in the left ventricle (LV). T = interval counting system between LV and RV recordings.

the earliest endocardial activation. There were 16 patients in the coronary and all patients in the "non coronary" group with catheter ablation at the earliest endocardial activation. In 9/16 (56%) patients with coronary artery disease we could induce multiple morphologies of ventricular tachycardia compared to 8/16 patients (50%) in the "non coronary" group (p = ns). In patients with coronary artery disease earliest endocardial activation was recorded in a range of 35 to 190 msec (mean 67 ± 11 msec) prior to the onset of surface ECG. In the "non coronary" group earliest endocardial activation ranged from 10 to 55 msec (mean 31 ± 8 msec) prior to the QRS complex.

During the ablation procedure we delivered a mean of 4.3 ±1.1 DC shocks per patient (range 1 to 10 shocks) in patients with coronary artery disease compared to a mean of 5.9 ± 1.3 DC shocks per patient (range 1 to 10 shocks) in the "non coronary" group.

After the ablation procedure a ventricular tachycardia was still inducible in 3/16 patients (19%) with coronary artery disease and in 2/16 patients (13%) in the "non coronary" group (p = ns).

Catheter ablation at the area of slow conduction. In 12/44 patients catheter ablation of ventricular tachycardia foci was performed at the area of slow conduction. All patients had an old myocardial infarction and we could not identify mid-diastolic potentials in any of the patients with "non coronary" disease.

There were 3/12 patients (25%) with multiple ventricular tachycardia morphologies during the ablation procedure. At the area of slow conduction we delivered a mean of 3.2 ± 1.1 DC shocks per patient (range 1 to 7 shocks). After catheter ablation a sustained monomorphic ventricular tachycardia was still inducible in 2/12 patients (17%).

Follow-up

The mean follow-up of our patients who underwent endocardial catheter ablation of ventricular tachycardia foci is now 18 ± 7 months (range 6 to 45 months). During the follow-up there were 2/44 patients (5%) dying suddenly, 6 and 9 months after the ablation. In addition, there were 3/44 patients (7%) who died from cardiac causes. During the follow-up there were 29/44 patients (66%) with non fatal ventricular tachycardia recurrences (Table 2): 17/28 patients (61%) with an old myocardial infarction and 12/16 patients (75%) with "non coronary" disease (p = ns). Ventricular tachycardia recurrences occurred more frequently in patients with catheter ablation at the earliest endocardial activation (26/32 patients, 81%) compared to patients with catheter ablation at the area of slow conduction (3/12 patients, 25%) (p < 0.01) (Table 2).

Table 2. Incidence of non fatal ventricular tachycardia recurrences after catheter ablation.

REC of VT	EEA (n = 32)	ASC (n = 12)	TOTAL (n = 44)
CAD (n = 28)	14 (50%)	3 (11%)	17 (61%)
Non CAD (n = 16)	12 (75%)	—	12 (75%)
Total (n = 44)	26 (81%)	3 (25%)	29 (66%)

Abbreviations: EEA = catheter ablation at the earliest endocardial activation, ASC = catheter ablation at the area of slow conduction, CAD = coronary artery disease, REC = ventricular tachycardia recurrences, VT = ventricular tachycardia

Mapping guided surgery of ventricular tachycardia foci

In 1978/79 electrophysiologically guided surgery for ventricular tachycardia was introduced by Guiraudon [6] and Harken [7]. Subsequently various operative procedures have been described to treat patients with recurrent episodes of ventricular tachycardia refractory to antiarrhythmic drug therapy

[8, 9, 10]. At our institution, mapping guided surgery is established since 1980 and now performed in 108 patients.

Patients

One hundred and eight patients (98 males and 10 females, mean age 53 ± 11 years) underwent mapping guided surgery for their antiarrhythmic drug refractory ventricular tachycardia. There were 97 patients (90%) with coronary artery disease, all of them with an old myocardial infarction (Table 1). The majority of these patients had an anterior myocardial infarction (64 patients, 66%), while the incidence of an inferior myocardial infarction (19 patients, 19%) or multiple myocardial infarctions (12 patients, 12%) was markedly lower. All patients underwent cardiac catheterization with left, right and coronary angiography. Most of the patients had single vessel disease (65 patients, 67%), 20 patients (20%) double and 12 patients (12%) three vessel disease. The mean left ventricular ejection fraction was 36 ± 11%.

Eleven patients had recurrent episodes of ventricular tachycardia without coronary disease ("arrhythmogenic ventricles"). In 10 patients (90%) the angiography revealed right and/or left ventricular dysplasia and the remaining patient developed ventricular tachycardia after surgical therapy of a Fallot' tetralogy.

All 108 patients had recurrent episodes of sustained monomorphic ventricular tachycardia, refractory to antiarrhythmic drug therapy prior to the surgical approach.

Operative procedure

Prior to surgery, all patients underwent an electrophysiologic study to determine morphology, mode of initiation and termination and the origin of ventricular tachycardia.

Intraoperatively we perfomed an electrophysiological study and a sustained monomorphic ventricular tachycardia was inducible in 91 patients (84%). In 3 patients (3%) we could induce only non sustained ventricular tachycardia and in 14 patients (13%) there were no arrhythmias inducible. In these patients the endocardial resection was directed by the preoperative electrophysiologic catheter mapping.

The surgical procedure was an encircling endocardial ventriculotomy according to the Guiraudon procedure [6] in the initial 14 patients, whereas a localized endocardial resection according to the Harken technique [7] was performed in the remaining patients. In patients in whom endocardial resection could not be performed due to anatomic or functional reasons, the additional cryolesion or cryolesion alone was used [11]. These are patients mostly with inferior or posterior scars or patients with an origin of their ventricular tachycardia around the area of the papillary muscle or the AV valve ring.

Results

During the mean follow-up of 29 ± 27 months (range 1–95 months) 31 patients (29%) died (Figure 3). There were 8 patients (7%) who died suddenly (within one hour after beginning of symptoms) (Figure 4) and 21 patients (19%) died from cardiac causes (Figure 5): 4 patients died from cardiogenic shock and 17 patients from heart failure. In addition, there were 2 patients dying from non cardiac causes: one patient died from suicide and the other one from pulmonary insufficiency.

There were 10 patients who died within the first 4 weeks after surgery, thus given an *early or in-hospital mortality* rate of 9%. The cause of death was low cardiac output in 8 patients and sudden death in the remaining 2 patients. After this period of time 21 patients died, giving a *late mortality* of 19%. The cause of death was heart failure in 13 patients and sudden death in 6 patients. The remaining 2 patients died from suicide or from pulmonary insufficiency.

There were no significant differences in the cardiac mortality (CM) or the incidence of sudden death (SD) between patients with coronary artery

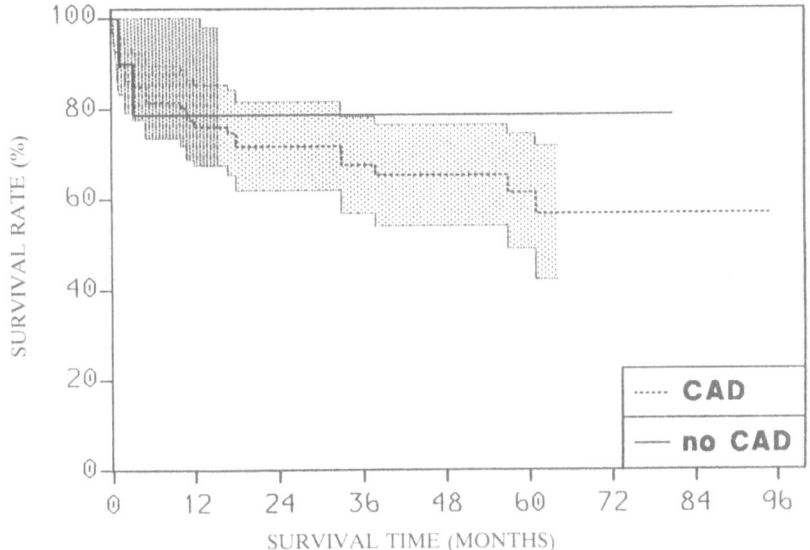

Figure 3. Kaplan-Meier survival curves (total mortality) in patients who underwent mapping guided surgery in relation to the underlying etiology. *Abbreviations:* CAD = coronary artery disease, no CAD = arrhythmogenic ventricles.

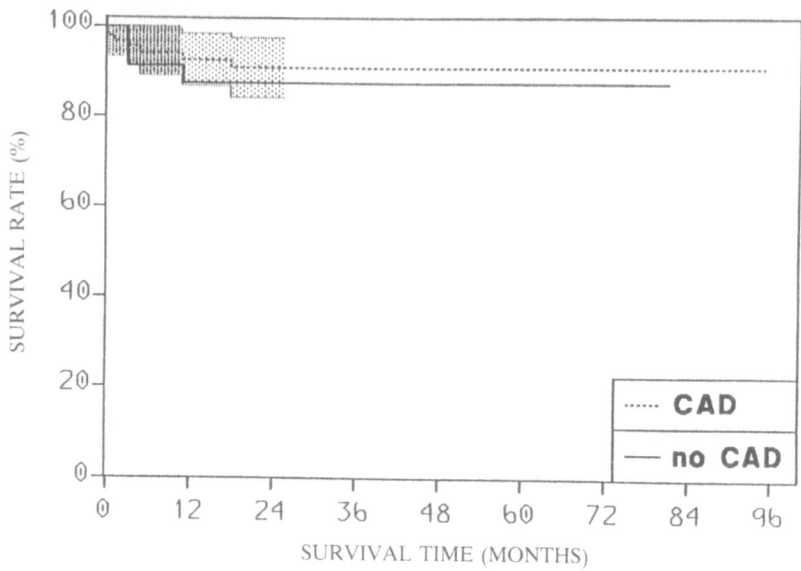

Figure 4. Kaplan-Meier survival curves (sudden death rate) in patients who underwent mapping guided surgery in relation to the underlying etiology. *Abbreviations:* CAD = coronary artery disease, no CAD = arrhythmogenic ventricles.

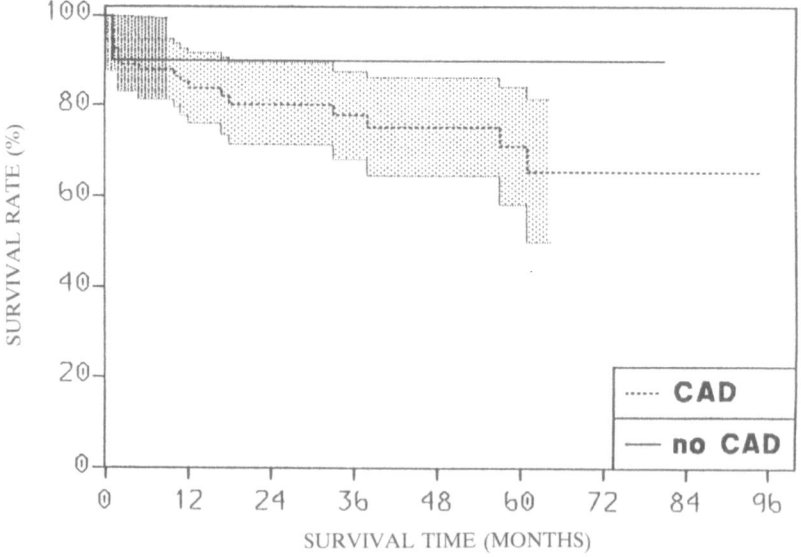

Figure 5. Kaplan-Meier survival curves (cardiac mortality) in patients who underwent mapping guided surgery in relation to the underlying etiology. *Abbreviations:* CAD = coronary artery disease, no CAD = arrhythmogenic ventricles.

disease (CM: 20/97 patients, 21%; SD: 7/97 patients, 7%) and those with "non coronary" disease (CM: 1/11 patients, 9%; SD: 1/11 patients, 9%) (Figures 4, 5).

Follow-up

During the follow-up there were 22/108 patients (20%) with ventricular tachycardia recurrences. There were significant differences in the incidence of recurrences between patients with coronary disease (16/97 patients, 16%) and those with arrhythmogenic ventricles (6/11 patients, 55%) (p < 0.01).

Eight of 22 patients (36%) had fatal recurrences (sudden death) while 14/22 patients (64%) survived their recurrences (non fatal recurrences). Sudden death occurred in 7/97 patients with coronary artery disease and in 1/11 patients (9%) in the "non coronary" group (p = 0.59) (Figure 4). In contrast, non fatal recurrences were observed more frequently in patients with arrhythmogenic ventricles (5/11 patients, 45%) compared to patients with coronary artery disease (9/97 patients, 9%) (p < 0.01).

Automatic implantable cardioverter defibrillator

In 1983, the automatic implantable cardioverter defibrillator (AICD) went into broad clinical application [12—14]. The value of life-threatening tachyarrhythmias has been reported in previous studies [15—17]. Our own experience with the automatic implantable cardioverter defibrillator started in January 1984 and until now we implanted the AICD in 94 patients.

Patients

Since January 1984, we implanted the AICD in 94 patients (85 males and 9 females, mean age 56 ± 11 years). The underlying etiology was coronary artery disease in 74 patients (79%) and "non coronary" disease in 20 patients (21%).

All patients with coronary artery disease had a history of a myocardial infarction (anterior in 38 patients 51%), inferior in 24 patients (32%) and multiple myocardial infarctions in the remaining 12 patients (17%) (Table 1). All patients underwent hemodynamic evaluation of their cardiac situation and an electrophysiologic study. There were 12 patients (16%) with single vessel disease, 25 patients (34%) with double and 37 patients (50%) with three vessel disease. The mean left ventricular ejection fraction was 25 ± 11% (range 12—45%) (Table 1).

There were 20 patients without coronary artery disease and malignant tachyarrhythmias: 9 patients (45%) had arrhythmogenic right and/or left ventricles and 11 patients (55%) cardiomyopathies (8 patients congestive and 3 patients hypertrophic cardiomyopathies).

All patients suffered from malignant tachyarrhythmias and underwent cardiac arrests with successful resuscitations. This occurred with a mean of 3.9 ± 1.1 (range 2—12) per patient. Antiarrhythmic drug treatment was performed in all patients prior to the implant. A mean of 4.1 ± 1.3 antiarrhythmic drug was given to the patients prior to the AICD.

Operative procedure

Previous studies have reported various operative procedures for implantation of the AICD [18, 19].

At our institution only the "patch-patch" technique was used. Following median sternotomy the pericardium was opened and after evaluation of the lowest defibrillation threshold with repeated induction of ventricular tachycardia or ventricular fibrillation, the patch electrodes were attached to the epicardium using fibrin glue. The larger of the two patch electrodes was placed over the epicardium of the left ventricle and the smaller patch electrode was placed over the epicardium of the right ventricle.

After gluing of the patch electrodes we again induce ventricular tachycardia or ventricular fibrillation to measure the final defibrillation threshold. We then connect the electrodes to the generator and again induce the arrhythmia to check the appropriate termination of the induced arrhythmia by the AICD. Thirty of our patients (32%) received an AIDB/BR, 45 patients (48%) an Ventak 1500 and the remaining 19 patients (20%) a Ventak P (CPI, St. Paul, Minneapolis, USA).

Results

The mean follow-up is now 21 ± 10 months (range 1—46 months). During this period of time 13 patients died (14%) (Figure 6), one of them suddenly (1%) (Figure 7). So far, 3 patients died after the AICD implantation (6, 12 and 48 hours after the opeation). The remaining 9 patients died from cardiac failure (4 patients), 2 patients from depleted battery and 3 patients from non cardiac causes.

During the follow-up 20 patients (21%) underwent generator replacement of the AICD due to battery depletion or due to a prolongation of the charging time. The mean time interval between implantation and generator replacement was 19 ± 5 months. Six patients (6%) had another generator replacement with a mean of 21 ± 6 months later. We could observe that there was no significant increase in the defibrillation threshold between implantation, first order second generator replacement. However, there were significant differences in the defibrillation threshold between patients with

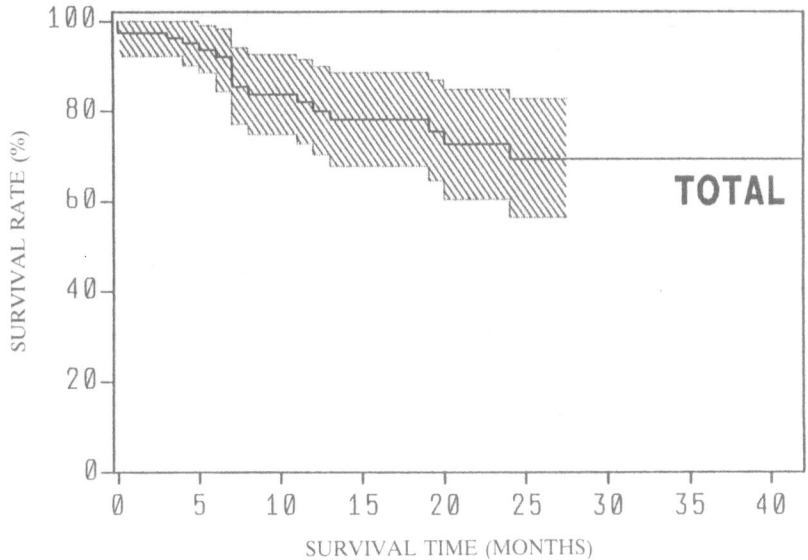

Figure 6. Kaplan-Meier survival curves (total mortality) in patients with an automatic implantable cardioverter defibrillator.

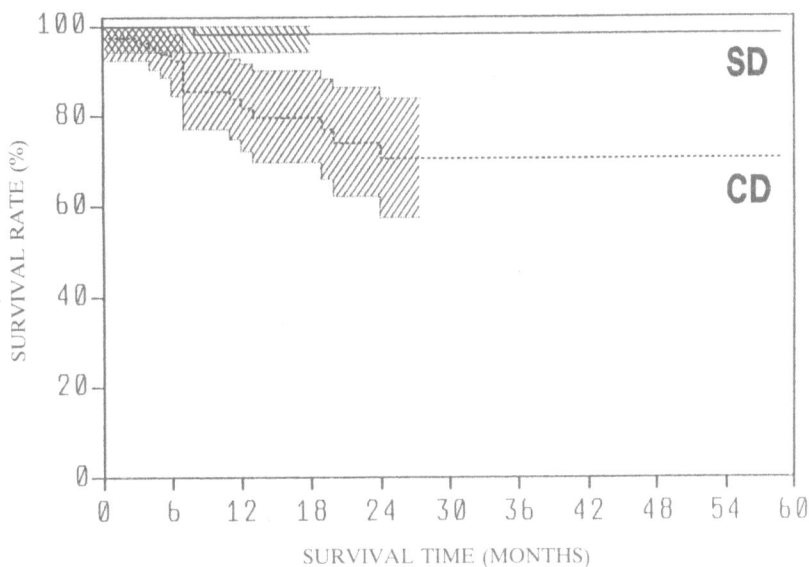

Figure 7. Kaplan-Meier survival curves (cardiac mortality and sudden death rate) in patients with an automatic implantable cardioverter defibrillator. *Abbreviations*: SD = sudden death, CD = cardiac death.

induced ventricular tachycardia compared to patients with induced ventricular fibrillation (Table 3).

Follow-up

All patients were studied in the outpatient clinic two monthly to test the number of delivered shocks and the charging time of the ACID.

At the present time there were 65/94 Patients (69%) with AICD-discharges. Three patients (3%) experienced recurrent shocks due to sudden onset of so far unknown atrial fibrillation with rapid ventricular response. In 3 patients we had to explant the device due to the pouch infection.

Discussion

Identification of patients at risk for sudden death remains a difficult problem in cardiology. In addition, patients with recurrent episodes of sustained ventricular tachycardia or ventricular fibrillation have a poor prognosis, in particular when ventricular arrhythmias occurs in the context of coronary artery disease [20]. In the present study we reported our experience of non pharmacological treatment in those patients with recurrent episodes of ventricular tachycardia or ventricular fibrillation.

At the present time *endocardial catheter ablation* of ventricular tachycardia has a success rate of about 50% or less [21—23].

In our study there were 29/44 patients (66%) with ventricular tachycardia recurrences after the ablation procedure; only 13 patients (34%) had no recurrences during the follow-up.

Studies from El Sherif *et al.* [24] and Morady *et al.* [25] revealed the importance of the area of slow conduction to treat (ablate) ventricular tachycardia. Recently, we could also demonstrate, in accordance with other reports, a better success rate of catheter ablation at the area of slow conduction compared to ablation at the earliest endocardial activation [26]. The present data showed that 26/32 patients (81%) had ventricular tachy-

Table 3. Defibrillation thresholds at implant, first or second generator replacement of the AICD.

(Joule)	VT	VF	VT/VF
Implantation (n = 94)	11 ± 8	21 ± 10	25 ± 12
1. Replacement (n = 20)	12 ± 7	18 ± 10	15
2. Replacement (n = 6)	10	20 ± 12	—
		p < 0.05	

Abbreviations: VT = ventricular tachycardia, VF = ventricular fibrillation

cardia recurrences when catheter ablation was performed at the earliest endocardial activation compared to 3/12 patients (25%) with recurrences when catheter ablation was performed at the area of slow conduction (p < 0.01).

In addition, we could show that the underlying etiology is important to predict the success of endocardial catheter ablation of ventricular tachycardia: the incidence of recurrences was higher in patients with "non coronary" disease (12/16 patients, 74%) compared to patients with an old myocardial infarction (17/28 patients, 61%).

Therefore, we believe that method and technique of catheter ablation of ventricular tachycardia need to be improved before ventricular tachycardia ablation can be generally recommended [22].

Surgical methods (*mapping guided surgery*) to treat patients with ventricular tachycardia are well known and are in general accepted [6—9].

It has been reported that about 80% of all patients undergoing ventricular tachycardia surgery become free of ventricular tachycardia [27, 28]. Miller *et al.* [29] reported an overall recurrence rate of 11%.

Our data are in accordance with these results: Twenty-two patients (20%) had ventricular tachycardia recurrences, while 86 patients (80%) became free of these arrhythmias. In addition to these acceptable results, only 8/108 patients (7%) died suddenly.

It is important to note that the underlying etiology and the origin of ventricular tachycardia allows an identification of patients with recurrences after surgery. Patients with an old myocardial infarction and resectable scars had less frequently recurrences (16%) than patients with arrhythmogenic ventricles (55%). Therefore, we believe that the surgical ablation is not a satisfactory approach for patients with arrhythmogenic ventricles.

The risk of sudden death is high in patients with coronary heart disease, low left ventricular function and ventricular tachyarrhythmias [20]. This group of patients is extremely difficult to treat medically and has a poor prognosis [30, 31]. In such patients who underwent ventricular tachycardia surgery and became free of recurrences we could demonstrate a total mortality rate of 29% with a rate of 12.5% per year. The majority of the patients (21/29 patients, 72%) died from cardiac causes, mainly due to left ventricular dysfunction. Similar results have been reported by the multicenter Surgical Alblation Registry [32] with a 72% survival after 2 years. Ostermeyer *et al.* [33] described 1987 a survival rate of 89% after 1 year and demonstrated the extent of the underlying heart disease to be the most important predictor of survival.

Therefore, in accordance with these reports, we believe that the "ideal" candidate for surgical treatment of ventricular tachycardia should have a single vessel coronary artery disease with circumscribed *anterior* akinetic or dyskinetic area with a left ventricular ejection fraction > 30%. In addition, these patients should have a reproducible inducibility of a sustained monomorphic ventricular tachycardia with only *one* ventricular tachycardia origin.

We already mentioned that antiarrhythmic drug treatment is often ineffective to prevent sudden death or ventricular tachycardia recurrences. Catheter ablation of ventricular tachycardia is still an "experimental" approach that needs to be improved and mapping guided surgery is only suitable in highly selected patients (single vessel disease, EF > 30%, one ventricular tachycardia origin).

However, there is a group of patients with severe left ventricular dysfunction (EF < 25%), three vessel disease, disparate sites of ventricular tachycardia origins and/or ventricular fibrillation. Most of these patients survived one or more episodes of circulatory arrest. For those patients no other non pharmacological approaches than the *automatic implantable cardioverter defibrillator* will be appropiate [12, 13, 14, 16].

Our experience and that of others showed as well that the sudden death rates dropped below 2% in patients with an AICD [12, 13, 14, 16, 17]. Therefore, we believe that the AICD is or will become the *therapy of choice* in patients with severe left ventricular dysfunction and life-threatening tachyarrhythmias. However, despite the excellent results to prevent sudden death one have to consider that most patients with an AICD have a poor left ventricular function and need careful surveillance of their heart disease.

Conclusions

Identification of patients at high risk for sudden death and the decision of the adequate therapy in those patients remains a difficult problem in cardiology 1990. Careful selection of patients for an antiarrhythmic regime is absolutely necessary, i.e. complete evaluation of the underlying heart disease, of the hemodynamic and electrophysiologically situation.

Antiarrhythmic drug treatment alone or in combination with non pharmacological approaches has still a place in the treatment of tachyarrhythmias. Endocardial catheter ablation of ventricular tachycardia is an "experimental" approach and needs more "tune up". Mapping guided surgery needs careful patient selection with an acceptable left ventricular function and only one ventricular tachycardia origin. The automatic implantable cardioverter defibrillator will become the therapy of choice in patients with severe left ventricular dysfunction and life-threatening tachyarrhythmias. Indications for the AICD will growing when future devices of the the AICD will be available.

References

1. Steinbrunn W, Lichtlen PR: Complete 5-year cumulative survival rates in 244 unselected, unoperated coronary patients undergoing angiography. Circulation 1977; 46: 174.
2. Burggraf GW, Parker JO: Prognosis in coronary artery disease: Angiographic, hemodynamic and clinical factors. Circulation 1975; 41: 146.

3. Deal BJ, Miller SM, Scagliatti D, Prechel D, Gallastegi JL, Hariman RJ: Ventricular tachycardia in a young population without overt heart disease. Circulation 1986; 73: 1111.

4. Marcus FI, Fontaine GH, Guiraudon G, Frank R, Laurenceau JL, Malergue C, Grosgogeat Y: Right ventricular dysplasia: A report of 24 adult cases. Circulation 1982; 65: 384.

5. Trappe HJ, Brugada P, Talajic M, Lezaun R, Wellens HJJ: Clinical course and prognostic value of ventricular tachycardia or ventricular fibrillation in patients without coronary artery disease. Z Kardiol 1989; 78: 500.

6. Guiraudon G, Fontaine G, Frank R, Escande G, Etevient P, Cabrol C: Encircling endocardial ventriculotomy. A new surgical treatment for life-threatening ventricular tachycardia resistant to medical treatment following myocardial infarction. Ann Thorac Surg 1978; 92: 438.

7. Harken AH, Josephson ME, Horowitz LN: Surgical endocardial resection for the treatment of malignant ventricular tachycardia. Ann Surg 1979; 190: 456.

8. Klein GJ, Harrison L, Ideker RF, Smith WM, Kasell J, Wallace AG, Gallagher JJ: Reaction of the myocardium to cryosurgery: Electrophysiology and arrhythmogenic potential. Circulation 1979; 59: 364.

9. Frank G, Klein H, Lichtlen P, Borst HG: Direct surgical therapy of ventricular arrhythmias in coronary heart disease. Thorac Cardiovasc Surg 1981; 29: 315.

10. Saksena S, Gadhoke A: Laser therapy for tachyarrhythmias: a new frontier. PACE 1986; 9: 531.

11. Frank G, Lowes D, Baumgart D, Haverich A, Klein H, Trappe HJ, Abraham C, Borst HG: Surgical alternatives in the treatment of life-threatening ventricular arrhythmias. Europ J Cardio Thorac Surg 1988; 2: 207.

12. Mirowski M, Reid PR, Mower MM, Watkins L, Gott VL, Schauble JF, Langer A, Heiman S, Kolenik SA: Termination of malignant ventricular arrhythmias with an implanted automatic defibrillator in human beeings. N Engl J Med 1980; 303: 322.

13. Reid PR, Mirowski M, Mower M, Platia EV, Griffin LS, Watkins L Jr, Bach SM Jr, Imran M, Thomas A: Clinical evaluation of the internal automatic cardioverter defibrillator in survivors of sudden cardiac death. Am J Cardiol 1983; 51: 1608.

14. Reid PR, Griffith LSC, Platia EV, Mower MM, Veltri EP, Mirowski M, Guarnieri T, Singer I, Juanteguy J, Watkins L: The automatic implantable cardioverter defibrillator: Five-year clincial results. In: Breithardt G, Borggrefe M, Zipes DP, (eds), Nonpharmacological therapy of tachyarrhythmias. Futura publishing company, Mount Kisco, New York, 1987; 477.

15. Klein H, Frank G, Trappe HJ, Hartwig CA, Kühn E, Jüppner L, Lichtlen PR: Implantierbarer automatischer Defibrillator bei malignen Kammerarrhythmien. In: Naumann d'Alnoncourt, editor.: Herzrhythmusstörungen. Springer-Verlag, Berlin, Heidelberg, New York, 1986; 221.

16. Winkle RA, Mead RH, Ruder MA, Gaudiani VA, Smith NA, Buch WS, Schmidt P, Shipman T: Long-term outcome with the automatic implantable cardioverter-defibrillator. J Am Coll Cardiol 1989; 13: 1353.

17. Kelly PA, Cannom DS, Garan H, Mirabal GS, Harthorne W, Hurvitz, RJ, Vlahakes GJ, Jacobs ML, Ilvento JP, Buckley MJ, Ruskin, JN: The automatic implantable cardioverter-defibrillator: efficacy, complications and survival in patients with malignant ventricular arrhythmias. J Am Coll Cardiol 1988; 11: 1278.

18. Lawrie GM, Griffin JC, Wyndham CRC: Epicardial implantation of the automatic implantable defibrillator by left subcostal thoracotomy. PACE 1984; 7: 1370.

19. Watkins L Jr, Mirowski M, Mower MM: Implantation of the automatic defibrillator: The subxiphoid approach. Ann Thorac Surg 1982; 34: 515.

20. Trappe HJ, Brugada P, Talajic M, Della Bella P, Lezaun R, Wellens HJJ: Prognosis of patients with ventricular tachycardia and ventricular fibrillation: Role of the underlying etiology. J Am Coll Cardiol 1988; 12: 166.

21. Breithardt G, Borggrefe M, Karbenn U *et al.*: Therapie refraktärer ventrikulärer Tachykardien durch transvenöse, elektrische Ablation. Z Kardiol 1986; 75: 80 (abstract).
22. Scheinmann MM: Catheter ablation for patients with cardiac arrhythmias. PACE 1986; 9: 551.
23. Tonet JL, Fontaine G, Frank R, *et al.*: Treatment of refractory ventricular tachycardias by endocardial fulguration. Circulation 1985; 72; 388.
24. El-Sherif N, Scherlag B, Lazarra R, Hope PR: Reentrant ventricular arrhythmias in the late myocardial infarction period. 1. Conduction characteristics in the infarction zone. Circulation 1977; 55: 686.
25. Morady F, Scheinman MM, DiCarlo LA, Davis JC, Herre JM, Griffin JC, Winston SA, De Biutleir M, Hantler CB, Wahr JA, Kon WH, Nelson SD: Catheter ablation of ventricular tachycardia with intracardiac shocks: results in 33 patients. Circulation 1987; 75: 1037.
26. Trappe HJ, Klein H, Schröder E: Where to ablate ventricular tachycardia? Circulation 1988; 78: 300 (abstract).
27. Ostermeyer J, Breithardt G, Borggrefe M, Godehardt E, Seipel L, Birks W: Surgical treatment of ventricular tachycardias. Complete versus partial encircling endocardial ventriculotomy. J Thorac Cardiovasc Surg 1984; 87: 517.
28. Swerdlow CD, Mason JW, Stinson EB, Oyer PE: Results of map-guided surgery in 103 patients with ventricular tachycardia. J Am Coll Cardiol 1985; 5: 409.
29. Miller JM, Hargrove WC, Josephson ME: Significance of "nonclinical" ventricular arrhythmias induced following surgery for ventricular tachyarrhythmias. In: Breithardt G, Borggrefe M, Zipes DP (eds), Nonpharmacological treatment of tachyarrhythmias. Futura publishing company, Mount Kisco, New York, 1987; 133.
30. Miller JM, Kienzle MG, Harken AH, Josephson ME: Subendocardial resection for ventricular tachycardia: predictors for surgical success. Circulation 1984; 70: 624.
31. Swerdlow CD, Winkle RA, Mason J: Determinants of survival in patients with ventricular tachyarrhythmias. N Engl J Med 1983; 308: 1436.
32. Borggrefe M, Podczek A, Ostermeyer J, Breithardt G and the Surgical Ablation Registry: Long-term results of electrophysiologically guided antitachycardia surgery in ventricular tachyarrhythmias: A collaborative report on 665 patients. In: Breithardt G, Borggrefe M, Zipes DP, (eds), Nonpharmacological treatment of tachyarrhythmias. Futura publishing company, Mount Kisco, New York, 1987; 109.
33. Ostermeyer J, Borggrefe M, Breithardt G, Podczek A, Goldmann A, Schroenen JD, Kolvenback R, Godehardt E, Kirklin JW, Blackstone EH: Direct operations of life-threatening ischemic ventricular tachycardia. J Thorac Cardiovasc Surg 1987; 94: 848.

16. Fulguration of chronic ventricular tachycardia

Results on 53 consecutive cases with a follow-up
ranging from 8 to 70 months

G. FONTAINE, R. FRANK, J. TONET, I. ROUGIER, G. FARENQ,
G. LASCAULT and Y. GROSGOGEAT

Introduction

Endocardial catheter fulguration is a new technique used by our group since more than 5 years in order to attempt at the radical treatment of ventricular tachycardia. Up to now it has completely replaced the surgical approach when we are dealing with a purely electric myocardial disease. Dramatic successes were obtained with this method whatever the etiology of VT [1]. Therefore the technique is no longer considered as a last resort approach when other less agressive methods proved ineffective. Fulguration is now extended to young patients with normal hearts, and non life-threatening arrhythmias associated with severe symptoms.

Endocardial fulguration is based on high voltage electrical shocks delivered to the tip of an endocardial catheter, located in the arrhythmogenic zone. Energy in the range of 3—4 Joules/kg body weight is generally produced by the electrical discharge of a defibrillator circuit. This therapeutic approach has been used originally in the treatment of supraventricular tachycardia and has been applied for the 1st time for the treatment of ventricular tachycardia in 1982 by Dr Hartzler in USA and in France, by Puech and Coll in a patient suffering from right ventricular dysplasia [2, 3].

Clinical series

We have now an experience of 61 consecutive cases with this technique. The purpose of this report is to present the results concerning the first 53 patients, fulgurated with a follow-up ranging from 8 to 70 months beginning in May 1983. This group is taken from a large series of 218 consecutive cases who represent the total amount of major ventricular arrhythmias observed at the Jean Rostand Hospital during the same period. We have excluded 9 survivors of cardiac arrest. Therefore, 156 cases of ventricular tachycardia have been treated by anti-arrhythmic drugs and 52 have been

A. Bayés de Luna et al. (eds.): *Sudden Cardiac Death*, 163–177.
© 1991 Kluwer Academic Publishers, Dordrecht.

fulgurated. This latter sub-group is the study population for this work of which shorter series have been already published [4—7].

Most of these patients were referred from other University Centers where they had been considered as resistant to drug therapy. The vast majority has been restudied at Jean Rostand Hospital according to the protocols developed by our group. This includes amiodarone therapy, used alone or in combination with Class I anti-arrhythmic agents, particularly class I-c and/or beta-blocking agents. Only patients resistant to this drug protocol have been considered candidates for the fulguration procedure. All these cases are consecutive, there was no exclusion due to age, clinical condition or other factors.

Our series consists of 45 men and 8 females, with an age ranging from 14 to 76 years, and a mean value of 44 ± 18 years. Their clinical characteristics are presented on Table 1.

The etiology of ventricular tachycardia includes 19 myocardial infarction, 15 arrhythmogenic right ventricular dysplasia, 8 idiopathic cardiomyopathy, 7 ventricular tachycardia sensitive to verapamil, 3 idiopathic infundibular ventricular tachycardia, 1 VT occuring 7 years after infundibular resection. In this series, no form of therapy other than fulguration or its association with drug therapy, has been used with the exception of one case referred to surgery.

Equipment

The approaches used in our hospital were mainly based on equipment originally aimed at the surgical treatment of WPW and ventricular tachycardia. The techniques have evolved along the years and have been published elsewhere. Therefore we will just review in this paper the main steps of the technical protocol currently used [8].

Catheters are selected after an in-vitro electrical non destructive test using voltages similar to those applied during fulguration shocks [9]. These catheters are introduced by either veins or arteries inside right or left ventricular cavities, under fluoroscopic guidance. Catheters are generally tri or quadripolar, USCI 7-F. Those introduced in the left ventricular cavities are guided through a plastic sheeth originally used for endocardial biopsies.

The fulgurator is a special equipment 'Fulgucor' developed on our design by the ODAM Company, Wissembourg, France. The energies can vary from 160 to 320 delivered Joules. This equipment incorporates two independant high voltage generators, one used for the fulguration procedure, the other for cardioversion or defibrillating shocks. This could be used either immediately after the fulguration shocks, or in case of deterioration of ventricular tachycardia, after programmed pacing.

Two tape recorders are used; the first records the fluoroscopic events on a video tape, the second, the ECG tracings from four surface leads as well as

Table 1.

N°	Age	SX	LOC	FC	EF	TI	NM	NE	LI	SI	INC	Nb	ENERG	RIP	AR	MT	10D	FOL
Arrhythmogenic right ventricular dysplasia																		
1	35	M	DIAPH	1	–	>20	1	>20	M	–	–	II	240*1	–	–	–	NP	DCOD
2	62	F	DIAPH	2	–	36	2	>20	M	W	–	I	160*5	RM	O	O	RM	64M
3	74	M	INFUN	2	52%	12	1	3	M	M	–	I	160*1	NI	AMIO	PRO	NI	62M
4	37	M	DIAPH	1	58%	6	1	3	M	<D	+	II	240*6	M	O	O	NP	61M
5	27	M	DIAPH	4	25%	120	4	6	Y	L	–	I	160*17	RM	O	O	NP	DC8D
6	41	F	INFUN	1	59%	48	2	16	M	M	–	II	240*1	TL	O	O	RM	59M
7	32	M	INFUN	1	–	4	1	2	W	<D	–	I	210*4	NI	AMIO	PRO	NI	58M
8	56	M	LV	1	45%	84	5	>20	Y	M	–	III	240*4	R	A+Pr	TH	IN	58M
9	30	M	F.W.	1	56%	12	2	2	M	M	–	II	240*2	TL	AMIO	TH	IN	57M
10	38	M	INFUN	–	–	–	2	>20	<Y	D	+	II	240*3	NP	–	–	–	DCOD
11	37	M	INFUN	2	–	408	3	>20	–	–	+	II	240*9	TL	A+Fl	TH	NC	DC7M
12	27	M	RV FW	2	50%	120	3	>20	–	–	–	II	240*4	M	Bb+QD	TH	NC	44M
13	23	F	SEPTRV	1	51%	24	1	>20	L	L	+	II	240*3	NI	Dis	TH	NI	44M
14	26	M	SEPTRV	2	59%	96	1	12	Y	M	–	II	280*3	–	O	O	NI	30M
15	40	M	INFUN	1	64%	60	1	5	Y	M	–	I	240*3	NI	AMIO	PRO	IN	19M
Myocardial infarction																		
16	60	M	ANTSEP	2	12%	1	2	>20	W	D	+	II	260*1	NI	AMIO	PRO	NP	70M
17	29	M	INF	1	42%	24	3	4	M	M	–	II	260*7	RM	A+Pr	TH	NP	65M
18	73	M	ANTSEP	2	22%	1	2	>20	M	L	+	II	160*1	NP	AMIO	PRO	NP	63M
19	55	M	INF	1	–	12	1	10	M	M	–	IV	240*2	NI	AMIO	PRO	NI	61M
20	65	M	ANTSEP	2	<30%	1	3	2	W	<D	–	I	160*5	NI	O	O	NI	61M
21	60	M	ANTSEP	3	<25%	24	3	10	M	M	–	I	240*2	NP	–	–	–	DC4D
22	67	M	ANTSEP	3	<25%	1	1	2	D	D	–	I	240*2	NP	AMIO	PEO	NP	DC1M
23	74	M	ANTSEP	1	<30%	–	2	10	M	D	–	I	240*2	NI	AMIO	TH	NI	55M
24	64	M	ANTSEP	2	46%	–	2	14	M	D	+	I	240*2	NC	AMIO	TH	IN	DC22M
25	62	F	ANTSEP	3	26%	4	6	>20	W	L	+	IV	240*3	R	A+Bb	TH	NP	DC9M
26	53	M	ANTPOST	1	<30%	3	2	7	W	M	–	I	240*2	NC	AMIO	TH	IN	DC4M

Table 1 (continued)

N°	Age	SX	LOC	FC	EF	TI	NM	NE	LI	SI	INC	Nb	ENERG	RIP	AR	MT	10D	FOL
27	64	M	INF	3	25%	16	2	>20	Y	D	−	I	240*2	NC	A+PM	TH	NP	DC18M
28	55	M	INF	1	<30%	2	3	7	W	D	−	I	280*3	NI	AMIO	PRO	NI	50M
29	52	M	ANTPOST	2	40%	12	2	>20	Y	M	−		240*3	NI	AMIO	PRO	NI	33M
30	65	M	LV	3	25%	36	2	>20	M	L	−	II	240*8	NI	A+Bb	TH	NI	27M
31	76	M	LV	1	48%	5	2	5	M	W	−	I	240*1	NI	A+Bb	TH	NP	26M
32	88	M	LV		52%	8	1	2	−	−	−	I	240*3		A+Bb	PRO	NI	17M
33	64	M	SEPTUM		<30%	60	1	>20	M	D	−	II	280*19	TL	AMIO	TH	NP	11M
34	44	M	SEPTLV	3	<30%	11	2	4	M	D	−	I	320*2	NI	A+Bb	TH	NI	8M
Idiopathic cardiomyopathy																		
35	18	M	ANTSEP	2	<30%	12	1	>20	M	L	+	I	260*5	O	AMIO	TH	NI	DC14M
36	14	F	SEPTLV	3	<20%	168	1	>20	L	L	+	I	168*3	O	O	O	NP	DC2M
37	56	M	LV	2	20%	36	1	6	Y	M	−	I	240*3	NI	AMIO	PRO	NI	DC16M
38	28	M	RV	1	48%	−	3	>20	<Y	D	+	III	240*1	NC	FLEC	TH	IN	55M
39	58	M	RV+LV	1	48%	120	2	>20	M	D	−	III	280*3	NC	QD+Bb	TH	NI	50M
40	21	M	RV APX	1	−	3	1	4	M	D	−	I	240*1	NC	A+Bb	TH	IN	45M
41	16	M	SEPTRV	3	<30%	24	1	>20	−	D	+	I	240*1	O	−	−	NP	DC1D
42	35	M	APEXRV	3	26%	120	1	>20	Y	D	−	I	320*1	NI	AMIO	TH	RM	12M
Idiopathic ventricular tachycardia																		
43	53	F	INFUN	1	59%	96	1	>20	M	D	+	II	240*2	NI	O	O	NI	59M
44	26	F	SEPTRV	1	50%	48	1	>20	Y	D	−	I	240*6	TL	QD	TH	NP	49M
45	58	F	INFUN	1	56%	8	1	>20	M	D	−	II	260*4	NI	FLEC	TH	NI	12M
Verapamil sensitive ventricular tachycardia																		
46	22	M	POSTSEP	1	−	60	1	>20	M	W	−	II	240*2	NI	O	O	NP	58M
47	17	M	SEPTLV	1	70%	40	1	6	Y	D	−	II	240*4	NI	O	O	NI	43M
48	38	M	SEPTLV	1	47%	252	1	>20	W	D	−	I	240*1	NI	O	O	NI	40M
49	22	F	SEPTLV	1	60%	120	1	>20	M	D	−	III	240*2	NI	O	O	NI	28M
50	42	M	LV	1	63%	23	1	>20	Y	L	−	I	240*1		O	O	NI	20M
51	25	M	SEPTLV	1	64%	96	1	10	M	M	−	I	240*1	NI	O	O	NI	12M
52	42	M	SEPTLV	1	70%	320	1	>20	M	W	−	I	280*1	NI	O	O	NI	11M

166 G. Fontaine et al.

Table 1 (continued)

N°	Age	SX	LOC	FC	EF	TI	NM	NE	LI	SI	INC	Nb	ENERG	RIP	AR	MT	10D	FOL
Corrected congenital disease																		
53	21	M	INFUN	1	61%	120	4	10	M	D	–	I	240*4	NI	AMIO	PRO	NP	63M

Dx: Cardiac diagnosis
  ARVD   Arrhythmogenic right ventricular dysplasia
  MI   Myocardial infarction
  IDCM   Idiopathic dilated cardiomyopathy
  IDIO   Idiopathic VT (no structural heart disease)
  CONG   congenital malformation.

LOC: Location of abnormality.
  DIAPH   Diaphragmatic
  INFUN   infundibulum
  LV   left ventricle
  F.W.   free wall
  ANTSEP   anteroseptal
  ANTPOST   anterior and posterior
  INF   inferior
  SEPTLV   left ventricular septum
  RV   right ventricle
  POSTSEP   posteroseptal

FC: Functional class (NYHA)
EF: Ejection fraction (echography, angiography, scintigraphy)
TI: Time interval since the first attack of VT (months).
NM: Number of clinical morphologies of VT.
NE: Total number of VT episodes prior to fulguration.
LI, SI: Longest and shortest interval between two episodes of VI.
  I, incessant; D, day; W, week; M, mmth; Y, year.
INC: Incessant VT in the electrophysiological laboratory.
Nb: Number of fulguration sessions.

ENERG: Joules delivered : 160*5 = discharges of 160 Joules
  (value concerning the last procedure).
RIP: Reasons for interrupting the procedure
  R   changes in rate; M: changes in morphology
  NP   programmed pacing not performed.
  TL   time limit
  NC   Nonclinical VT
  NI   VT not inducible

AR: Anti-arrhythmic prescription upon hospital discharge.
  AMIO   Amiodarone
  A+Pr   Amiodarone + propafenone
  A+Fl   Amiodarone + flécainide
  FLEC   Flecainide
  A+Bb   Amiodarone + beta-blockers
  A+PM   Amiodarone + pacemaker
  QD   Quinidine
  Dilt   Dilthiazem

MT: Mode of treatment
  PRO, TH   prophylactic or therapeutic treatment.

10D: provocative test performed 10 days after fulguration.
  NP   Provocative test not performed.
  NI   VT not inducible.
  IN   Inducible by programmed stimulation.
  RM   Change in rate and morphology of VTmorphology.

FOL: Follow-up   DC   Death

endocardial signals. Comments given by the 5 most important investigators who are wearing microphones and head sets are also recorded on the same tape. This proved to be of great value in case of major complications.

The radial blood pressure is continuously monitored during the procedure and a Swan-Ganz catheter is used to record the pulmonary wedge pressure and to perform cardiac output measurement by thermodilution technique. The activation times are measured on an Electronic for Medicine VR12 recorder for the first approach of the appropriate electrophysiological parameters and during the final approach by a three channel digital Tektronix 5116 oscilloscope.

Before the fulguration session, Class I antiarrhythmic drugs are interrupted during a period at least equal to or longer than 5 half-lives. Amiodarone is not interrupted. A preliminary electrophysiological study is frequently performed in order to determine the ease of induction of ventricular tachycardia, how they are tolerated, the number of morphologies of the clinical and non-clinical ventricular tachycardias. Their behavior is also evaluated: sustained, non sustained, polymorphic. Only sustained monomorphic ventricular tachycardias are considered for fulguration. Fulguration is made under general anesthesia, because it is generally necessary to deliver several shocks during each session. When VT is not incessant when the patient is entering the laboratory, tachycardia is generally induced by programmed pacing.

The 'classical' approach was to record the so called *site of origin* of ventricular tachycardia as it was previously demonstrated effective during surgery after epicardial mapping. The technique of pacemapping is also used and should reproduce in 12 leads QRS complexes which should be rigorously identical to the spontaneous ventricular tachycardia QRS complexes. Pacing in such case is better achieved by a slight overdrive during VT by the same catheter which will be used for delivering the electrical shocks. In most recent studies we have paid a particular attention to *the area of slow conduction* which is frequently represented by fragmented potentials located between two ventricular QRS complexes [10, 11].

When the check list is completed, a count-down is started during which any relevant equipment is put into action. If the tachycardia is not incessant, the shock synchronised on the QRS complexes is finally delivered during sinus rhythm for better hemodynamic [12] and rhythmologic [13] tolerance. The shock is delivered between the distal electrode which is working as an anode, and an indifferent electrode of large surface covered by a conductive jelly located in the back. From 1 to 17 shocks (mean 3.5) are delivered during each session (143 in the right ventricule, 112 in the left ventricular and 2 transeptal shocks). Just after the shock, a complete transient atrioventricular block could be observed and ventricular pacing is achieved by a catheter which has been previously located in the apex of the right ventricle. This catheter should be located at least 3 cm away from the fulgurating electrode. In case of rapid VT or VT degenerating into VF, a cardioversion shock is delivered to the patch electrode placed on the anterior aspect of the thorax. This shock is delivered by the safety defibrillator which is a part of the Fulgucor. The second electrode is the same as the electrode used for delivering the electrical shock. Therefore, it is not necessary to remove the sterile fields or the X-ray equipment, defibrillation being performed in the anterio-posterior direction. Low energies in the range of 40 to 160 J are generally sufficient.

After delivering the shock, the patient being in sinus rhythm, all the electrophysiological manoeuvres are interrupted during a rest period of 10 minutes, which are necessary for the electrical, as well as the hemodynamical stabilization of myocardium. After that time, programmed pacing is resumed to try to reinduce ventricular tachycardia or to try to induce a different morphology. The session is over when it is no longer possible to induce ventricular tachycardia, or if the necessary protocol has been modified. The session is also interrupted if episodes of ventricular fibrillation or unstable ventricular tachycardia are induced or for technical reasons.

The immediate follow-up

The in-hospital follow-up period is performed with monitoring of the radial blood pressure and central venous pressure during a period of 24 hours. A sub-clavian catheter located at the apex of the right ventricle is left during a period which could go to ten days. At this time a new electrophysiological study could be performed, generally at the bedside, in order to know if the tachycardia is or not reinducible. During this follow-up period of 10 days, the ECG is monitored by a computerized Hewlett Packard monitoring equipment with the Nadia software, the patient being connected by cable or telemetry.

When a ventricular tachycardia identical or similar to the previous attacks in rate, as well as in morphology, occurs spontaneously, or is inducible, new pharmacological attempts are made, which could be sometimes effective. The same dosage and drugs as before the fulguration procedure are tried. When this drug treatment is effective, it is called 'therapeutic' because it is indispensable to prevent ventricular arrhythmias after fulguration which has only partially modified the arrhythmogenic substrate. However, in order to simplify, we have included in this group, some patients in whom antiarrhythmic treatment different from those used before the fulguration led to the control of the cardiac arrhythmia.

The treatment is called 'prophylactic' when non inducible patients need to take these medicines for safety reasons, in case of unpredicted relapses or to treat ventricular or supraventricular extrasystoles. Effectiveness of fulguration is reassessed before discharge by Holter recording, stress test, programmed pacing going up to 3 extrastimuli on a cycle length going from 600 to 400 ms.

After the hospital stay, the follow-up of these patients is made with the help of the computer system, based on a DEC PDP 11/23+ and a specialized software developed in our Institution. The follow-up is made by the general practitioner, the cardiologist, and the referring hospital, as well as by direct phone calls to the patient. In this series of fulgurated cases, no patient has been lost of follow-up.

Results

Considering that 5 patients were moribund when the fulguration procedure was performed and that 2 were already unconscious, results are impressive. However, 5 early deaths (during the procedure or within one month after the procedure) have been observed. None was related to malignant arrhythmia or tamponade, or has been observed as a direct consequence of the fulguration itself. For reasons which will be explained later, we have chosen to express the results at 3 months after discharge from the hospital. These results are expressed schematically on Figure 1.

Their classification has been made in 4 categories: 'death', 'success' when the patient does not take antiarrhythmic drugs to prevent relapses, or is taking them for prophylactic reasons, 'partial' success when the drug therapy is necessary to prevent relapses or ventricular tachycardia, and 'failure' when the same attacks of VT in rate and morphology which have been previously fulgurated could not be controlled by drugs, and need a new fulguration procedure.

On the series of 53 patients who have been submitted to a first session, we have observed 2 early deaths, 17 success, 12 partial success, and 22 failures, which correspond to a success rate of 47% after a single session. On the 22 patients who have not been controlled by the fulguration procedure alone or combined with antiarrhythmic drugs and in whom a second session has been

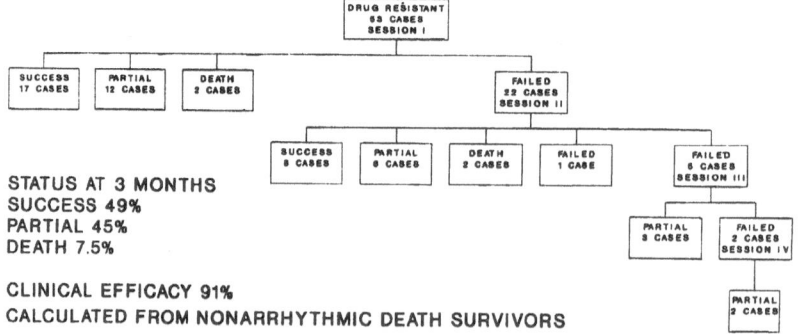

Figure 1. Ventricular tachycardia fulguration taken from the Jean Rostand series of 53 cases resistant to antiarrhythmic therapy and submitted to one to four procedures (see text for definitions).

performed, we have observed 2 deaths during the session, 8 success, 6 partial success and 6 failures. After 2 sessions, it is therefore possible to obtain on this population of survivors, 81% of clinical efficacy. In 5 patients in whom two sessions were not effective, used alone or in combination with antiar-rhythmic drugs, a third session has been performed leading to a partial success in three cases since antiarrhythmic drugs proved to be necessary, and a failure in two cases. These two patients needed a fourth fulguration session leading to two partial success.

However, in this series, two patients had relapses of ventricular tachycardia after hospital discharge. They had been at the beginning considered as fulguration failure. However, with time, the attacks became less and less frequent, and after 3 months, these patients no longer experienced relapses leading to the reduction or even almost complete suppression of drug treatment. This is why our results are expressed at 3 months after discharge. The remaining patient did not accepted another procedure.

Finally, from the patients who survived the initial phase, ventricular tachycardias have been controlled in all cases except one by a single or multiple fulguration sessions. No form of therapy other than the fulguration procedure used alone or associated with drug therapy has been used in this study. However, half of them need to take antiarrhythmic drugs after partially effective fulguration sessions.

During the overall period of study with a mean value of 43 months, 13 deaths have been observed, none of them seemed to be related to the fulguration itself.

Early deaths
Five patients died during or within one month after the fulguration procedure.

Cardiac deaths
They have been observed in 2 cases at the beginning of our experience when monitored hemodynamic surveillance was not performed in one case. In the other it occured after a progressive and irreversible decrease of the cardiac output, while the patient needed external cardiac massage after a defibrillation shock for an increase in the tachycardia rate.

Non cardiac deaths
They were observed in three cases: the first one had arrhythmogenic right ventricular dysplasia and was referred after multiple episodes of ventricular tachycardia after angio-coronarography, and was unconscious at arrival. Despite effective fulguration session, the patient died 8 days later of refractory hypoxia due to extensive pulmonary infection, which was already

observed before the fulguration procedure. The 2nd case was a patient who had a poor ejection fraction after an old myocardial infarction, who has been considered as beyond surgery. During the fulguration procedure, a delay in the cardiopulmonary ressuscitation led to irreversible cerebral damage and the patient died four days later of this complication.

The 3rd case had a very poor myocardial function and was at the terminal phase of a dilated idiopathic cardiomyopathy. He had pulmonary hypertension and was in permanent VT since two years. A poor hemodynamic function was observed during induction of anesthesia and the situation being under control, a single shock was delivered and was well tolerated. During the following night, when the hemodynamic situation was satisfactory, the patient developed an abrupt septic shock of unknown mechanism leading to hyperkalemia and death.

Autopsy and histological study have been performed in all cases except the two last ones. It showed the effect of shocks on myocardium similar to the modification observed in the experimental laboratory, these histological pictures being superimposed to the particular histological structure of the underlying cardiac disease [14].

Late mortality

Cardiac mortality

Sudden deaths. Three cases could be classified as sudden deaths: they were observed 4, 14 and 22 months after the fulguration procedure (Figure 2). All could be considered as the result of recurrence of ventricular tachycardia. This event was predicted in two cases, but the tachycardia being well tolerated, a new attempt or another form of therapy was finally not decided.

Congestive heart failure. Two patients died one month and 18 months after hospital discharge from pulmonary edema without recurrence of ventricular tachycardia. Both of them had a severe form of coronary artery disease, a poor ejection fraction, cardiomegalia and left ventricular failure, making them non appropriate candidate for surgery.

One case of dilated idiopathic cardiomyopathy died three months after the fulguration of pulmonary edema without recurrence of cardiac arrhythmia. One case died of cardiac insufficiency 10 months after the fulguration when he was successfully treated by therapeutic antiarrhythmic agents.

Two patients died of a non cardiac cause
All these patients died outside the hospital, therefore autopsy was not possible.

Complications. Pulmonary edema has been observed in three cases, occur-

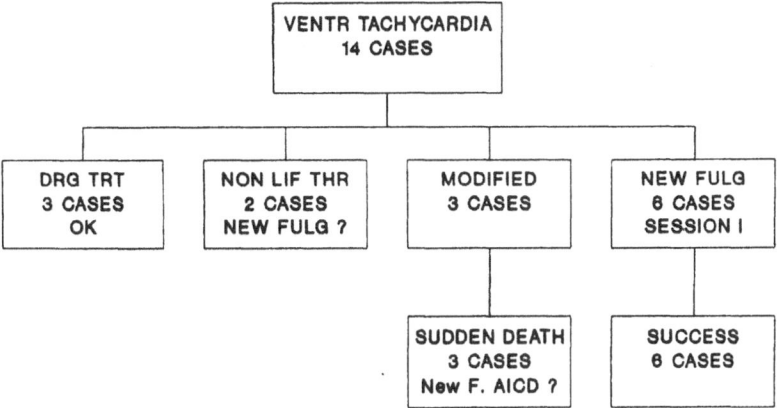

Figure 2. Ventricular tachycardias observed during the follow-up with a mean value of 43 months.

DRG TRT   Drug treatment
NON LIF THR   Non life-threatening ventricular tachycardia
MODIFIED   New episodes of probable ventricular tachycardia were better tolerated.
NEW FULG   A new fulguration session or implantation of an AICD should have been considered.

ring generally 10 minutes after fulguration procedure. However, this situation has always been controlled using routine techniques. In one case, during the second fulguration session, the patient experienced angina during endocardial mapping performed before the beginning of anesthesia and this was observed in conjunction with modifications of the ST segment and transient bundle branch block. In this patient, the CPK MB fraction got up to 140 IU, definitely larger than the mean value obtained with the remaining part of the series (37 ± 15). Atrioventricular block has been also frequently observed during the sessions (17% out of 167 shocks) and in two cases, AV block disappeared only after a period of 2 hours. Short lasting intraventricular blocks and 5 cases of right bundle branch block were observed in the same group of 167 shocks. Acceleration of ventricular tachycardia or ventricular fibrillation have been observed in 12% of the shocks, generally occurring immediately after the electrical discharge. In all cases, these arrhythmias have been easily converted or defibrillated through the patch electrode, except two cases in whom one was in major hemodynamic failure, and the other in hypoxia. However, no malignant arrhythmia, resistant to medication has been observed during or immediately after the fulguration procedures. One patient in whom the shock was delivered close to the pacing electrode of the permanent pacemaker, needed generator replacement [15].

Late relapses. According to the previous definition concerning the analysis of results, long time relapses have been observed 3 months after hospital discharge. Their classification could fall in different categories (Figure 2):

Relapses better tolerated
Three patients (already mentioned) in whom cardiac arrhythmias were less severe and better tolerated probably because of modification of the arrhythmogenic substrate died suddenly, for one after episodes of palpitations, for the other two with less suggestive troubles, as dyspnea, fatigue, or gastrointestinal problems. In one of these cases, systematic Holter recording exhibited an incessant asymptomatic VT at 110/mn. In these patients, and despite a change in drug treatment made in the last one, sudden death was not prevented.

Relapses controlled by drugs
This has been observed in 3 patients, and was considered as the result of decrease of therapeutic antiarrhythmic treatment. This drug regimen was reinstituted and proved to be effective at the appropriate level.

Relapses controlled by a new session of fulguration
This situation has been observed in 6 cases and has always been successfully managed after the new session. However, in one patient, fewer spontaneous episodes were observed and decreased progressively thereafter. This situation suggested the evolution previously indicated concerning early relapses.

Relapses not refulgurated
One patient who was controlled during a period of one year and a half in whom new extrasystoles and VT were observed, did not want to undergo a new session. VT occurred on a 'normal heart', attacks were incapacitating, but not life-threatening.

Case who failed completely
This was observed in one case of non life-threatening arrhythmia which was slightly improved by the combination of DDD overdrive pacing, amiodarone and beta-blocking agent.

Discussion

These results demonstrate the effectiveness of fulguration on a significant series of patients suffering from chronic ventricular tachycardia of various origins. Some deaths were observed during the learning phase of our experience, each case has been investigated retrospectively from the different tape recorders. In all cases except the patient with sepsis, it was possible to understand the mechanism of the catastrophe leading to modification of the protocol, and the same problems did not recur thereafter.

If we include the case of death observed during the learning phase, for a mean follow-up of 45 months, the percentage of death per year is 7.4%. If we withdraw from this series the three patients whose death was due to a poor protocol, and the case of unevitable death by pulmonary infection, and unconsciousness, the series consists of 38 cases in whom a mortality rate of 10 cases has been observed we obtain the same mortality rate of 7.4 per year. However, the main goal of fulguration is prevention of a cardiac arrhythmia, which is potentially lethal. It should therefore be judged on the occurrence of sudden death during the follow-up period. This event has been in fact observed only in 3 cases in this series leading to a death rate of 1.6% (calculated on the 38 survivors followed during a mean follow-up period of 43 months). In this subgroup, the risk of sudden death has been strongly predicted in two patients and in the last one it could not be assumed that the therapeutical management was the most appropriate.

Taking into account that 64% of cases of the series had attacks of VT at a rate equal to or superior than one per month, these patients were not candidate for the implantable defibrillator, and we were therefore led to favourable opinion concerning the use of fulguration for the control of ventricular tachycardia and sudden death in this particular subgroup. It is also interesting to speculate that the fulguration procedure could be indicated in patient with implantable defibrillator who has received frequent discharges leading to psychological distress [16].

Being considered the small quantity of CK MB isoenzyme released after the fulguration session in which several shocks had been delivered, it is possible to think that this method finally induces modifications of myocardium on very small areas, therefore a precise localisation of the arrhythmogenic focus seems mandatory, or the need of repeated shocks on a large zone.

In the most recent developments, we tried to fulgurate not the site of origin but earlier in the tachycardia cycle, in the area of slow conduction. The most difficult approach is to deliver the shock on the area of slow conduction which is *indispensable* for the perpetuation of ventricular tachycardia, because there are inside the arrhythmogenic substrate, other areas of slow conduction which are only bystanders [17].

A particular problem is related to the morphology of ventricular tachycardia which could be induced by programmed pacing. It is now well accepted that non sustained or polymorphic ventricular tachycardias, induced by programmed pacing have no clinical significance [18]. This explains why only sustained monomorphic VT have been considered for the fulguration procedure.

However, programmed cardiac pacing could also induce episodes of VT which have not been previously documented, the so called 'non clinical VT'. As all the class I antiarrhythmic drugs have been interrupted several days before the fulguration session, it is not possible to consider that these different VT morphologies are the result of these drug treatments. Therefore, we think that in most cases, it is necessary to fulgurate clinical VT as well as non clinical VT. A rigorous approach to the study of fulguration results should be assessed on its effectiveness on each VT morphology [1, 19]. It could be possible to tolerate some ventricular tachycardias which are hemodynamically stable, provided that they have symptoms that the patient could recognize as recurrences of VT. A reliable implantable equipment for long-term follow-up is mandatory in this line.

During this study which extends on a period of 5 years, concepts and protocols have envolved with time. The selection of cases also has changed. At the origin, the fulguration was applied as a last resort procedure, for the most severe cases, some patients being even moribund. When it was demonstrated that the technique was safe and effective, it was extended to young subjects with invalidating but not life-threatening tachycardias.

With time and a better experience of the technique of endocardial mapping, the number of sessions per patient has decreased. It is now rare to use more than two sessions per patient, and finally that antiarrhythmic drugs are frequently needed.

This situation could be explained by the small quantity of myocardium which is modified during the procedure, as suggested by the small variation of CPK MB. We have recently demonstrated in a subgroup of patients fulgurated for ventricular tachycardia after arrhythmogenic right ventricular dysplasia, that non effective fulguration session was correlated with a small release of CKMB [20—21].

New studies are on the way to try to increase the size of tissue modified during the shock, and to apply the energy to the area of slow conduction which could be the optimal zone to deliver the fulguration shocks.

References

1. Tonet JL, Fontaine G, Frank R, Grosgogeat Y: Treatment of ventricular tachycardias by endocardial catheter fulguration: further experience and long-term follow-up (abstract). Circulation 1988; 78: Supp-II, 306.
2. Hartzler GO: Electrode catheter ablation of refractory focal ventricular tachycardia. J Am Coll Cardiol 1983; 2: 1107—1113.
3. Puech P, Gallay P, Grolleau R, Koliopoulos N: Traitement par électrofulguration endocavitaire d'une tachycardie ventriculaire récidivante par dysplasie ventriculaire droite. Arch Mal Coeur 1984; 77: 826—835.
4. Fontaine G, Frank R, Tonet JL, Gallais Y, Touzet I, Todorova M, Baraka M, Grosgogeat Y: Treatment of resistant ventricular tachycardia with endocavitary fulguration and antiarrhythmic therapy, compared to antiarrhythmic therapy alone: experience in 111 consecutive cases with a mean follow-up of 18 months. Texas Heart Inst 1986; 13: 401—418.
5. Fontaine G, Tonet JL, Frank R, Rougier I: Electrode catheter ablation of ventricular tachycardia by fulguration and antiarrhythmic therapy. Experience of 43 patients with a mean follow-up of 29 months. Chest 1989; 95: 785—797.
6. Fontaine G, Tonet JL, Frank R, Touzet I, Farenq G, Dubois-Rande JL, Baraka M, Abdelali S, Grosgogeat Y: Traitement des tachycardies ventriculaires rebelles par fulguration endocavitaire associe aux anti-arythmiques. Arch Mal Coeur 1986; 79: 1152—1162.
7. Fontaine G, Tonet JL, Frank R, Touzet I, Dubois-Rande JL, Gallais Y, Grosgogeat Y: Treatment of resistant ventricular tachycardia by endocavitary fulguration associated with antiarrhythmic therapy. Eur Heart J 1987; 8: Supp-D, 133—141.

8. Fontaine G, Cansell A, Tonet JL, Frank R, Gallais Y, Rougier I, Grosgogeat Y: Techniques and methods for catheter endocardial fulguration. Pace 1988; 11: 592—602.

9. Fontaine G, Cansell A, Lampe L, Baraka M, Tonet JL, Frank R, Grosgogeat Y: Endocavitary fulguration (electrode catheter ablation): equipment-related problems. In: Ablation in Cardiac Arrhythmias — Fontaine G, Scheinman MM (eds), Futura Publ. Co., Mount Kisco, NY 1987: 85—100.

10. Fontaine G: Du lieu d'origine á la zone á conduction lente. Application au traitement de la tachycardie ventriculaire. Arch Mal Coeur 1988; 81: 145.

11. Frank R, Tonet JL, Kounde S, Farenq G, Fontaine G: Localization of the area of slow conduction during ventricular tachycardia. In: Cardiac Arrhythmias: Where to Go from Here?, Brugada P, Wellens HJJ (eds), Futura Publ. Co., Mount Kisco, NY 1987: 191—208.

12. Gallais Y, Touzet M, Gateau O, Maneglia R, Frank R, Fontaine G, Cousin M Th:Anesthesie et surveillance dans la fulguration endocavitaire pour le traitement radical des tachycardies ventriculaires. Ann Cardiol Angeiol 1986; 35: 539—549.

13. Baraka M, Tonet J, Fontaine G, Abdelali S, Menezes-Falcao L, Frank R, Grosgogeat Y: Les troubles du rythme et de la conduction au decours immediat de la fulguration ventriculaire. Arch Mal Coeur 1988; 81: 269—275.

14. Fontaine G: The effects of high-energy DC shocks delivered to ventricular myocardium. In: Catheter Ablation of Cardiac Arrhythmias. Scheinman MM (ed), Martinus Nijhoff Pub., Boston 1988: 97—114.

15. Fontaine G, Lemoine B, Frank R, Tonet JL, Maendely R, Grosgogeat Y. Effects of fulguration on the permanent pacemaker. In: Ablation in Cardiac Arrhythmias. Fontaine G, Scheinman MM (eds), Futura Publ. Co., Mount Kisco, NY 1987: 367—378.

16. Brodsky AM, Miller MH, Cannom DS, Ilvento J, Mirabal GS, Carillo R: Psychosocial adaptation to the automatic implantable cardioverter defibrillator. Circulation 1988; 78: Supp-II, 155.

17. Morady F, Frank R, Kou WH, Tonet JL, Nelson SD, Kounde S, De Buitleir M, Fontaine G: Identification and catheter ablation of a zone of slow conduction in the reentry circuit of ventricular tachycardias in humans. J Am Coll Cardiol 1988; 11: 775—782.

18. Brugada P, Green M, Abdollah H, Wellens HJJ: Significance of ventricular arrhythmias initiated by programmed ventricular stimulation: the importance of the type of ventricular arrhythmia induced and the number of premature stimuli required. Circulation 1984; 69: 87—92.

19. Tonet JL, Baraka M, Frank R, Fontaine G, Gallais Y, Abdelali S, Grosgogeat Y: Endocardial catheter fulguration of ventricular tachycardias: pitfalls of the clinical and nonclinical approach (abstract). Circulation 1985; 72: Sup-III, 388.

20. Fontaine G, Frank R, Rougier I, Tonet JL, Gallais Y, Farenq G, Lascault G, Lilamand M, Fontaliran F, Chomette G, Grosgogeat Y: Electrode catheter ablation of resistant ventricular tachycardia in arrhythmogenic right ventricular dysplasia. Experience of 13 patients with a mean follow-up of 45 months. Eur Heart J 1989; 10 (suppl D): 74—81.

21. Fontaine G, Volmer W, Nienaltowska E, Aaddaj S, Cansell A, Grosgogeat Y: Approach to the physics of fulguration. In: Ablation in Cardiac Arrhythmias. Fontaine G, Scheinman MM (eds), Futura Publ. Co., Mount Kisco, NY 1987: 101—116.

17. Transcoronary chemical ablation of tachycardias

PEDRO BRUGADA, HANS DE SWART, JOEP L.R.M. SMEETS and
HEIN J. J. WELLENS

Cardiac arrhythmias can be successfully controlled nowadays in a remarkable percentage of patients. We have at our disposal new antiarrhythmic
drugs with high efficacy and acceptable side-effect profiles [1]. Selected
patients with selected arrhythmias not controllable with antiarrhythmic drugs
[2] can be treated with electrical devices. Refined surgical techniques for the
treatment of supraventricular [3—4] and ventricular arrhythmias [5—6] are
available. The implantable defibrillator has become a reality [7]. Percutaneous electrical ablation is effective to create atrio-ventricular block in patients
with atrial fibrillation with uncontrollable rapid ventricular rates [8]. Unfortunately, we are still far from controlling cardiac arrhythmias in all patients.
Not all respond to antiarrhythmic drugs. Many are not amenable to
antitachycardia pacing or control by an implantable defibrillator. Because of
the important myocardial damage present in many patients surgery for
ventricular tachycardia has a high perioperative mortality. Percutaneous
electrical ablation of accessory pathways is still experimental and electrical
ablation of ventricular tachycardia [9] has not offered the expected results
[10]. This technique creates lesions with a small size. Extensive myocardial
damage can result when multiple shocks are given. However, surgery and
percutaneous electrical ablation are forms of treatment that can destroy or
remove the arrhythmia substrate, offering a definitive cure when successful.
Antiarrhythmic drugs and electrical devices are palliative therapies. Techniques able to destroy the arrhythmia substrate overcoming the problems of
percutaneous electrical ablation and surgery would represent an important
addition to our antiarrhythmic armentarium.

Inoue *et al.* have shown in the experimental laboratory suppression of
aconitine-induced arrhythmias by transcoronary administration of alcohols
[11]. Radiologists have effectively ablated with absolute ethanol renal tumors
in humans [12—13]. Any arrhythmogenic area or pathway in the heart
requires a blood supply. Blood supply is necessary for the cells to generate
and maintain electrical activity. If cells are deprived of their blood supply or
destroyed an arrhythmia where these cells participate as a necessary link will
be impossible. In the border zone of the infarction surviving cells with

A. Bayés de Luna et al. (eds.): *Sudden Cardiac Death*, 179–190.

normal action potentials but bad intercellular connections create the area of slow conduction and reentry [14—15]. Surviving cells in the border zone require a blood supply to generate and conduct electrical activity. We developed a new technique with the following aims:

a) demonstrate it is possible to identify and catheterize a small coronary artery giving blood supply to an arrhythmogenic area or pathway ('tachycardia-related coronary artery');

b) if a 'tachycardia-related coronary artery' can be identified destroy the arrhythmogenic substrate with ethanol given in that coronary artery

A. Acute transcoronary termination of tachycardias

Eighteen patients with regular tachycardias and two patients with atrial fibrillation were studied to develop the technique. All gave informed consent. Clinical characteristics are summarized in Table 1. First, a complete programmed electrical stimulation study was first performed. Previously described methodology was used [16]. Mapping of electrical activity was done

Table 1. Clinical characteristics of patients studied.

Patient	Age	Sex	Clinical diagnosis
1	32	F	WPW — CMT
2	44	F	WPW — CMT
3	36	F	Incessant atrial tachycardia
4	19	F	Incessant idiopathic VT
5	35	F	Incessant idiopathic VT
6	63	M	Inferior MI, paroxysmal VT
7	45	M	Posterior MI, paroxysmal VT
8	42	M	Anterior MI, paroxysmal VT
9 *	61	M	Anterior/Inferior MI, incessant VT
10	47	F	Inferior MI, paroxysmal VT
11 *	44	M	Anterior/Inferior MI, incessant VT
12	71	M	Anterior/Inferior MI, paroxysmal VT
13	44	M	Anterior MI, paroxysmal VT
14 *	62	M	Anterior MI, incessant VT
15	61	M	Anterior MI, paroxysmal VT
16 *	58	M	Anterior MI, incessant VT
17 *	59	M	Anterior MI, incessant VT
18 *	62	M	Anterior/Inferior MI, incessant VT
19 **	70	F	atrial fibrillation
20 **	64	F	atrial fibrillation

Abbreviations: CMT = circus movement tachycardia, F = female, M = male, MI = myocardial infarction, VT = ventricular tachycardia, WPW = Wolff-Parkinson-White syndrome, * = patients in whom transcoronary chemical ablation of ventricular tachycardia was performed. ** = Transcoronary chemical ablation of the artioventricular node.

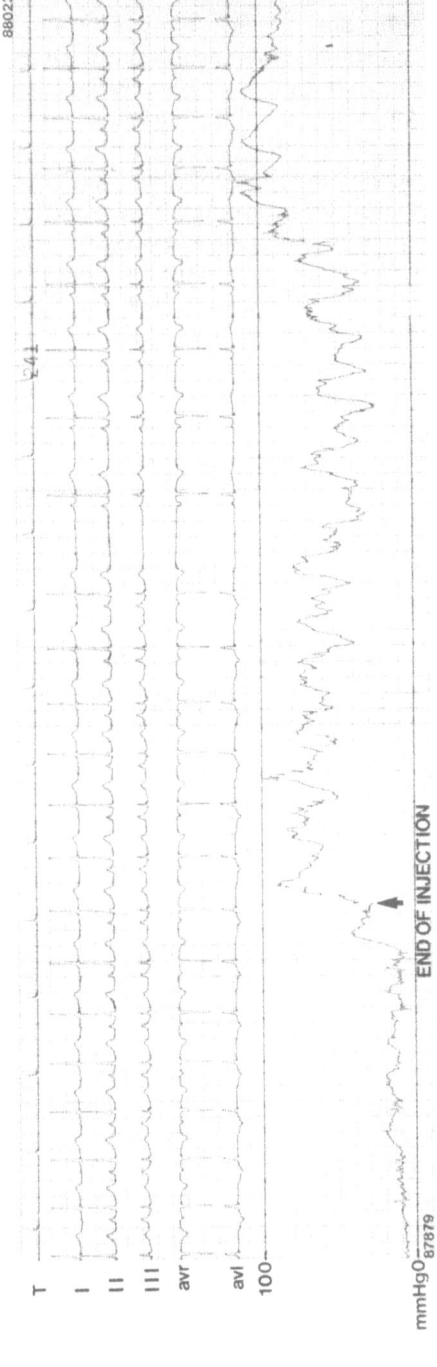

Figure 1. Termination of incessant atrial tachycardia by adminstration of isotonic saline given in a left atrial branch. Five surface ECG leads are shown. Note the negative P wave in lead aVL indicating the left atrial site of origin of the arrhythmia (left atrial appendate). After transient termination of atrial tachycardia the arrhythmia reinitiates spontaneously in the right part of the figure. A pressure recording is simultaneously shown. From Brugada P *et al.* Am J Cardiol 1988; 62: 387–392.

during sinus rhythm and tachycardia using uni- and bipolar recordings. The diagnosis of the arrhythmia was confirmed and the site of origin of ventricular and atrial tachycardia and the site of implantation of accessory pathways was studied. Pace-mapping was also done in patients with ventricular tachycardia. To localize the site of origin of ventricular tachycardia, the locatization of myocardial infarction, when present, and the axis and morphology of the QRS complex on the 12-lead surface electrocardiogram were considered [17—19] along results of mapping and pace-mapping. In patients with the Wolff-Parkinson-White syndrome, the patient with incessant atrial tachycardia and one patient with ventricular tachycardia data during arrhythmia surgery confirmed the preoperatively localized site of origin of the arrhythmia or implantation of the accessory pathway. After the electrophysiologic study a coronary angiography was performed by the Judkins technique. Data from programmed stimulation and coronary angiography were correlated to identify a possible 'tachycardia-related coronary artery'. The artery was selectively catheterized with an angioplasty steerable guidewire (0.014 inch). A 2.5 F lumen catheter with a distal metalic marker was thereafter introduced as far as possible in the 'tachycardia-related coronary artery'. With this catheter coronary flow was interrupted and iced isotonic saline and the 96% ethanol given.

Administration of iced isotonic saline and interruption on blood flow to the arrhythmogenic area or pathway

Iced isotonic saline was first given aselectively during tachycardia at a dose of 10 ml and as fast as possible (usually 1.5—2.5 sec) in the left main coronary artery and ostium of the right coronary artery. That had no effects in any tachycardia except in one patient with incessant idiopathic ventricular tachycardia. That arrhythmia originated high in the interventricular septum and terminated transiently. The iced saline was thereafter given in the 'tachycardia-related artery'. Reproducible termination of ventricular tachycardia was obtained in all patients with incessant tachycardias. The effect lasted for a few seconds in the patient with incessant atrial tachycardia (Figure 1) and for a variable length in the patients with incessant ventricular tachycardia. The same effects were obtained when ischemia was produced by wedging the catheter or by inflating a balloon catheter in two patients. In patients with paroxysmal ventricular terminated in all but one. In one patient with the Wolff-Parkinson-White syndrome transient block of anterograde conduction over the accessory pathway during sinus rhythm was obtained by giving iced saline through the circumflex coronary artery. In the other patient circus movement tachycardia was terminated by iced saline given in the atrioventricular nodal artery.

B. Transcoronary chemical ablation of ventricular tachycardia

Once the 'tachycardia-related coronary artery' was identified chemical ablation of the arrhythmia was undertaken in 6 patients with incessant ventricular
tachycardia after myocardia infarction. All 6 patients had no other therapeutic alternatives and were in incessant ventricular tachycardia for 1 to 4
months. All patients had incessant ventricular tachycardia after myocardial
infarction. Three had suffered from two infarctions. The left ventricular
ejection fraction ranged from 11 to 20%. Three had had aneurysmectomy
with placement of a patch. Available antiarrhythmic drugs (including experimental ones) failed to control incessant ventricular tachycardia and/or
caused severe depression of the hemodynamic condition with pulmonary
oedema. Five patients were in functional class III for dyspnea of the New
York Heart Association and one patient in class IV.

In patient 1 (Figure 2) ventricular tachycardia was reproducibly terminated by administration of saline through the first septal branch. Spontaneous
asymptomatic occlusion of that septal branch occurred during the procedure.
Incessant ventricular tachycardia disappeared and was not inducible by
programmed stimulation. Four weeks after discharge, the patient had again
incessant ventricular tachycardia. A repeat coronary angiography demonstrated retrograde collateral flow to the left anterior descending coronary
artery from a right ventricular and conus branch. Selective catheterization
and administration of saline through the conus branch repeatedly terminated
the arrhyhtmia. Administration of a total of 6 ml 96% ethanol through that
branch resulted in occlusion of the artery and cure of incessant ventricular
tachycardia. After 17 months follow-up recurrences of the arrhythmia have
occurred.

In patient 2 transcoronary chemical ablation was performed after repeat
demonstration of termination of incessant ventricular tachycardia by giving
saline through the first septal branch (Figure 3). The arrhythmia terminated
abruptly after administration of 1.5 ml of 96% ethanol. Complete atrio-
ventricular block developed at that time and lasted for three days. Although
atrio-ventricular conduction recovered, a permanent on demand pacemaker
was implanted. At twelve months follow-up no recurrences of the arrhythmia
have occurred and anterograde conduction is preserved.

In patient 3 incessant ventricular tachycardia could repeatedly terminated
by saline given in the distal posterior descending coronary artery. The
arrhythmia originated in the distal septum. Chemical ablation was performed
by giving 1.5 ml 96% ethanol in that artery (Figure 4). After six months
follow-up no recurrences of the arrhythmia have occurred.

Patient 4 had incessant ventricular tachycardia that could be terminated
by giving saline in a right ventricular branch giving collateral blood supply to
the left descending anterior coronary artery. Administration of 1.5 ml of 96%
ethanol in that branch resulted in disappearance of ventricular tachycardia.

184   *P. Brugada et al.*

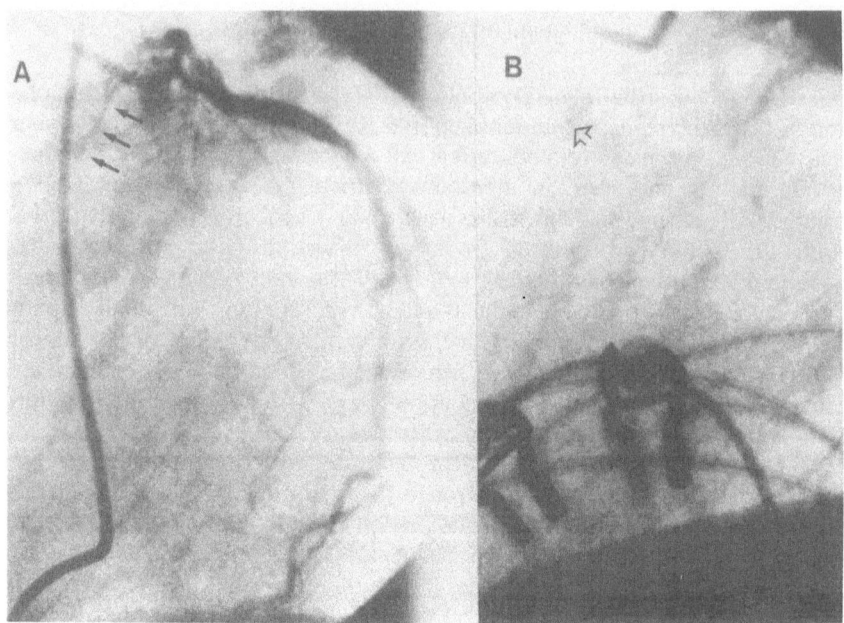

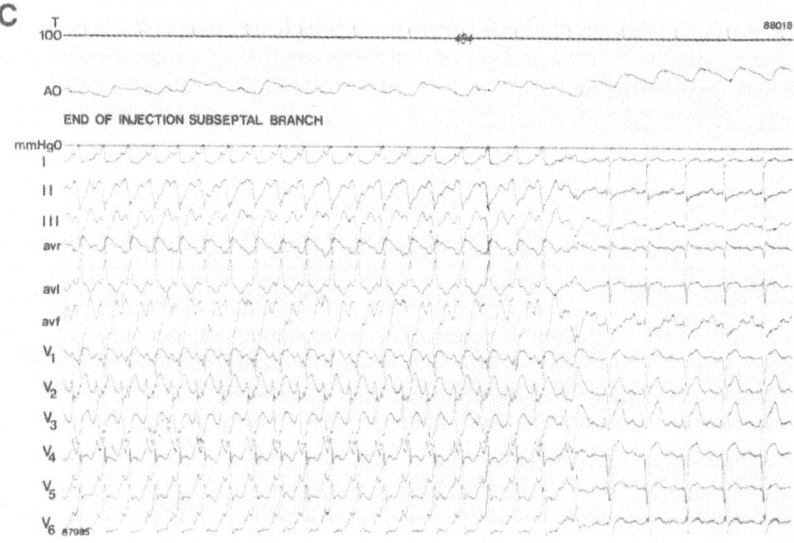

Figure 2. Left anterior oblique projection during left coronary angiorgraphy showing an occluded left anterior descending coronary artery and a small septal branch before the occlusion (arrow) (panel A). In panel B the septal branch has been selectively catheterized. Note the metalic marker of the 2.5 F lumen catheter (open arrow) (panel B). Panel C illustrates termination of a ventricular tachycardia with a left bundle branch block morphology and left axis in the frontal plane. That arrhythmia originated from the apical-inferior septum. Twelve surface ECG leads are shown. From Brugada P *et al.* Circulation 1989.

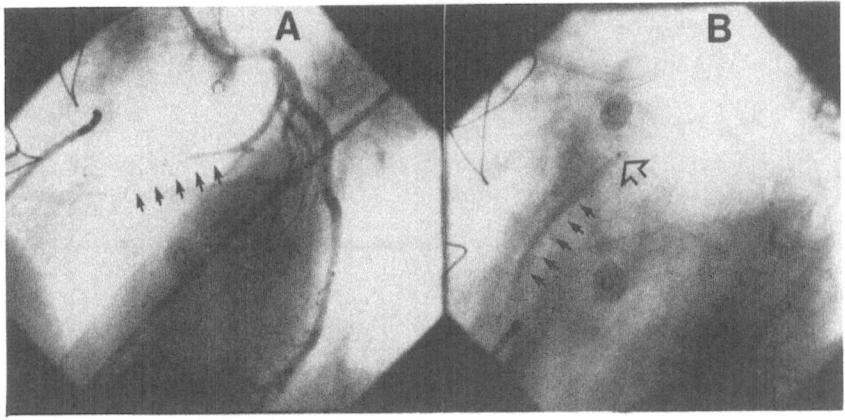

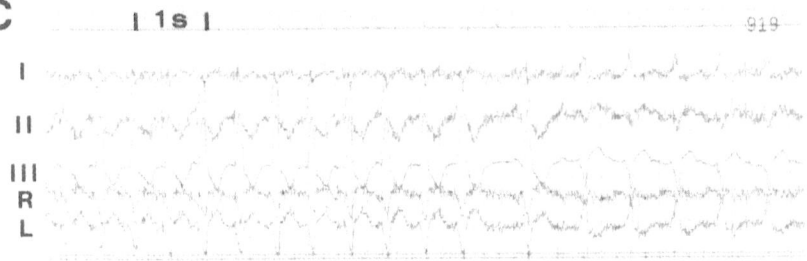

Figure 3. Panel A shows the left anterior oblique projection during left coronary angiography. A septal artery is observed (arrow) before an occluded left anterior descending coronary artery. In panel B the septal branch has been selectively catheterized. In panel C termination of the incessant ventricular tachycardia by iced saline is shown. Administration of ethanol resulted in cure of the arrhythmia. From Brugada P *et al.* Circulation 1989.

Interestingly, in this patient the vessel did not occlude after giving the ethanol. After 5 months follow-up the patient is asymptomatic.

In patients 5 and 6 a similar procedure was followed to cure incessant ventricular tachycardia by giving ethanol in the distal left anterior descending coronary artery and the distal part of a posterior marginal branch from the circumflex coronary artery.

Five patients complained of chest pain during administration of ethanol. The chest pain was, however, very short-lasting (a few seconds) probably because of immediate destruction of the nerve terminals by the ethanol. The oxalactic transaminase rose to 180 units in patient 1, to 89, 80, 190, 140 and 120 in patients 2 to 6 respectively (normal value less than 40 units). A technetium pyrophosphate scan did not show an area of infarction in any patient but patient 4. After cure of incessant ventricular tachycardia the functional class improved in all patients. Patient 1 is in functional class II, patients 2 and 3 have resumed work and are in functional class I. Patient 4 is in functional class II. Patient 5 died of a drug intoxication and patient 6 remains in functional class III.

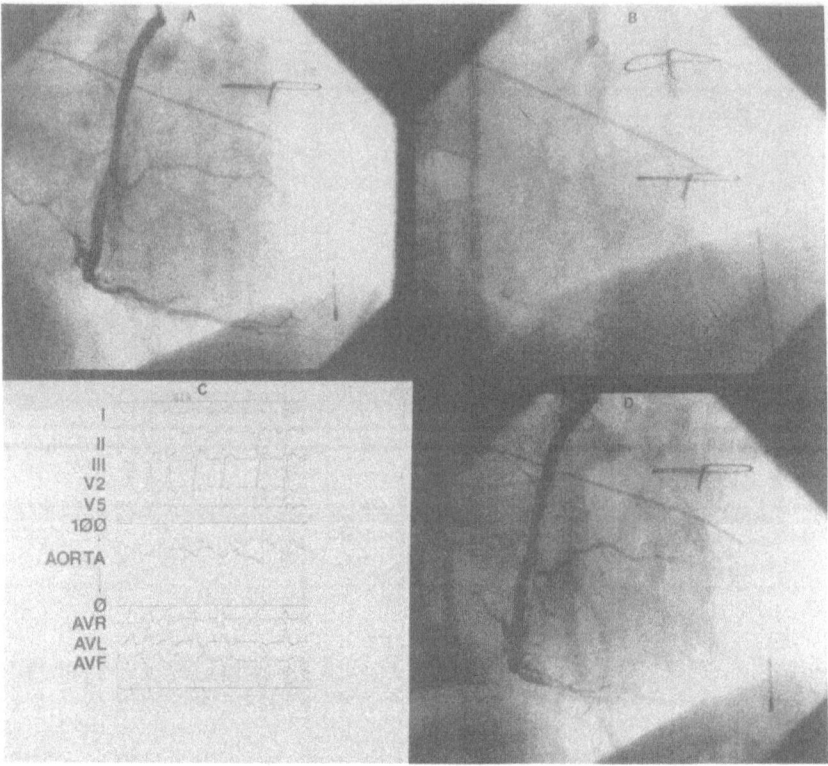

Figure 4. Right anterior oblique projection during right coronary angiography (panel A) and after selecting catheterization of the distal posterior descending coronary artery (panel B). Panel C shows the abrupt termination of ventricular tachycardia with ethanol. Panel D illustrates occlusion of the distral posterior descending coronary artery. From Brugada P *et al.* Circulation 1989.

C. Transcoronary chemical ablation of the atrioventricular node

In two patients with uncontrollable ventricular rates during atrial fibrillation transcoronary chemical ablation of the atrioventricular node was performed after various attempts to ablate the bundle of His with an electric shock had failed. Using the described techniques the atrio-ventricular nodal artery was selectively catheterized. The administration of 1 ml ethanol resulted in permanent complete atrio-ventricular block (Figure 5).

Complication during transcoronary termination and ablation of tachycardias

Selective catheterization of the coronary arteries is not devoid from complications. Manipulation of the catheters resulted in coronary spasm in two patients. The spasm was solved without further consequences. The enzyme

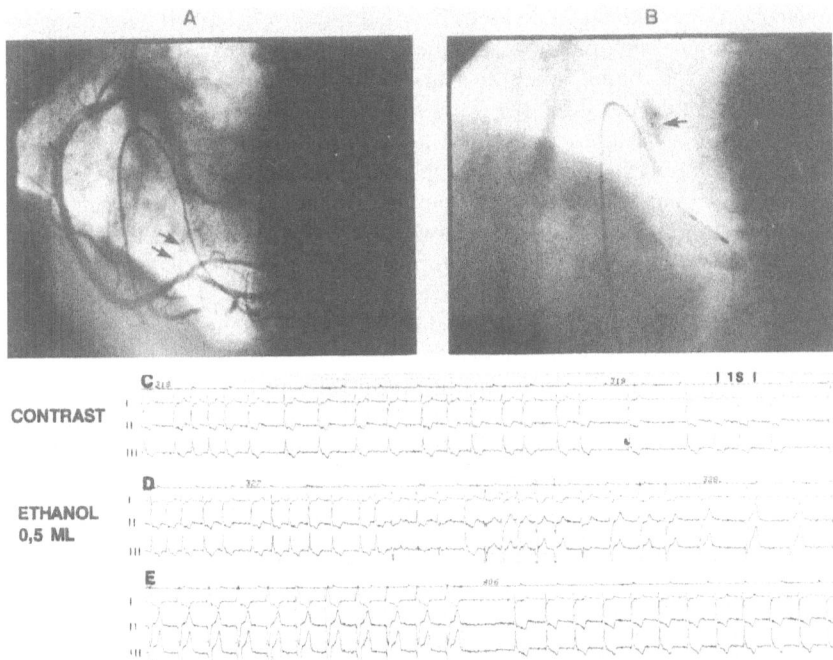

Figure 5. Panel A shows the left anterior obligue projection and the right coronary angiography. The arrows point to the atrio-ventricular nodal artery selectively catheterized in panel B (arrow). Panel C shows the effect of contrast material with transient atrio-ventricular block in the right part. Panel D shows complete atrio-ventricular block after administration of ethanol. Panel E shows ventricular pacing being terminated to illustrate the high regular escape rhythm developing in these patients.

rise after ethanol was expected. It has to be realized that chemical ablation results in a myocardial infarction. In our eight patients destruction of a small myocardial area had enormous benefits in terms of control of their arrhythmia and improvement of their functional class. However, in other patients the benefit may be only marginal (arrhythmias with a better prognosis) or the damage too large (larger infarctions resulting in an overall poorer quality of life). The risk to benefit ratio has to be carefully considered on each individual patient. It seems warranted to presently reserve this technique only for patients without any other therapeutic option until much more information becomes available on the benefits and risks and how to becomes available on the benefits and risks and how to assess its balance in a particular individual.

Discussion

The results of this study demonstrate that there exists a 'tachycardia-related coronary artery' which can be identified and selectively catheterized using the present refined angioplasty techniques. This 'tachycardia-related coronary artery' provides blood flow to the arrhythmogenic area or a critical tachycardia pathway (like the atrio-ventricular node). This 'tachycardia-related' coronary artery can be used to administer chemicals (ethanol in our study) to destroy the arrhythmia substrate or tachycardia pathway. There remain many challenges and open questions for the further refinement of this technique. Findings during transcoronary termination with iced saline may help us better understand many pathophysiologic aspects of arrhythmias in man. A major reconsideration of the concepts utilized during electrical mapping and pacemapping of ventricular tachycardia may be required if one considers the discrepancies between 'electrical' and 'anatomical mapping' findings. We realize, however, that the specificity of the 'tachycardia-related artery' was not completely assessed in our study. Only successful ablation of incessant ventricular tachycardia in our six patients and of the atrio-ventricular node in other 2 support that we localized a critical anatomic area for perpetuation of the arrhythmia. This technique has been developed at a time when major disappointment exists on the results of percutaneous electrical ablation of ventricular tachycardia [10]. Results from transcoronary termination with iced saline may help better define the indications and the technique to be used during percutaneous electrical ablation of arrhythmias. In that way they may become complementary rather than excluding each other.

Further refinement of presently available catheters and guide wires and available radiology tachniques will be required to allow catheterization of still smaller coronary arteries and to unable us reaching in infarct-related vessel retrogradely from collaterals. That will help reduce the amount of myocardial damage while still obtaining the desired effect. It should not be forgotten, however, that chemical ablation is aimed to destroy the arrhythmia substrate, thus a myocardial infarction will always be created. The further success of this technique will depend upon the ability to successful control the arrhythmia while creating less damage than surgery but more damage than unsuccessful percutaneous electrical ablation (which damages less tissue but at the wrong site).

Important questions are also the mechanisms of action of both saline and ethanol from which not much is known at the present time. Also whether saline and ethanol are the best options for the selected purposes is unknown. Saline allows confirmation of the identification of the 'tachycardia-related artery' before definitive ablation is undertaken. In that way, it allows the investigator performing the procedure to anatomically 'map' the area where definitive ablation will be performed. Injection of radioisotopic or contrast material may allow estimation of the mass of myocardium that may eventually be destroyed by the ethanol.

As shown by our fourth patient, successful ablation with ethanol does not necessarily require occlusion of the 'tachycardia-related coronary artery'. As illustrated by our first patient occlusion of the 'tachycardia-related coronary artery' without chemical ablation may by insufficient to destroy the arrhythmia substrate if collateral flow develops. From the theoretic point of view destruction of the 'tachycardia cells' by a chemical without occlusion of the coronary artery should offer the best results.

Successful transcoronary chemical ablation of tachycardia (TCAT) has been performed in our six patients with incessant ventricular tachycardia and two patients with uncontrollable rates during atrial fibrillation. We have not attempted to ablate other types of arrhythmias at the present time. Although we successfully terminated one circus movement tachycardia by means of iced saline given in the atrio-ventricular nodal artery, chemical ablation in patients with an acccessory pathway should ideally be directed to destroy the accessory pathway. One has to realize, however, that we have no information at the present time about blood supply to accessory pathways. This will require extensive pathologic investigation of the normal and abnormal atrioventricular groove. Similarly, extensive investigation of the blood supply to the border zone of an infarction, atrial myocardium and conduction system will further refine and possibly extend the applications of this technique. The basic concept behind this technique is, however, simple: there is a blood supply to any area of the heart capable to generate and/or conduct electrical activity. If the artery providing that blood supply is recognized and selectively catheterized that area can be destroyed using the appropriate chemical. When that area plays a critical role as site of origin or pathway of an arrhythmia, destruction of that area should cure the arrhythmia.

References

1. Brugada P, Lemery R, Talajic M, Della Bella P, Wellens HJJ: Treatment of patients with ventricular tachycardia or fibrillation: First lessons from the 'Parallel Study'. In: Brugada P, Wellens HJJ (eds), Cardiac Arrhythmias: Where to go from here?' Mount Kisco, New York, Futura Publ. Col., 1987, 435—456.
2. Zipes DP, Heger JJ, Miles WH, Mohamed Y, Brown JW, Spielman SR, Prystowski EN: Early experience with an implantable cardiovertor. N Engl J Med 1984; 311: 485—490.
3. Cobb FR, Blumenschein SD, Sealy WC, Boineau JP, Wagner GS, Wallace AG: Successful surgical interruption of the bundle of Kent in patient with Wolff-Parkinson-White syndrome. Circulation 1968; 38: 1018—1029.
4. Guiraudon GM, Klein GJ: Closed heart sugery for Wolff-Parkinson-White syndrome. Int J Cardiol 1984; 5: 387—391.
5. Harken AH, Josephson ME: Surgical management of ventricular tachycardia. In: Josephson ME, Wellens HJJ (eds) Tachycardias: Mechanisms, Diagnosis and Treatment. Philadelphia, Lea and Febiger, 1984, p. 475—487.
6. Kron I, Lerman B, Dimarco J: Extended subendocardial resection: A surgical approach to ventricular tachyarrhythmias that cannot be mapped intraoperatively. J Thorac Cardiovasc Surg 1985; 90: 580—591.
7. Mirowski M, Reid PR, Watkins L, Wesifeldt ML, Mower MM: Clinical treatment of life-threatening ventricular tachyarrhythmias with the automatic implantable defibrillator. Am Heart J 1981; 102: 265—270.

8. Scheinman MM, Evans TG Jr.: Catheter electrical ablation of cardiac arrhythmias. In ref. 1, p. 529—538.
9. Hartzler GO: Electrode catheter ablation of refractory focal ventricular tachycardia. J Am Coll Cardiol 1983; 2: 1107—1113.
10. Evans TG Jr., Scheinman MM and the Executive Committee of the Registry. The percutaneous cardiac mapping and ablation registry: Final summary of results. PACE 1988; 11: 1621—1626.
11. Inoue H, Waller BF, Zipes DP: Intracoronary ethylic alcohol or phenol injection ablates aconitive-induced ventricular tachycardia in dogs. J Am Coll Cardiol 1987; 10: 1342—1349.
12. Ellman BA, Parkhill BJ, Curry III TS, Marcus PB, Peters PC: Ablation of renal tumors with absolute ethanol: A new technique. Radiology 1981; 141: 619—626.
13. Ellman BA, Parkhill BJ, Marcus PB, Curry TS, Peters PC: Renal ablation with absolute ethanol: Mechanism of action. Invest Radio 1984; 19: 416—423.
14. Friedman PL, Steward JR, Fenoglio JJ Jr., Wit AL: Survival of subendocardial Purkinje fibers after extensive myocardial infarction in dogs: In vitro and in vivo correlations. Circ Res 1973; 33: 597—611.
15. Wit AL, Dillon S, Ursell PC: Influence of anisotropic tissue structure on reentrant ventricular tachycardia. In: ref. 1, p. 27—50.
16. Brugada P, Wellens HJJ: Standard diagnostic programmed electrical stimulation protocols in patients with paroxysmal recurrent arrhythmias. PACE 1984; 7: 1121—1128.
17 Josephson ME, Horowitz LN, Farshidi A, Spear JF, Kastor JA, Moore GV: Recurrent sustained ventricular tachycardia: II. Endocardial mapping. Circulation 1978; 57: 440—447.
18. Miller J, Harken AH, Hargrove C, Josephson ME: Pattern of endocardial activation during sustained ventricular tachycardia. J Am Coll Cardiol 1985; 6: 1280—1287.
19. Coumel P: Diagnostic significance of the QRS form in patients with ventricular tachycardia. In: Barold SJ (ed), Cardiology Clinics, August 1987. 12-lead Electrocardiography. Philadelphia, WB Saunders Co., 1987; 527—540.

18. Sudden death and the autonomic nervous system
The prognostic value of heart rate variability

PHILIPPE COUMEL and JEAN-PIERRE DESCHAMPS

Numerous markers have been proposed to evaluate the prognosis of patients having suffering from a myocardial infarction (MI). They range from parameters as simple as age to complex investigations including hemodynamic studies, coronary angiography and programmed electrical stimulation. Non-invasive approaches naturally tend to have the clinicians' preference, and particularly data derived from Holter recordings, so that an abundant, rather controversial and frequently revised literature deals with the prognostic value of ventricular arrhythmias. The discussion is still active about the definition of the most sensitive and specific criteria that should be considered. There is some evidence that relying on a limited view of arrhythmic events to assess the long-term prognosis of a disease that by definition concerns many aspects of the cardiac functions would be illusory, and progressively most of the initially proposed criteria have been abandoned or the emphasis on their value has been tempered. The number of ventricular premature beats, their distribution into isolated extrasystoles with or without bigeminy, with or without repetitive activity, the coupling interval have been claimed to constitute valuable markers of low- or high-risk groups of patients. It is now largely admitted that a common primary condition to any prognostic index is an impaired myocardial function, the most convenient if not the most reliable way for its evaluation being a left ventricular ejection fraction of less that 30 or 40 p. 100.

Post-Mi prognosis: the HRV approach

Heart rate variability (HRV) has been considered since a long time as the possible marker of an impaired heart status conditioning a poor prognosis, but with the remarkable exception of some pioneers [1, 2] it did not provoke a large interest from clinicians. Among many reasons including the difficulty of clearly understanding the complexity of the physiology [3] of the autonomic nervous system (ANS), a real obstacle was the difficulty of standardizing the techniques of evaluation. They require specially oriented

A. Bayés de Luna et al. (eds.): *Sudden Cardiac Death*, 191–207.

laboratory investigations, mainly based on the measurement of the respiration- or blood pressure-related variations of the heart rate on a short term basis. In essence, monitoring continuously the heart rate on a long-term basis during normal activity rather than on the occasion of somewhat experimental and time-limited conditions was the main obstacle. Curiously however the introduction of the Holter technique did not provoke a renewed attention to this problem. The difficulty of evaluating and quantifying HRV certainly was a technical obstacle, but the fact is that the interest of cardiologist was focused on arrhythmias for determining the prognosis of MI. Some disappointment in this area, and overall the demonstrated beneficial effect of beta-blockers in the prevention of sudden death most probably explain the resurgence of interest for the methods exploring the ANS through HRV.

The heart rate variations are dependent upon the ANS and its different components, that not only differ in their function of accelerating or decelerating the heart, but in their neurogenic or humoral origin which conditions the time constant of their influence. When defining the mechanism of the different types of heart rate variations, it is essential not to be manichean because most phenomena depend on a balance rather than on the effect of a single action of a part of the system. Of course, roughly speaking the main function of the vagus nerve is to slow the heart rate whereas the sympathetics accelerate it. However, these functions in fact depend on the starting balance of the system and the decrease of the sympathetic tone or the increase of the vagal drive may slow the heart without producing the same pattern of HRV. The vagal drive is responsible for short-term heart rate changes [4], and the respiratory RR interval variations are easily visible on beat-by-beat tachograms of Holter recordings (Figure 1). According to the reference method formed by the power spectral analysis [5], these fluctuations associated with breathing are responsible for the high-frequency peak centered at values of 0.20 to 0.40 Hz. The significance becomes less and less easy to interpret as the wavelength increases: heart rate oscillations covering 10, 15, 20 second, the so-called Mayer waves [6, 7] certainly have to do with the sympathetic innervation, a fact that does not imply that they only reflect the neurogenic sympathetic activity and that the vagal drive is not concerned. This mid-frequency peak centered between 0.08 and 0.12 Hz was in fact initially related to the frequency effects of the basoreceptor reflex. Much longer oscillations covering up to one or two minutes (Figure 2) can also be observed [8], and they are most probably caused by humoral rather than neurogenic modulations that can involve not only catecholamines but also the renin-angiotensin system [5].

HRV and the post-MI prognosis: a personal experience

Our experience with sudden prediction comes from the retrospective analysis of baseline 24-hour tapes of 20 patients belonging to the IMPACT study

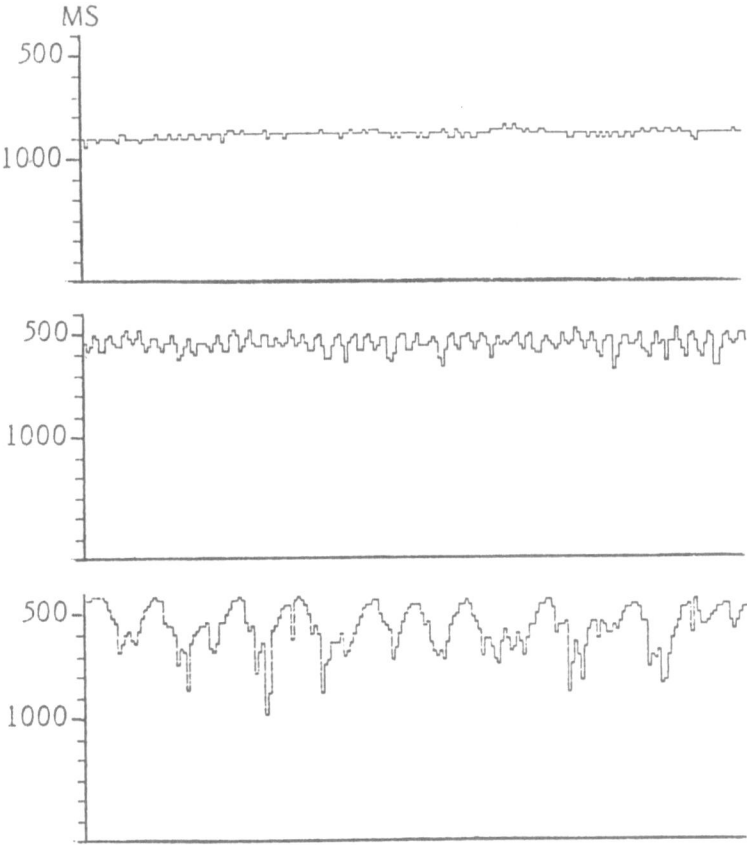

Figure 1. Beat-by-beat visualization of HRV. Cycle-to-cycle changes are clearly visible in the tachograms of Holter recordings. The upper tracing shows a very stable rate. It is in sharp contrast with the middle panel displaying typical respiratory-related heart rate oscillations, whereas the bottom panel shows variations of adrenergic origin, of much longer duration and larger amplitude. Note that the level of heart rate has nothing to do with these different patterns. This tracing was recorded in a 3-year old child.

data bank [9]. Two sets of 10 tapes were matched in such a way that the classically considered arrhythmic events ('simple' and 'complex' arrhythmias . . .) were equivalent. The initial part of our study was conducted blindly and its aim was to detect which 10 patients had died suddenly or survived during the 1-year follow-up of this intervention trial using mexiletine. Just taking into account an increased sinus rate, frequent sudden changes detected at the audio-visual processing of tapes (Figure 2), and the occurrence of any arrhythmias (atrial as well as ventricular) in the context of a sinus tachycardia, we were able to find out 8 of the ultimately dead patients (true positives), 8 of the surviving patients (true negatives), with only 2 false positives and 2

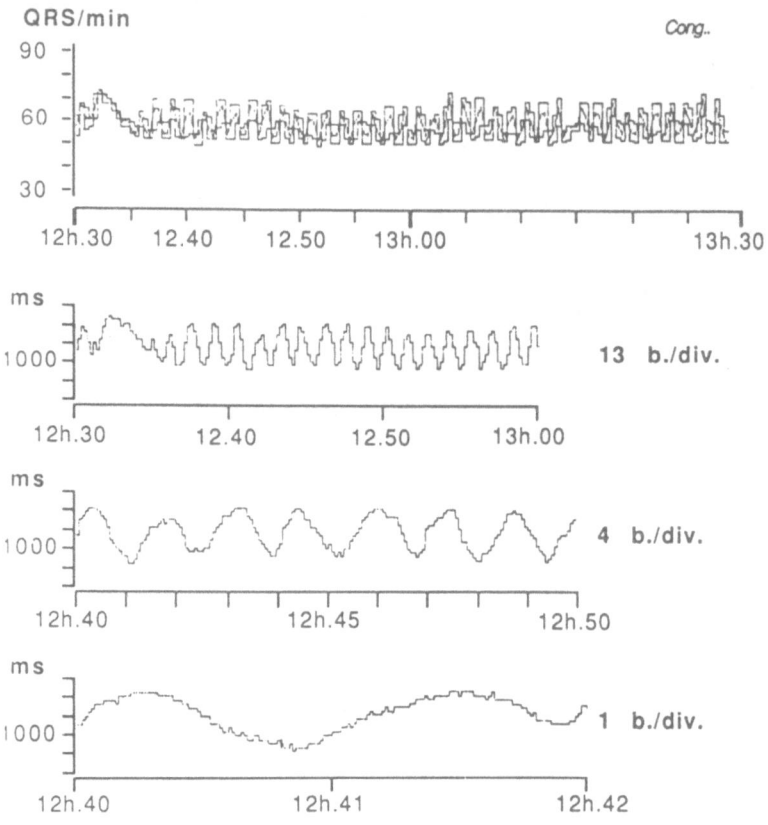

Figure 2. Heart rate oscillations of humoral origin. Heart rate oscillations may involve tens of seconds or minutes, so that using different scales may be useful to evidence them. From bottom to top the the steps of the tracings represent from 1 to 13 beats per division (b./div.), thus giving a more flexible evaluation than the upper usual heart rate trend.

false negatives. The probability of obtaining such a result just by chance was less than 2% at the exact test. It is important to underline that the absence of heart failure was required for inclusion in the IMPACT study.

This experience led us to concentrate on HRV rather than arrhythmia behavior, and the study was continued openly using our method of HRV evaluation. It is based on the detection of oscillatory heart rate changes over a certain number of RR intervals. If, for instance, a sequence of 2 to 4 progressive shorter and shorter (or longer and longer) cycles is preceded and followed by 2 cycles having the opposite trend, this oscillation is stored and its amplitude, i.e., the difference between the longest and the shortest cycle is measured. This category of short, respiration-related heart rate variations corresponds to the high-frequency peak in the frequency domain [5, 7, 10]. Longer oscillations involving a central sequence of acceleration or decelera-

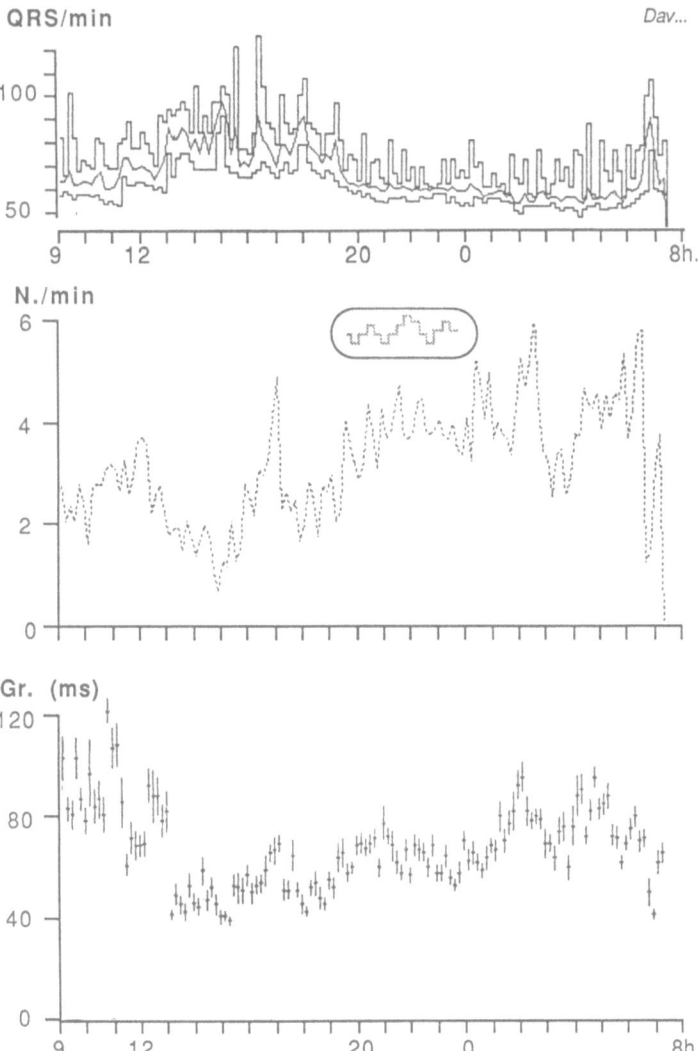

Figure 3. Analysis of respiratory heart rate oscillations. In this 24-hour recording of a normal patient (maximal, mean and minimal heart rate trends in the upper diagram), the short-term cycle length oscillations have been targetted by the computer. They involve shorter and shorter sequences of 2 to 4 cycles preceded and followed by 2 cycles displaying the opposite trend. Oscillations having a minimal amplitude (gradient between the longest and the shortest cycle of the sequence) of 40 ms are quantified in number per minute in the middle diagram, as well as their amplitude ('Gr' for gradient, mean ± SEM) in the lower diagram. The numbers are higher at night than at daytime, whereas the amplitudes are variable.

tion over 8 to 12 cycles surrounded by opposite trends over 5 cycles correspond to the mid-frequency peak, and even longer sequences of 15—30 cycles form the low-frequency peak. The number and the amplitude of each type of oscillation can be considered separately (Figures 3 and 4), or the product of the two expressed in milliseconds, and we verified that it was equivalent to the power spectrum in the frequency domain [11]. The main difference is that our method of valuation can be used in the time domain. The whole 24-hour tracing can be processed in about 20 minutes rather than being restricted to stationary sequences of 256 or 512 beats or seconds, as it is.usually the case with methods based on the fast Fourier transform.

We compared 3 groups of 10 patients, and the data are displayed in Figures 5 and 6. In addition to the two preceding groups of 'survivors' and 'dead' IMPACT patients, we formed a reference cohort of 10 normal subjects. The raw data clearly show large interindividual variations in each group (Figure 5). Not only the relative importance of 'short', 'mean' and 'long' oscillations largely vary from case to case, but the relative importance of each category cannot be standardized. In Figure 6 the results are given for the groups, and if one can easily distinguish some trends, it is by no means possible to separate dead patients from survivors. Interestingly, the best performance is obtained by considering the short, vagally-mediated oscillations. Their 'product' (number times amplitude) is 5282 ± 2358 ms (mean ± SD) in normals, 2812 ± 2026 in survivors, 2152 ± 1667 in dead patients. The difference is significant for the 3 groups (p < 0.01, analysis of variance). However, it is essentially related to the difference between subjects and patients, not between the two groups of patients. Considering the other types of oscillations does not show any significant differences whatsoever between the groups. One can only distinguish trends of diminution from normal to survivors and dead patients for mean (4327 ± 1433 ms, 3828 ± 4151, 2621 ± 1447, respectively) and long (3489 ± 988, 2939 ± 1976, 2129 ± 976) oscillation products. Clearly these trends would have become significant if confirmed over a much large number of cases, but it was not less clear that it would not be possible to individualize further the patients that are really at risk. At this stage the analysis had to be refined.

A very frequent characteristic of patients in comparison to subjects is the alteration of the normal day and night distribution of the different types of oscillations. Figure 3 and 4 displayed the typical pattern in a normal subject, with a predominance of vagally-mediated oscillations at night, and a predominance of sympathetics-related oscillations at daytime. This pattern is very frequently altered in patients, in whom the curves tend to parallel (Figure 7). Considering the two trends of a decreased HRV (whatever the category of oscillations) and altered circadian behavior, we defined an HRV index as the sum of the different types of oscillations, each being weighted by its own circadian behavior: night/day ratio for the short, day/night ratio for the mean and long oscillations. This sensitized HRV index was higher than the basic values in survivors (15349 ± 9745 ms vs. 14654 ± 9712). What

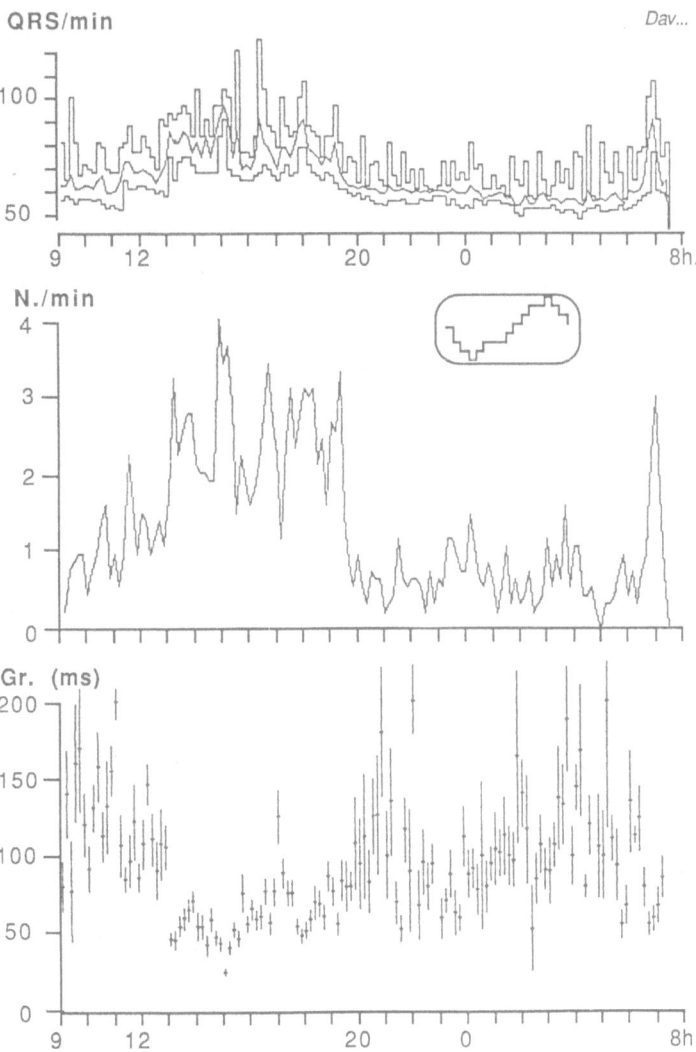

Figure 4. Analysis of adrenergic heart rate oscillations. In the same patient as in Figure 3, longer sequences including 8 to 12 accelerating or decelerating cycles are analyzed in terms of number and amplitude. Their behavior differs from that of short oscillations: they are more numerous at daytime than at night. The same would apply to longer oscillations involving more than 15 cycles. The absolute value of the amplitude of the two categories obviously differ, but their relative changes throughout the 24-hour period are parallel.

was only a trend between the two groups became a significant difference clearly displayed in Figure 8 using the χ^2 test: with a cut-off value of 14000 ms, only 3 survivors, and 9 out of 10 dead patients were individual-

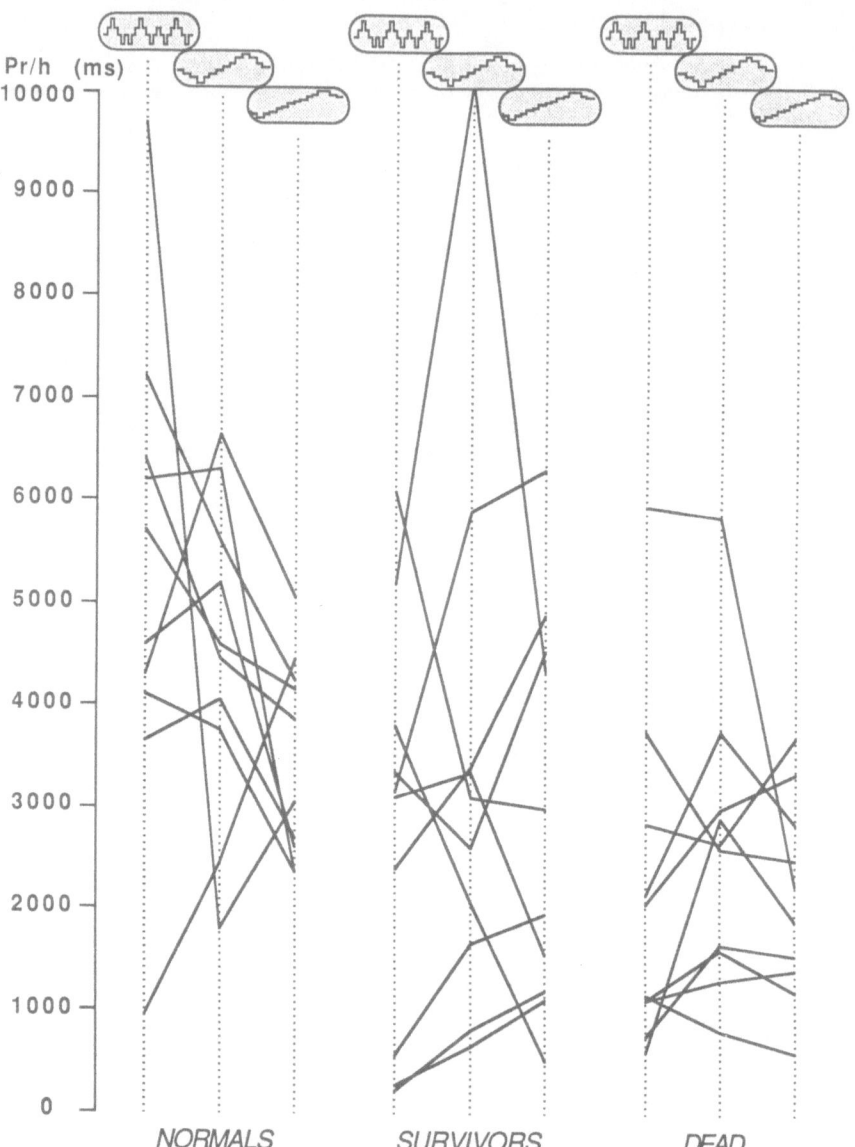

Figure 5. Individual data of survivors and dead patients of the IMPACT study, compared to normals. The groups are composed of 10 cases. Tapes of normal subjects are compared to baseline tapes of 20 patients divided into two groups according to the outcome during the 1-year follow-up: 10 survivals and 10 sudden deaths. The quantification of short, mean and long oscillations according to the numbers of beats of the central sequence (2—4, 8—12, 15—30 respectively) are expressed by the product (per hour) of amplitude times number (in ms). The magnitude of interindividual variations is striking, even though a general trend of decreasing values can be distinguished from left to right.

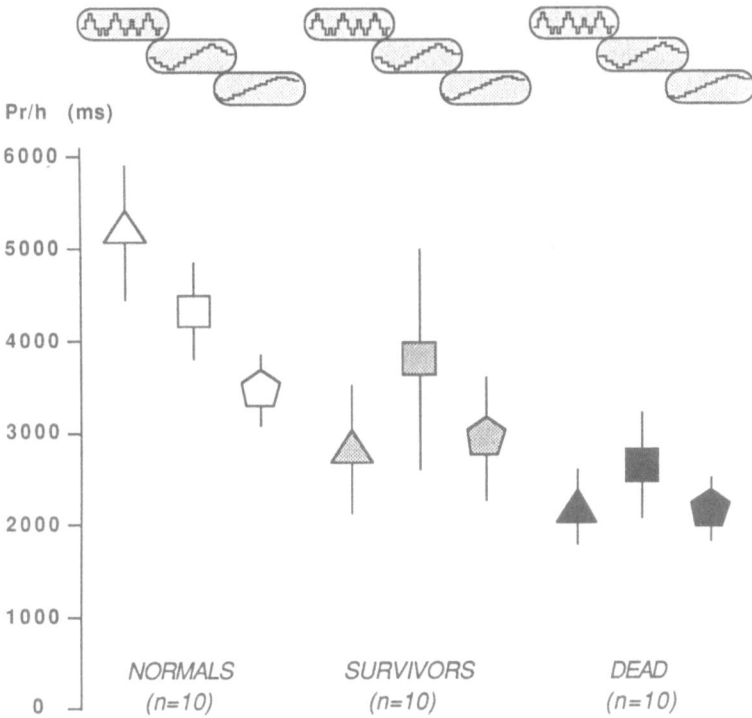

Figure 6. Averaged data of survivors and dead patients compared to normals. The mean values (± SEM) of short (triangles), mean (squares) and long (pentagones) oscillations are given for the groups of 10 normal (open symbols), 10 survivors (grey symbols) and 10 patients dead during the 1-year follow-up (solid symbols). There is a clear trend of decreasing values from normal subjects to survivors and dead patients. However, a significant difference was only evidenced for the short oscillations, and it was restricted to separating subjects from patients.

ized, a significant difference between the two groups ($p < 0.01$). Of course all the 10 normal subjects were above this cut-off value.

This experience shows that we can indeed demonstrate a prognostic value of HRV which in the present case permits to designate the patients at risk not as a group but as individuals. However, there are at least two limitations of this study. One is that the HRV index we finally chosed after others was carefully tuned for these groups, and it remains to be verified if it would be as effective in other randomly selected tapes, a process we are presently carrying out. Another limitation is that the tapes initially selected had been matched in terms of arrhythmias, not in age, and a significant difference between the two groups appeared when the code was open, the survivors being younger by more than 6 years ($p < 0.05$). As it is well established that HRV diminishes with age, clearly this bias favors the HRV index performance for detecting high-risk patients. On the other hand, it can be argued

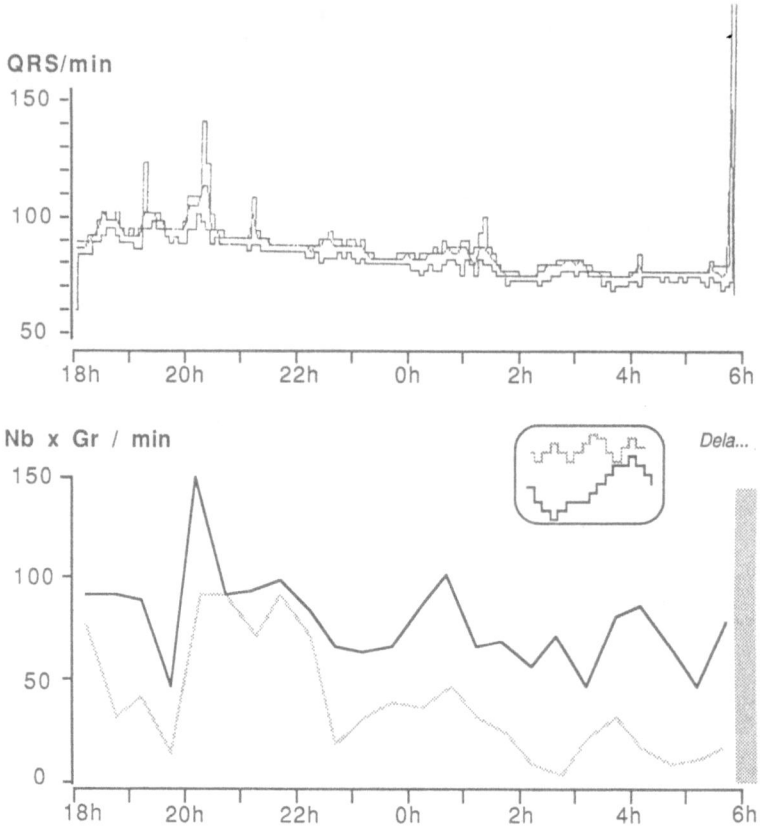

Figure 7. Trends of hourly values of oscillations in a patient dying suddenly. The product (number times gradient) is expressed in milliseconds per minute of recording for the vagally-mediated and adrenergic types of oscillations in the ambulatory recording of a severely diseased patient who actually died suddenly at the end of the recording. Not only the values are less than half the normality, but the distribution is particular: the parallelism between the two curves is in contrast with the behavior observed in normal (compare with Figure 3 and 4). Another evidence of the globally decreased HRV is given by the pattern of the heart rate trends: the difference between the maximal and minimal heart rates is very much reduced.

that age itself is indeed a classical factor of poor prognosis in the MI follow-up, so that it is correct to include implicitely in any index this factor, as probably others that are not clearly individualized.

Methods, experiences and significance of HRV evaluation

A number of methods have now been described for assessing HRV. They are not equivalent, but they do concur to emphasize the poor prognosis included in decreased HRV. It is not easy to understand why methods that are

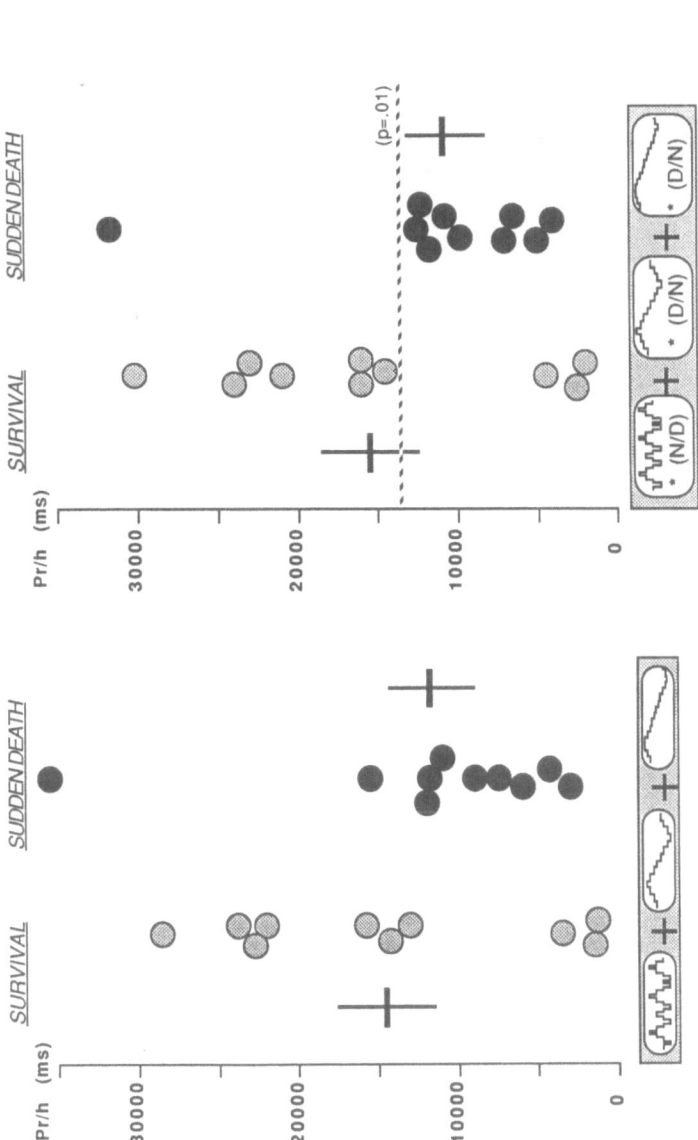

Figure 8. Sudden death prediction and the HRV index. In the left diagram, summing up the basic values displayed in figures 5 and 6 for the groups of survivors and dead patients does not allow to find any significant difference in terms of groups (analysis of variance) or individuals. On the right diagram, an HRV index was weighted according to the normal day (D) and night (N) distribution of the various types of short, mean and long oscillations. The effect of sensitizing this HRV quantification was to obtain at the chi2 test (cut-off value of the product at 14000 ms) a p value of 0.01 between the survivors and dead patients, thus permitting to individualize high-risk patients with a good probability.

addressing very different aspects of HRV are finally so consistent in the message they deliver.

Methods of evaluation of HRV

The power spectral analysis is generally accepted as the reference for the development of other approaches of HRV quantification, even though after all using time-series techniques in the frequency domain (Fourier analysis) may not be the most appropriate method: in particular it supposes the stationarity of the data and the symmetry of heart rate oscillations, two conditions that are never strictly respected [12]. The consequence is that the possibilities are limited by the necessity of studying short, carefully selected periods which may not reflect totally the clinical reality. These limitations explain in part why, in the recent resurgence of interest concerning the HRV [7], other methods have been proposed [13—16] that must be replaced in the context of the more classical ones [1, 2, 17, 18]. Figure 9 situates some of the methods that were recently critically reviewed [10] with respect to the three high-mid- and low-frequency peaks of the frequency domain, or the short, mean and long oscillations used in the time domain with our or other [12] methods. The most global evaluation certainly is provided by the standard deviation of RR intervals during long periods of up to 24 hours [19]: obviously this method excludes any approach of the dynamicity of the ANS because it realizes a mixture of the different types of HRV occuring over seconds to hours. The result is the impossibility to distinguish any type of dysfunction of the ANS. The counterpart of this limitation is the robustness of the method which is particularly easy to handle and in fact already exists more or less in many commercially available Holter processing systems. Unsurprisingly, strong correlations can be evidenced between this method and others that are all dealing with the low- or extremely low-frequencies like the day-night difference in mean heart rate or the 'heart rate spikes' [4], because all these approaches have in fact nothing to do with the short-term HRV. Considering the mean of standard deviations of RR intervals over 5 min segments [20] acts as a high-pass filter in the Fourier domain, suppressing in particular the day-to-night variations, the heart rate spikes and oscillations of the type we showed in figure 2 for instance. The contrary applies to the standard deviation of the means of 5 min segments that for Myers [10] represents a low-pass filter of approximately 0.006 Hz. A very original method proposed by Ewing [13] was to count the number of beat-to-beat transitions greater than 50 ms ('BB 50'), and because it compares adjacent cycles, by definition it concerns the high-frequency peak of the power spectrum. The same applies to the 'mean circular resultant' [16], particularly directed to exploring the repiration-related cycle length variations. Finally, the baroreflex sensitivity [18] explores a complex reflex arc [21] in which the vagus is certainly the efferent route, whereas the afferent nerves are of sympathetic as well as parasympathetic nature.

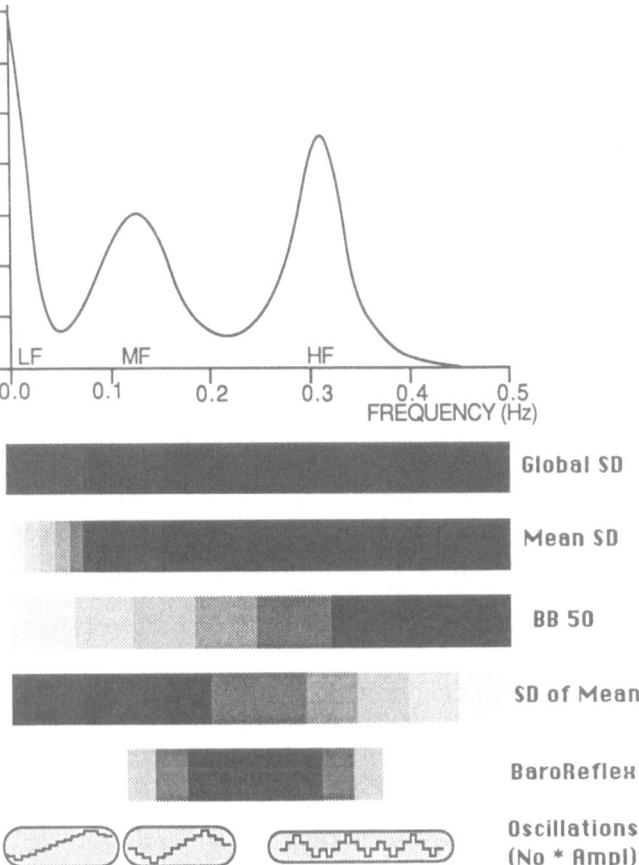

Figure 9. Various indices of HRV in the frequency domain. The power spectral analysis is figured in the upper part of the diagram as the reference, including the 3 classical high- (HF), mid- (MF) and low-frequency peaks, expressed in Hz (the scale in the vertical axis is arbitrary). These peaks correspond to the short, mean and and long oscillations of the heart rate in the time domain. Other methods of evaluation are represented in terms of sensitivity to this or that type of HRV in the frequency domain, the darker areas figuring the most sensitive to any type of frequency, and to a lesser extent this also applies to the 'mean SD' (mean of the standard deviations of 5-min segments). The 'BB 50' (number of > 50 ms differences between adjacent cycles) only deals with high-frequency variability, whereas the contrary applies to the 'SD of the mean' (standard deviation of the means of 5-min segments). Finally, the baroreflex sensitivity deals with a complex reflex involving the neurogenic vectors of the vago-sympathetic balance (high- and mid-frequency peaks) but not the humoral adrenergic stimulation (low frequency).

To summarize this rapid review it is clear that the various methods do not explore the same components of HRV, hence comparable aspects of the ANS functions. If we try to express it in physiological terms, some approaches obviously focus on the vagal drive by exploring essentially the respiratory HRV, and some only explore the adrenergic influences of humoral origin that have wavelengths of the order of one minute to several hours. The baroreflex sensitivity are somewhere in-between these extremes whereas the power spectral analysis, the peak-trough method [12] or our method of quantification of oscillations have the ambition of exploring selectively all the various components of the system.

HRV and the prognosis of cardiopathies

The general experience is that HRV decreases as the cardiopathy progresses [1, 2, 10, 16, 19, 20, 22—25]. Not only heart failure [1, 24] but the simple existence of a coronary heart disease [22], contribute to diminish the HRV, and the evolution of the changes that follow MI can be traced [23, 26]. Studies aiming at a more accurate evaluation of prognosis, particularly the prediction of death and sudden death provide consistent results. Statistically significant features are documented either thanks to the large number of cases [19] or to the sensitivity of the method [8, 10, 25], and our personal experience we have just reported is in accordance.

What is striking in this rapidly increasing literature is the fact that it is consistent no matter the method used. One would expect that exploring selectively the different types of HRV would provide a better sensitivity than a global approach. This is partly verified by the fact that the high-frequency HRV dealing essentially with the parasympathetics is more effective to separate the groups or the individuals than less selective methods. This was true in our experience where short oscillations distinguished normals from patients whereas other types did not, and the same applies to the baroreflex method [25]. Still, incrementing the number of cases and the follow-up duration remains the best way to overcome the important dispersion of individual data (Figure 5). In this sense, considering the global HRV makes the statistical analysis easier even though it leaves some frustration about the practical interest of more selective evaluations. Refining the use of the latter is certainly the best way to improve the predictive value of the studies, as we did for defining our HRV index. However, what we really need is a better understanding of the significance of the various types of oscillations, their relationships with the complex physiology of the ANS. Just to take the example of the method we are presently using, it is by far not demonstrated that expressing its results in terms of product 'amplitude times number' is the best way to exploit it. We simply did so because by analogy with the power spectrum, but it may well be that the two components of the product do not have the same physiological significance. The amplitude of the heart rate oscillations may be an image of the flexibility of the sinus response through the various types of receptors, whereas the number may reflect in some way the neural traffic.

Significance of HRV

There must be fundamental reasons explaining the decreased HRV and its very different modalities from patient to patient. Heart failure is well-known for diminishing the beta-adrenergic receptor density [27, 28]. This is supposed to explain the decreased sensitivity to catecholamines [27] that contrast with an enhanced sinus rate sensitivity to beta-blockers, and coexists with a decreased sensitivity to atropine that has been demonstrated as well [1]. These blunted sensitivities coexist with a dramatically increased traffic in the sympathetic nerves [29]. What we are evaluating with HRV is the global result of the very complex interplay of a chain of components forming the ANS. Neural and humoral vectors are permanently interacting behind a sort of curtain formed by the receptors that transmit the balanced influences to the sinus node. The existence of a patent heart failure is otherwise not the common explanation of a decreased HRV: this was not the Kleiger's experience [19], and it is not ours with the IMPACT patients who were supposed not to have this condition to be included in the study. Even in the absence of a cardiac insufficiency that by definition indicates the failure of compensatory mechanisms, the intermediate stage of myocardial dysfunction provokes the ANS reactions we are able to evaluate. A decreased flexibility of the ANS indicates that it is stressed for reasons that may not be patent. HRV measures this flexibility, which may be altered at the expense of this or that of its components, thus probably explaining why its features may be different from patient to patient, but with the common result of an impaired adaptive function.

References

1. Eckberg DL, Drabinsky M, Braunwald E: Defective cardiac parasympathetic control in patients with heart disease. New Engl J Med 1971: 285; 877—883.
2. Hinkle LE, Carver ST, Plakun A: Slow heart rates and increased risk of cardiac death in middle-aged men. Arch Int Med 1972: 129; 732—750.
3. Levy MN: Sympathetic-parasympathetic interactions in the heart. Circulation Res 1971: 29; 437—445.
4. Katona PG, Jih F: Respiratory sinus arrhythmia: noninvasive measure of parasympathetic cardiac control. J Appl Physiol 1975: 39; 801—805.
5. Askelrod S, Gordon D, Ubel FA, Shannon DC, Barger AC, Cohen RJ: Power spectrum analysis of heart rate fluctuations: a quantitative probe of beat-to-beat cardiovascular control. Science 1981: 213; 220—222.
6. Preiss G, Polosa C: Patterns of sympathetic neuron activity associated with Mayer waves. Am J Physiol 1974: 226; 724—730.
7. Pagani M, Lombardi F, Guzzetti F, Rimoldi O, Furlan R, Pizzinelli P, Sandrone G, Malfatto G, Dell'Orto S, Piccaluga E, Turiel M, Baselli G, Cerutti S, Malliani A: Power spectral analysis of heart rate and arterial pressure variabilities as a marker of sympatho-vagal interaction in man and conscious dog. Circulation Res 1986: 59; 178—193.

8. Goldberger AL, Rigney DR, Berman AD, Mietus J, Weistein JS, Moody GB, Antman EM, Greenwald S. Periodic heart rate dynamics in sudden cardiac death syndrome: spectral analysis (abst). J Am Coll Cardiol 1988: 11; 199A.

9. IMPACT RESEARCH GROUP: International Mexiletine and Placebo Antiarrhythmic Coronary Trial I. Report on arrhythmia and other findings. JACC 4; 1148—1984.

10. Myers GA, Martin GJ, Magid NM, Barnett PS, Schaad JW, Weiss JS, Lesch M, Singer DH: Power spectral analysis of heart rate variability in sudden cardiac death: comparison to other methods. IEEE Trans Biomed Eng 1986: BME 33; 1149—1156.

11. Kauffmann F, Maison-Blanche P, Cauchemez B, Deschamps JP, Clairambault J, Coumel P, Henry J, Sorine M: A study of non stationary phenomena of HRV during 24-hour ECG ambulatory monitoring. Med & Biol Eng & Comput 1988: 26 (in press).

12 Schechtman VL, Kluge KA, Harper RM: Time-domain system for assessing variation in heart rate. Med & Biol Eng & Comput 1988: 26 (in press).

13. Ewing DJ, Neilson MM, Travis P: New method for assessing cardiac parasympathetic activity using 24-hour electrocardiograms. Br Heart J 1982: 52; 396—402.

14. Bigger JT, Kleiger RE, Fleiss JL, Rolnitzky LM, Steinman RC, Miller JP, the Multicenter Post-Infarction Research Group: Components of heart rate variability measured during healing of acute myocardial infarction. Am J Cardiol 1988: 61; 208—215.

15. Schwartz PJ, Vanoli E, Stramba-Badiale M, De Ferrari GM, Billman GE, Foreman RD: Autonomic mechanisms and sudden death. New insights from analysis of baroceptor reflexes in conscious dogs with and without a myocardial infarction. Circulation 1988: 78, 969—979.

16. Genovely H, Pfeifer MA: RR-variation: the automonic test of choice in diabetes. Diabetes/Metabolism Reviews 1988: 4; 255—271.

17. Opmeer CHJM: The information content of successive RR interval times in the ECG. Preliminary results using factor analysis and frequency analysis. Ergonomics 1973: 16; 105—112.

18. Smyth HS, Sleight P, Pickering GW: Reflex regulation of arterial pressure during sleep in man: a quantitative method of assessing baroreflex activity. Circulation Res 1969: 24; 109—121.

19. Kleiger RE, Miller JP, Bigger JT, Moss AJ, the Multicenter Post-Infarction Research Group: Decreased heart rate variability and its association with increased mortality after acute myocardial infarction. Am J Cardiol 1987: 59; 256—262.

20. Magid NM, Martin GJ, Kehoe RF, Zheutlin A, Eckberg DL, Myers GA, Barnett PS, Murray EA, Gonzales SK, Weiss JS, Lesch M, Singer DH: Diminished heart rate variability in sudden cardiac death. Circulation 1985: 72.

21. Smith SA, Stallard TJ, Salih MM, Littler WA: Can sinoaortic baroreceptor heart rate reflex sensitivity be determined from phase IV of the Valsalva manoeuvre? Cardiovasc Res 1987: 21; 422—427.

22. Airaksinen KEJ, Ikäheimo MJ, Linnaluoto MK, Niemelä M, Takkunen JT: Impaired vagal heart rate control in coronary artery disease. Br Heart J 1987: 58; 592—597.

23. Lombardi F, Sandrone G, Pernpruner S, Sala R, Garimoldi M, Cerutti S, Baselli G, Pagani M, Malliani A: Heart rate variability as an index of sympathovagal interaction after acute myocardial infarction. Am J Cardiol 1987: 60; 1239—1245.

24. Saul JP, Arai Y, Berger RD, Lilly LS, Colucci WS, Cohen RJ: Assessment of autonomic regulation in chronic congestive heart failure by heart rate spectral analysis. Am J Cardiol 1988: 61; 1291—1299.

25. La Rovere MT, Specchia G, Mortara A, Schwartz PJ: Baroreflex sensitivity, clinical correlates, and cardiovascular mortality among patients with a first myocardial infarction. A prospective study. Circulation 1988: 78; 816—824.

26. Schwartz PJ, Zaza A, Pala M, Locati E, Beria G, Zanchetti A: Baroreflex sensitivity and its evolution during the first year after myocardial infarction. J Am Coll Cardiol 1988: 12; 629—636.

27. Bristow MR, Ginsburg MR, Minobe W, Cubiciotti RS, Sageman S, Luire K, Billingham ME, Harrison DC, Stinson EB: Decreased catecholamine sensitivity and beta-adrenergic receptor density in failing human hearts. New Engl J Med 1982: 307; 205—211.
28. Hertel C, Müller F, Portenlier M, Staehelin M: Determination of the desensitization of beta-adrenergic receptors by (3H)CGP 12177. Biochem J 1983: 216; 669—674.
29. Leimbach WN, Wallin BG, Victor RG, Aylward PE, Sundlöf G, Mark AL: Direct evidence from intraneural recordings for increased central sympathetic outflow in patients with heart failure. Circulation 1986: 73; 913—919.

19. Ventricular electrical instability
Markers and trigger mechanisms

GÜNTER BREITHARDT, MARTIN BORGGREFE and
ANTONI MARTÍNEZ-RUBIO

The underlying arrhythmia in most patients who die suddenly outside the hospital is some type of ventricular tachyarrhythmia, mostly monomorphic ventricular tachycardia degenerating into ventricular fibrillation. This has been shown in a multitude of long-ECG recordings in patients who died suddenly [1, 2]. In only a minority of patients, sudden cardiac death is due to bradyarrhythmias. Bayés de Luna *et al.* reported on 61 patients from the literature who died from ventricular fibrillation during ambulatory long-term ECG recording [1]. Though ventricular fibrillation was the initial rhythm in 28% of cases, the initial rhythm was a monomorphic ventricular tachycardia subsequently degenerating into ventricular fibrillation in 69% of cases. In the remaining 3% of cases, ventricular flutter degenerated into ventricular fibrillation. These initiating ventricular tachycardias frequently had a rate below 300 bpm [2].

The mechanisms that led to the development of ventricular tachyarrhythmias have been studied in animal models and in man [3—6]. From these studies, several mechanisms emerged that underly the occurrence of ventricular tachyarrhythmias and subsequent sudden cardiac death (Table 1). Since most cases of sudden cardiac death occur in patients with coronary artery disease, mainly after a previous myocardial infarction, this clinical spectrum has been studied most extensively. It has become apparent that the most important factors are the frequency and type of spontaneous ventricular

Table 1. Pathophysiological mechanisms of sudden cardiac death.

Chronic electrophysiological abnormalities
Transient ischemia
— acute coronary occlusion without/with a preceeding myocardial infarction
— coronary spasm
— unstable coronary artery plaques leading to embolization into the peripheral coronary system
— exercise induced ischemia
Changes in autonomous nervous innervation

A. Bayés de Luna et al. (eds.): *Sudden Cardiac Death*, 209–222.
© 1991 Kluwer Academic Publishers, Dordrecht.

arrhythmias, the degree of left ventricular dysfunction, the occurrence of ischemia, and the modulation by the autonomous nervous system.

In this paper, those factors and mechanisms that are presently considered as important for the genesis of ventricular tachyarrhythmias and, thus, sudden cardiac death will be discussed with the main focus on patients with coronary artery disease. Any description of the mechanisms leading to sudden cardiac death has to take into consideration those factors that have been shown to be important for assessing prognosis in patients with coronary artery disease, mainly after previous myocardial infarction [7, 8]. In addition, it should explain why some patients have frequent and complex ventricular arrhythmias during long-term ECG-recording after myocardial infarction but do not die suddenly whereas others who die suddenly, may have had less dramatic findings in their ECG.

It is now generally accepted that most episodes of ventricular tachyarrhythmias are due to reentry that may occur in small, circumscribed areas of the myocardium, mostly in areas of previous myocardial infarction. Alternatively, it may involve larger parts of the ventricles. Reentry mostly needs some area of abnormal tissue with the propensity to develop slow conduction and initiating factors (trigger factors) that start reentrant excitation. Trigger factors may be single premature ventricular beats, ventricular couplets or short runs of ventricular tachycardia (salvoes) or an episode of ischemia affecting the potential reentrant circuit. The tissue capable of developing reentry may be permanently abnormal or may change its electrophysiological characteristics transiently under the influence of ischemia.

The role of spontaneous ventricular arrhythmias as trigger factors for ventricular tachyarrhythmias has been shown in patients after myocardial infarction in whom the risk of subsequently dying suddenly was closely related to frequent and repetitive ventricular arrhythmias [8]. However, a substantial number of patients who die suddenly after myocardial infarction do not have frequent and complex spontaneous ventricular arrhythmias [7]. In the presence of an abnormal tissue with the propensity to ventricular tachyarrhythmias, also artificially induced premature beats using programmed ventricular stimulation may induce ventricular tachyarrhythmias [3, 9—14]. Changes in the activation properties within the potential reentrant circuit due to changes in basic heart rate may also cause reentrant excitation [6, 15]. These events may obviously be modulated by changes in autonomic nervous innervation [16, 17]. If there is no abnormal or potentially abnormal tissue in the ventricles, the same spontaneous ventricular arrhythmias will not initiate reentry. This explains why spontaneous ventricular arrhythmias are benign in otherwise healthy hearts [18].

Arrhythmogenic substrate

An abnormal tissue that may become the site for the genesis and maintenance of reentry, may be called an 'arrhythmogenic substrate'. Though this term is obviously not well defined, its use has some conceptual advantages as it suggests that the occurrence of high grade ventricular tachyarrhythmia is not due to an abnormal response of the whole ventricles but instead is due to an area with abnormal electrophysiological properties.

Experimental and clinical studies have provided evidence that myocardial infarction may leave a zone of electrically abnormal ventricular myocardium that may have the propensity to ventricular tachycardia, the 'arrhythmogenic substrate'. This tissue is mostly located at the border zone of a previous myocardial infarction. It is characterized by islands of relatively viable muscle alternating with areas of necrosis and later fibrosis. Such tissue may result in fragmentation of the propagating electromotive forces with the consequent development of high-frequency components that can be recorded directly from these areas [4–6, 19, 20] or noninvasively using signal-averaging techniques [9, 10, 21–30]. The fragmented signals that can be recorded from these areas have been called 'ventricular late potentials' [26]. The individual components of fragmented electrograms most probably represent asynchronuous electrical activity in each of the separate bundles of the surviving muscle under the electrode. The intrinsic asymmetry of cardiac activation due to fibre orientation (anisotropy) may be accentuated by infarction and may predispose to reentry [4, 20]. The slow activation of these areas might result from conduction over circuitous pathways caused by the separation and distortion of the myocardial fibre bundles. The low amplitude of the electrograms from these regions probably results from the paucity of surviving muscle fibres under the electrode because of the large amounts of connective tissue, and not from depression of the action potentials. Therefore, the anatomic substrate for reentry seems to be present in regions where fragmented electrograms can be recorded which, thus, indicates slow inhomogenous conduction.

In the chronic post-myocardial infarction phase, the 'arrhythmogenic substrate' is usually considered to be permanently present in form of myocardium interspersed with fibrosis. However, a zone with arrhythmogenic properties may also arise acutely and be present only transiently. The classical example of an acutely developing arrhythmogenic tissue is acute myocardial infarction that is frequently accompanied by ventricular fibrillation. The changes that occur in this situation are frequently transient in nature and may subside as soon as the tissue is completely necrotic.

Ischemia may also occur in the presence of a chronic 'arrhythmogenic substrate'. The importance of this combination is suggested by the high incidence of recurrent ventricular fibrillation and sudden cardiac death in survivors of out-of-hospital cardiac arrest where ischemic events in the presence of preexisting healed myocardial infarction, obviously, enhance the risk of the occurrence of fatal arrhythmias. The importance of this mechanism has been demonstrated in experimental studies where ventricular fibrillation could result from ischemia at a site remote from previous myocardial infarction [15, 31]. Other studies have shown that cat hearts with acute infarction superimposed on healed myocardial infarction have a greater incidence of spontaneous and induced ventricular arrhythmias than do hearts with acute infarction alone [32].

Ischemia may be confined to a small area of the myocardium that may be too small to sustain a reentrant tachycardia. However, it may be a site of origin for some type of abnormal automaticity that may act as a trigger factor modifying a chronic arrhythmogenic tissue after previous myocardial infarction in a way that it is able to sustain a tachyarrhythmia. Such acute (transient) changes in the electrophysiological properties of the arrhythmogenic substrate, either affecting it directly (hereby slowing conduction velocity and modifying refractory periods) or indirectly via ischemia-induced spontaneous repetitive ventricular activity acting as a trigger factor, may be an important mechanism for the occurrence of sudden cardiac death. Davies *et al.* [33], e.g., were able to show that in patients who died suddenly within 6 hours after onset of symptoms, 50% had either isolated multifocal microscopic necrosis or regional coagulative necrosis. This was frequently caused by unstable plaques in the proximal coronary arteries due to rupture with or without trombus deposition. Partly, this thrombotic material might have been washed downwards into the coronary system. Similar conclusions might be derived from a study by Falk [34] who reported on the significance of platelet microemboli in sudden cardiac death occurring within 24 hours. Further support for the role of intramyocardial platelet aggregates in survivors of cardiac arrest was recently presented by Lo *et al.* [35]. Ruptured atherosclerotic plaques manifested angiographically were more prevalent in patients without inducible monomorphic ventricular tachycardia (11 of 22 patients, 50%) than in those with it (5 of 27 patients, 19%, $p < 0.05$). Similarly, a higher incidence of ruptured plaques was found in patients without akinetic or dyskinetic segments (8 of 14 patients, 57%) than in those with them (8 of 34 patients, 24%, $p < 0.06$). Thus, ruptured plaques were more prevalent in patients without a demonstrable anatomic and/or electrophysiologic substrate for reentrant ventricular tachycardia.

Another factor that may cause transient episodes of regional ischemia serving as a trigger factor, may be the occurrence of coronary arterial spasm. Bertrand *et al.* [36] reported that 20% of patients with recent transmural myocardial infarction showed provocation of coronary spasm after intravenous injection of 0.4 mg methergine compared to only 6.2% in patients studied later after myocardial infarction.

The relatively small areas of necrosis as found in the studies by Davies *et al.* [33] and Falk [34] are themselves not sufficient to cause ventricular fibrillation. However, by acting as a trigger factor by locally inducing spontaneous ventricular activity, they might induce ventricular tachyarrhythmias at sites distant from the one of ischemia. This latter mechanism, though still hypothetical, would explain why these patients died suddenly from such small areas of necrosis without evidence of extended myocardial infarction.

This may present a link between anatomic and physiologic disturbances in sudden cardiac death [37]. Another apparent difference between the patient with the chronic arrhythmogenic substrate and the one with an acute ischemic syndrome due to a ruptured plaque obviously is the difference in time between onset of symptoms and death. In the latter situation, it is conceivable that focal necrosis needs some time to develop and expand during which the adequate conditions for triggering a ventricular tachyarrrhythmias are met.

Thus, on the basis of the data presented above, one might speculate that a previous myocardial infarction provides the 'arrhythmogenic substrate' which is then triggered by ischemia-induced ventricular arrhythmias occurring at a site distant from this infarction. This would be another explanation for the observation by Patterson *et al.* [15] that transient ischemia caused ventricular fibrillation only if there was a previous myocardial infarction. Though these hypothetical links between disturbances in coronary circulation due to regional occlusions and sudden death are attractive, they are not yet corroborated by data from clinical intervention studies.

In the recent preliminary report from the aspirin component of the ongoing Physicians Health Study [38], there was no significant difference in the prevalence of sudden cardiac death (JCD code 798) in those on placebo compared to aspirin. In contrast, data from the registry of the Coronary Artery Surgery Study (CASS) [39] suggest that recurrent ischaemia may play a role in sudden cardiac death. Freedom from sudden death (< 1 hour) in high risk patients (i.e. with 3-vessel disease and left ventricular dysfunction) was observed in 69% of medically treated patients, but in 91% of surgically treated patients (p < 0.0001). This may imply that prevention of recurrent ischemia by adequate revascularization may be the underlying mechanism responsible for the greater freedom from sudden death in these patients. With regard to the contradictory findings of these studies, more information is obviously needed before the definite role of ischemia in the mechanisms of sudden death can be established.

If the size of ischemic myocardium is sufficiently large, ventricular fibrillation in the absence of previous myocardial infarction may occur and cause sudden cardiac death. The true incidence of this mechanism is unknown. This mechanism would apply to persons who die suddenly without an antecedent myocardial infarction ('primary' sudden death). Long-term ECG recording is rarely performed if not at all, in these asymptomatic patients. Therefore, no information from patients studied out-of-hospital is available. However, as this situation resembles the very early stage of acute myocardial infarction, it can be assumed that in most of these cases, sudden cardiac death is initiated by ventricular fibrillation. This is obviously in contrast to the mechanism of sudden cardiac death in patients with previous myocardial infarction in whom the initiating event is mostly a sustained monomorphic ventricular tachycardia [1, 2].

Parameters to assess the presence of electrical instability

Since the mechanisms of sudden death in general as well as in post-myocardial infarction patients are complex (Figure 1 and Table 1), no single method will be able to identify the patient at risk. Therefore, several techniques have been developed (Figure 2).

For the analysis of *spontaneous ventricular arrhythmias* ambulatory long-term ECG recording has been used for many years. Multivariate statistical techniques have shown that frequent and complex ventricular arrhythmias can be considered as harbingers of sudden death in patients after myocardial infarction [8, 40, 41]. However, the large spontaneous variability of ventricular ectopic beats and above all of complex forms such as pairs, salvoes,

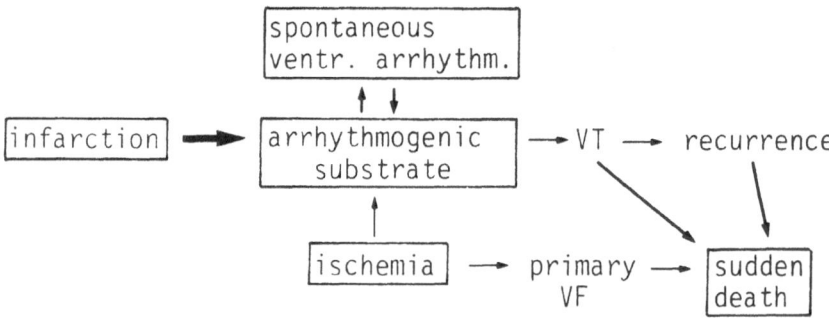

Figure 1. Factors that influence the arrhythmogenic substrate.

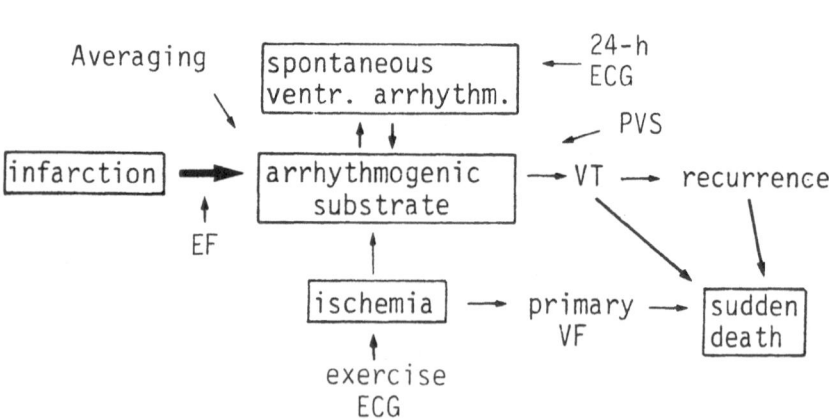

Figure 2. Methods for diagnostic assessment of the arrhythmogenic substrate and of those factors that may influence it. Abbreviations: EF = ejection fraction; PVS = programmed ventricular stimulation; VT = ventricular tachycardia; VF = ventricular fibrillation.

and runs of non-sustained ventricular tachycardia [42—45] demands extended periods of long-term ECG recording. Furthermore, the accuracy of the long-term ECG in correctly identifying high-risk patients has been questioned [46] as spontaneous ventricular arrhythmias also occur in a large proportion of patients who do not develop ventricular tachycardia or sudden death during follow-up. Thus, the large number of false-positive results limits the clinical value of spontaneous ventricular arrhythmias especially when the question is to decide who should or should not be treated with anti-arrhythmic drugs. In addition, long-term ECG recording, although non-invasive, is time-consuming, even if semi-automatic or automatic arrhythmia detection devices are used.

Another factor that may initiate arrhythmias is the occurrence of *ischemia*. A propensity to ischemia may be diagnosed using electrocardiographic exercise testing, thallium myocardial scintigraphy, gated-blood pool imaging, as well as coronary arteriography. However, though these methods may well be suitable to give an estimate of the propensity to ischemia in an individual patient at the time of the study, there is no way to predict whether and when a progression in the degree of stenosis or even the progression to occlusion will occur.

The effects of spontaneous ventricular arrhythmias and/or of ischemia may be modulated by the *autonomous nervous system*. We are still in an early stage of understanding its role in the genesis of lethal arrhythmias in patients with coronary artery disease [16, 17]. There is a need for appro-priate techniques that allow to analyse its role. Our knowledge of the contri-bution of increased sympathetic discharge to an ischemia-mediated increase in ventricular vulnerability has been based mainly on indirect observations. However, there is now growing evidence that autonomous reflexes likely play an important role in several clinical conditions such as transient myocardial ischemia and spontaneous or induced myocardial reperfusion [16, 17, 47]. Preliminary studies in uncomplicated post-infarction patients showed that measurable cardiac electrophysiological modifications occurred as a con-sequence of psycho-emotional stimulation even though this mental stress did not induce arrhythmias [17].

Spontaneous ventricular arrhythmias only represent the trigger factor that may influence the *arrhythmogenic substrate* and may induce sustained ventricular tachycardia in the presence of predisposing electrophysiological conditions. Presently used approaches include a more direct assessment of the electrophysiological ('arrhythmogenic') substrate. A promising approach that has been introduced during recent years, is the detection of ventricular *late potentials* on the body surface (Figure 3) [23]. These ventricular late potentials consist of low-amplitude fragmented electrical activity that occurs at the end of QRS or during the ST-segment and that probably originates from areas of regional slow conduction in the border zone of old myocardial infarction (see above) [23, 48]. Their presence is closely correlated with the propensity to ventricular tachycardia [10].

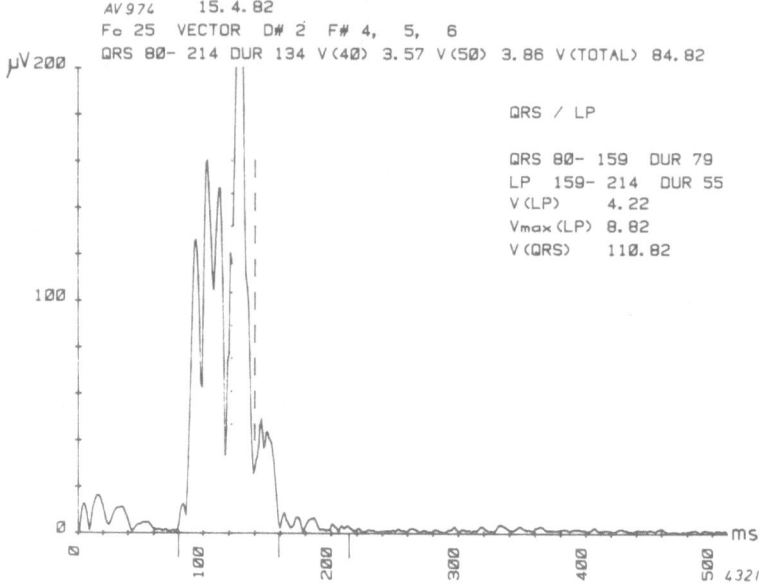

Figure 3. Signal-averaged and filtered recording of leads x, y, z, (vector magnitude) in a patient with ventricular tachycardia. QRS-duration in the highly amplified recording was 134 msec. Low-amplitude activity appeared between 159 and 214 msec (duration 55 msec). The program automatically identified the end of the total QRS-complex at 214 msec on the x-axis. The amplitude in the terminal 40 msec was low (V(40) = 3.57 microvolts) which was automatically measured by the program. Additionally, the onset of low-amplitude activity was automatically identified at 159 msec on the horizontal axis. The program also measured the mean voltage of the late potential (V(LP) = 4.22 microvolts), the maximal voltage of the late potential (Vmax(LP) = 8.82 microvolts), and the mean voltage of the true QRS-complex (V(QRS) = 110.82 microvolts).

Our own clinical experience is presently based on a total of 628 patients. Only patients without a history of sustained ventricular tachycardia or fibrillation outside the acute phase of myocardial infarction, without a history of syncope and without complete bundle branch block were included. During a mean duration of follow-up of 49 ± 15.0 months, the incidence of arrhythmic complications (sustained ventricular tachycardia or sudden cardiac death within one hour) increased as a function of the presence and duration of late potentials. The risk of major arrhythmic complications was 2.8 times greater in patients with late potentials of less than 40 ms duration compared to those without, and 9.3 times greater in those with a duration of 40 ms or more.

Similar results were reported by others though the methodology for recording, the algorithms used, and the entry criteria into the studies differed [25, 27, 49, 50].

Programmed electrical stimulation of the ventricles (Figure 4) represents another approach to assess the presence of an arrhythmogenic substrate. Since the pioneering work by Wellens *et al.* [14], it has been well-known for many years that in patients with previously documented ventricular tachycardia, identical tachycardias can be induced in a high proportion of cases by appropriate ventricular stimulation techniques. Furthermore, in patients resuscitated from out-of-hospital cardiac arrest, non-sustained and often sustained ventricular tachyarrhythmias can be induced by programmed ventricular stimulation in about two thirds of cases [51, 52, 53]. Recently, great interest has developed in the use of programmed ventricular stimulation not only for the diagnosis of ventricular tachycardia in patients with previously documented episodes but also for assessing the prognosis of patients with coronary artery disease.

Our own prospective study includes 548 patients. 402 patients had a history of previous mycardial infarction. In 269 patients, the study was done within 2 months after myocardial infarction. Using single and double premature stimulti at different cycle lengths of basic drive, non-sustained or sustained ventricular tachycardia was induced in 34 and 11% of patients, respectively. During a mean follow-up duration of 22 ± 18.5 months, 2.8% of patients died suddenly whereas a similar number of patients developed an episode of spontaneous symptomatic sustained ventricular tachycardia requiring emergency intervention. Sensitivity for predicting sudden death was 62%, and for predicting sustained ventricular tachycardia 92%. The highest predictive value for an abnormal result of programmed ventricular stimulation was found in patients in whom sustained ventricular tachycardia at a rate below 270 bpm was induced (predictive value: 39.3%). In contrast, induction

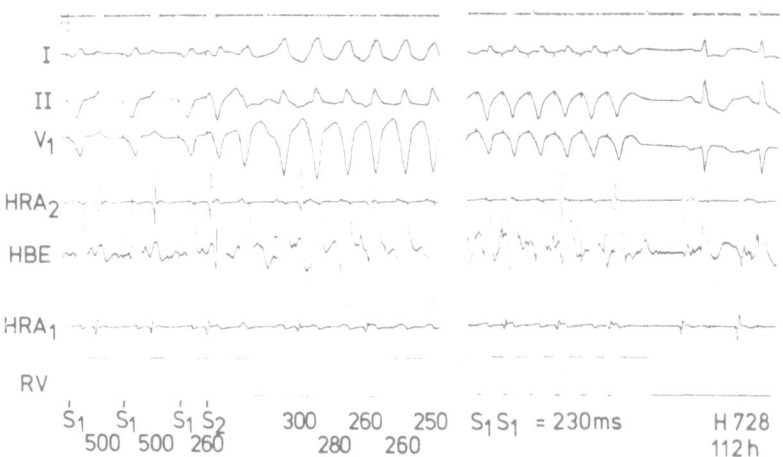

Figure 4. Programmed ventricular stimulation with induction and termination of monomorphic sustained ventricular tachycardia in a patient after recent myocardial infarction.

of either no ventricular echo beats or only non-sustained ventricular tachycardia indicated a good prognosis as only 8/198 cases experienced an arrhythmic event. Relating the induction of sustained ventricular tachycardia at a rate below 270 bpm to ejection fraction (cut-off point 40%), the predictive value of a positive test increased to 71%. No patient with inducible sustained ventricular tachycardia and an ejection fraction greater than 40% developed an arrhythmic event. A normal result of programmed stimulation (induction of less than 4 consecutive echo beats) predicted a high chance of being not at risk of sudden cardiac death or of symptomatic sustained ventricular tachycardia. Thus, the results of our prospective study in patients after recent myocardial infarction and in patients with chronic coronary artery disease has shown that the subsequent occurrence of sudden cardiac death (within one hour) or of symptomatic sustained ventricular tachycardia requiring some type of emergency intervention could be predicted by the results of programmed ventricular stimulation in a high percentage of patients. If the type of induced ventricular arrhythmia (non-sustained and sustained ventricular tachycardia), the rate of induced ventricular tachycardia, the interval between myocardial infarction and electrophysiological study, and the degree of left ventricular impairment (ejection fraction) is taken into account, the predictive value of the test can be increased.

Similar results were reported by Hamer et al. [54] and Richards et al. [11]. In contrast, Marchlinski et al. [55] as well as Santarelli et al. [56] were not able to predict the subsequent occurrence of arrhythmic events as they had a very low event rate in their small patient cohorts.

In these studies, the predictive value of an abnormal result of programmed stimulation (defined differently in the various studies) varied considerably. This partly depended on the fact that in some studies, there were no arrhythmic events or due to the small number of these events, no prediction could be made. The only two studies (besides our study) that actually were able to predict the subsequent occurrence of sudden cardiac death were those by Hamer et al. [54] and by Richards et al. [11]. These two studies included only patients after recent myocardial infarction. The predictive value of a positive test for sudden cardiac death was 33.3 and 21.1%, respectively. Similar to our study, Richards et al. [11] also observed the occurrence of sustained ventricular tachycardia after discharge from the hospital whereas Hamer et al. [54] did not report any episode of sustained ventricular tachycardia after hospital discharge.

Clinical approach to the evaluation of post-myocardial infarction patients

From the clinical point of view, non-invasive procedures are obviously desirable for screening purposes whereas it would be acceptable to use more aggressive invasive techniques in certain subsets of patients. A step-like approach using non-invasive recording of late ventricular potentials as the initial step would allow one to preselect patients for further evaluation by invasive electrophysiological techniques. Whether this approach might be feasible was tested in 132 postmyocardial infarction patients who were studied prospectively [9]. It could be demonstrated that the *combined use of signal averaging and programmed ventricular stimulation* helped to identify subgroups of patients at markedly different risk of developing spontaneous symptomatic sustained ventricular tachycardia. Patients at highest risk were characterized by, first, the presence of ventricular late potentials; second, an abnormal result of programmed ventricular stimulation; third, a rate of induced ventricular arrhythmia less than 270 bpm. With regard to establishing antiarrhythmic therapy, this might be a subgroup of postmyocardial infarction patients that might benefit most.

With respect to presently available information, signal averaging for the detection of late ventricular potentials seems to be a promising new technique for the identification of patients at risk of ventricular tachyarrhythmias. However, the relative value of this technique for the prediction of ventricular tachycardias in comparison to sudden cardiac death demands further prospective study. With regard to the significant number of false-positive results which is not only the case with signal averaging but also with, for instance, long-term ECG recording, it seems unjustified to expect any one method to be able to identify the individual patient at risk of sustained ventricular tachycardia and/or sudden death. In this context, long-term ECG recording and signal averaging might prove useful as screening methods whereas programmed ventricular stimulation might serve for further risk stratification. No definite answer can presently be given with regard to the future role of programmed ventricular stimulation for the identification of patients at risk of severe arrhythmic events after myocardial infarction. Though the results of prospective studies in large populations are encouraging and support the view that these arrhythmic events are obviously related to chronic electrophysiological abnormalities, confirmation of these data is urgently necessary.

References

1. Bayés de Luna A, Torner P, Guindo J, Soler M, Oca F: Holter ECG study of ambulatory sudden death, review of 158 published cases. New Trends in Arrhythmias 1985; I: 293–297.
2. Olshausen K, Pop T, Treese N, Meyer J: Sudden death during Holter monitoring. Eur Heart J 1985; 6: abstr. suppl I: 45.
3. Breithardt G, Seipel L, Loogen F: Der akute Herztod. Bedeutung elektrophysiologischer Stimulationsverfahren. Verh. Dtsch. Ges. Herz-. Kreislaufforschg. 1980; 46: 38–64.
4. Richards DA, Blake GJ, Spear JF, Moore EN: Electrophysiologic substrate for ventricular tachycardia: correlation of properties in vivo and in vitro. Circulation 1984; 69: 369–81.
5. Daniel T, Boineau J, Sabiston D: Comparison of human ventricular activation with canine model in chronic myocardial infarction. Circulation 1971; 44: 74–89.
6. El-Sherif N, Scherlag BJ, Lazzara R, Hope RR: Reentrant ventricular arrhythmias in the

late myocardial infarction period. I. Conduction characteristics in the infarction zone. Circulation 1977; 55: 686—702.

7.   Kostis JB, Byington R, Friedman LM, Goldstein S, Furberg C for the BHAT Study Group: Prognostic significance of ventricular ectopic activity in survivors of acute myocardial infarction. J Am Coll Cardiol 1987; 10: 231—42.

8.   Moss AJ: Clinical significance of ventricular arrhythmias in patients with and without coronary artery disease. Progr. Cardiovasc Dis 1980; 23: 33.

9.   Breithardt G, Borggrefe M, Haerten K: Role of programmed ventricular stimulation and noninvasive recording of ventricular late potential for the identification of patients at risk of ventricular tachyarrhythmias after acute myocardial infarction. In: Zipes DP, Jalife J (eds), Cardiac electrophysiology and Arrhythmias. Grune and Stratton 1985: 553—61.

10. Breithardt G, Borggrefe M, Quantius B, Karbenn U, Seipel L: Ventricular vulnerability assessed by programmed ventricular stimulation in patients with and without late potentials. Circulation 1983; 68: 275—81.

11. Richards DA, Cody DV, Denniss AR, Russell PA, Young AA, Uther JB: Ventricular electrical unstability: a predictor of death after myocardial infarction. Am J Cardiol 1983; 51: 75—80.

12. Breithardt G, Seipel L, Meyer T, Abendroth R: Prognostic significance of repetitive ventricular responses during programmed ventricular stimulation. Am J Cardiol 1982; 49: 693—698.

13. Han J: Ventricular vulnerability during acute coronary occlusion. Am J Cardiol 1969; 24: 857.

14. Wellens HJJ, Durrer DR, Lie KI: Observations on mechanisms of ventricular tachycardia in man. Circulation 1976; 54: 237—244.

15. Patterson E, Gibson JK, Lucchesi BR: Electrophysiologic actions of lidocaine in an canine model of chronic myocardial ischemic damage. Arrhythmogenic actions of lidocaine. J Cardio Pharmacolog 1982; 4: 925—934.

16. Lombardi F: Acute myocardial ischemia, neural reflexes and ventricular arrhythmias. Eur Heart J 1986; 7 (suppl A): 91—97.

17. Tavazzi L, Zotti AM, Rondanelli R: The role of psychologic stress in the genesis of lethal arrhythmias in patients with coronary artery disease. Eur Heart J 1986; 7 (supply. A): 99—106.50.

18. Kennedy HL, Whitlock JA, Sprague MK, Kennedy LJ, Buckingham TA, Goldberg RJ: Long-term follow-up of asymptomatic healthy subjects with frequent and complex ventricular ectopy. N Engl J Med 1985; 312: 193—7.

19. Flowers NC, Horan LG, Thomas JR, Tolleson WJ: The anatomic basis for high frequency components in the electrocardiogram. Circulation 1969; 39: 531—539.

20. Gardner PI, Ursell PC, Fenoglio JJ, Wit AL: Electrophysiologic and anatomic basis for fractionated electrograms recorded from healed myocardial infarcts. Circulation 1985; 72: 596—611.

21. Berbari EJ, Scherlag BJ, Hope RR, Lazzara R: Recording from the body surface of arrhythmogenic ventricular activity during the ST segment. Am J Cardiol 1978; 41: 697.

22. Breithardt G, Becker R, Seipel L, Abendroth RR, Ostermeyer J: Non-invasive detection of late potentials in man: a new marker for ventricular tachycardia. Eur Heart J 1981; 2: 1—11.

23. Breithardt G, Borggefe M: Pathophysiological mechanisms and clinical significance of ventricular late potentials. Eur Heart J 1986; 7: 364—85.

24. Breithardt G, Borggrefe M, Karbenn U, Abendroth RR, Yeh HL, Seipel L: Prevalence of late potentials in patients with and without ventricular tachycardia: correlation to angiographic findings. Am J Cardiol 1982; 49: 1932—1937.

25. Denniss AR, Cody DV, Fenton SM et al: Significance of delayed activation potentials in survivors of myocardial infarction. J Am Coll Cardiol 1983; 1: 582 (abstr).

26. Fontaine G, Frank R, Gallais-Hamonno F, Allali I, Phan-Thuc H, Grosgogeat Y:

Electrocardiographie des potentiels tardifs du syndrome de post-exitation. Arch Mal Coeur 1978; 71: 854.

27. Kacet S, Libersa C, Caron J, Boudoux B, d'Haute Feuille X, Marchand J, Dagano J, Lekieffre J: The prognostic value of averaged late potentials in patients suffering from coronary artery disease. In: Aliot E, Lazzara R (eds), Ventricular Tachycardias. Dordrecht-Boston-Lancaster: Martinus Nijhoff Publishers, (in press).

28. Kanovsky MS, Simson MB, Falcone RA, Dresden C, Josephson ME: The late potential is an independent marker for ventricular tachycardia. J Am Coll Cardiol 1983; 1: 582.

29. Kuchar D, Thorburn C, Sammel N: Natural history and clinical significance of late potentials after myocardial infarction. Circulation 1985 72: III—477.

30. Simson MB: Use of Signals in the Terminal QRS complex to identify patients with ventricular tachycardia after myocardial infarction. Circulation 1981; 64: 235—242.

31. Garan H, McComb JM, Ruskin JN: Spontaneous and electrically induced ventricular arrhythmias during acute ischaemia superimposed on two week-old canine myocardial infarction. JACC 1988; 11: 603—611.

32. Myerburg RJ, Epstein K, Gaide MS, Wong SS, Castellanos A, Gelband H, Bassett AL: Electrophysiologic consequences of experimental acute ischaemia superimposed on healed myocardial infarction in cats. Am J Cardiol. 1982; 49: 323—330.

33. Davies MJ, Path FRC, Thomas AC, Path MRC, Knapman PA, Hangartner JR: Intramyocardial platelet aggregation in patients with instable angina pectoris suffering sudden ischemic cardiac death. Circulation 1986; 73: 418—427.

34. Falk E: Unstable angina with fatal outcome: dynamic coronary thrombosis leading to infarction and/or sudden death. Autopsy evidence of recurrent mural thrombosis with peripheral embolization culminating in total vascular occlusion. Circulation 1985; 71: 699—708.

35. Lo YS, Cutler JE, Blake K, Wright AM, Kron J, Swerdlow ChD: Angiographic coronary morphology in survivors of cardiac arrest. Am Heart J 1988; 115: 781—5.

36. Bertrand ME, Lablanche JM, Tilmant PY, Thieuleux FA, Delforge MR, Carre AG, Asseman P, Berzin B, Libersa C, Laurent JM: Frequency of provoked coronary arterial spasm in 1089 consecutive patients undergoing coronary arteriography. Circulation 1982; 65: 1299—1306.

37. Gorlin R, Fuster V, Ambrose JA: Anatomic-physiologic links between acute coronary syndromes. Circulation 1986; 74: 6—8.

38. Steering Committee of the Physicians Health Study Research Group: Preliminary report: Findings from the aspirin component of the ongoing Physicians' Health Study. N Engl J Med 1988; 318: 262—6.

39. Holmes JDR, Davis KB, Mock MB, Fisher LD, Gersh BJ, Killip III T, Pettinger M: Participants in the Coronary Artery Surgery Study. The effect of medical and surgical treatment on subsequent sudden cardiac death in patients with coronary artery disease: a report from the Coronary Artery Surgery Study. Circulation 1986; 73: 1254—63.

40. Geltman EM, Ehsani AA, Campbell MK, Schechtman K, Roberts R, Sobel BE: The influence of location and extent of myocardial infarction on long-term dysrhythmia and mortality. Circulation 1979; 60: 805.

41. Ruberman, W, Weinblatt, E, Goldberg, JD, Frank, CW, Shapiro, S, Chaudary, BS: Ventricular premature complexes in prognosis of angina. Circulation 1980; 61: 1172.

42. Andresen D, von Leitner RV, Wegschneider K, Schröder R: Nachweis komplexer tachykarder ventrikulärer Rhythmusstörungen im Lang-Zeit-EKG. Dtsch med Wschr 1982; 107: 571.

43. Michelson El, Morganroth J: Spontaneous variability of complex ventricular arrhythmias detected by long-term electrocardiographic recording. Circulation 1980; 61: 690.

44. Morganroth J, Michelson EL, Horowity LN, Josephson ME, Pearlman AS, Dunkman WB: Limitation of routine long-term ambulatory electrocardiographic monitoring to assess ventricular ectopic frequency. Circulation 1978; 58: 408.

45. Winkle RA: Antiarrhythmic drug effect mimicked by spontaneous variability of ventricular ectopy. Circulation 1980; 61: 690.
46. Cats VM, Lie KL, van Capelle FJL, Durrer D: Limitations of 24 hour ambulatory electrocardiographic recording in predicting coronary events after acute myocardial infarction. Am J Cardiol 1979; 44: 1257.
47. Schwartz PJ, Zaza A: The rational basis and the clinical value of selective cardiac sympathetic denervation in the prevention of malignant arrhythmias. Eur Heart J 1986; 7 (suppl A): 107—118.
48. Wiener I, Mindlich B, Pitchon R, Pichard A, Kupersmith J, Estioko M, Jurado R, Camunas J, Litwak R: Epicardial activation in patients with coronary artery disease: effects of regional contraction abnormalities. Circulation 1982; 65: 154—60.
49. Höpp HW, Hombach V, Osterspey A, Deutsch H, Winter U, Behrenbeck DW, Tauchert M, Hilger HH: Clinical and prognostic significance of ventricular arrhythmias and ventricular late potentials in patients with coronary heart disease. 1985; 297—307 In: Holter Monitoring Technique. Technical Aspects and Clinical Applictions. Stuttgart-New York.
50. Von Leitner R, Oeff M, Loock D, Jahns B, Schröder R: Value of non-invasively detected delayed ventricular depolarizations to predict prognosis in post myocardial infarction patients. Circulation 1983; 68 (suppl III): III—83.
51. Borggrefe M, Breithardt G, Yeh HL: Klinisch-elektrophysiologische Befunde bei Patienten nach Kammerflimmern. Z Kardiol 1982; 71: 643.
52. Myerburg RJ, Conde CA, Sung RJ et al: Clinical, electrophysiologic and haemodynamic profile of patients resuscitated from prehospital cardiac arrest. Am J Med 1980; 68: 568.
53. Ruskin JN, DiMarco JP, Garan H: Out of hospital cardiac arrest. N Engl J Med 1980; 303: 607.
54. Hamer A, Vohra J, Hunt J, Sloman G: Prediction of sudden death by electrophysiologic studies in high risk patients surviving acute myocardial infarction. Am J Cardiol 1982; 50: 223—229.
55. Marchlinski FE, Buxton AE, Waxman HL, Josephson ME: Identifying patients at risk of sudden death after myocardial infarction: value of the response to programmed stimulation, degree of ventricular dysgunction. Am J Cardiol 1983; 52: 1190.
56. Santarelli P, Bellocci F, Loperfido F, MAzzari M, Mongiardo R, Montenero AS, Manzoli U, Denes P: Ventricular arrhythmia induced by programmed ventricular stimulation after acute myocardial infarction. Am J Cardiol 1985; 72: 487—494.

20. Risk factors of sudden cardiac death after acute myocardial infarction

Ventricular disfunction, ischemia and ventricular arrhythmias

FRANCISCO NAVARRO-LOPEZ

Introduction

It is well known that the risk of sudden cardiac death (SCD) increases in patients who have survived an acute myocardial infarction during the first months or years after the acute event. And it is also recognized that the SCD is basically an arrhythmic death due to ventricular fibrillation, preceded or not by ventricular tachycardia. The incidence of SCD has been estimated in 3.5—5% a year, representing the 60—80% of all deaths [1—4]. This group of patients may then be considered an excelent model to study 'risk factors' related to its occurrence.

The widespread interest on these studies is mainly due to the fact that the 'risk factors' are prognostic indicators. They may identify a 'high risk' group of patients that could benefit from a preventive approach, and a 'low risk' group of patients that may be spared of expensive workups and unnecessary treatment. In the second place, the identification of those risk factors with clear physiopathological meaning may help to clarify the mechanisms of SCD, its substrate or its precipitating factors. Furthermore, our understanding of its mechanisms may help to design a specific preventive strategy whose epidemiological importance can not be overenfasized, since this population represents the largest group of patients at risk of sudden death [4].

The aim of this short review is to analyse some of the lessons learned in the long term follow up of patients surviving an acute myocardial infarction.

Thanks to these studies we know that the factors that predispose to SCD are basically of three types [5] (Figure 1): the major factor is the left ventricular disfunction, related to the extent of the myocardial necrosis; lesser factors are the residual myocardial ischemia, reflecting the presence of severe coronary artery disease, and the ventricular arrhythmias.

It is commonly accepted that the risk factors related to SCD are no different from the factors of cardiac death.

A. Bayès de Luna et al. (eds.): *Sudden Cardiac Death*, 223–237.
© 1991 Kluwer Academic Publishers, Dordrecht.

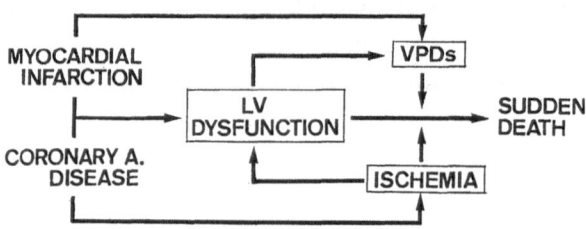

Figure 1. Major risk factors of SCD in post-infarction patients (Modified from Gotlieb [5]).

Statistical methods

A risk factor is a variable whose association with SCD has been documented by the Student 't' test, the χ^2 test or the 'log rank test' (univariate analysis). To determine the relative importance of the different risk variables, a multivariate analysis may be performed, such as multiple regression analysis or the discriminant analysis [6]. These statistical techniques (Table 1) usually identify, among a number of variables with an univariate prognostic value, the variable showing the strongrest association with the survival or death of the patients (in the case of multiple logistic regression) or with the length of survival (in the survival analysis of Cox). Once the variable with the strongest predictive value has been identified (X_1), the model selects next a second or a third variable $(X_2, X_3,$ etc.) with prognostic information not included in the previous one. This variable is said to have an 'independent' predictive value.

Table 1. Multiple regression analysis.

Lineal	$P = (B + B_1 \cdot X_1 + B_2 \cdot X_2 + \ldots B_n \cdot X_n)$
Logistic	$P = 1/1 + e^{(B + B_1 \cdot X_1 + B_2 \cdot B_2 + \ldots B_n X_n)}$
Survival (Cox)	$P = F(t) \, e^{(B + B_1 \cdot X_1 + B_2 \cdot B_2 + \ldots B_n \cdot X_n)}$

The methodology has important limitations and the variables selected depend largely on the population studied, on the variables included in the analysis, the dispersion of the data, and sometimes of a certain erratic nature of the statistical model [7]. Those circumstances might account for some of the discrepancies observed in the literature.

Left ventricular dysfunction

A number of studies have shown that left ventricular disfunction is the single more important factor determining cardiac and SCD [1—5, 8—16]. Patients with the highest risk of SCD are those with a severe residual impairment of left ventricular function due to an extensive necrosis. Many clinical and hemodynamic variables related to the ventricular function have been found to have univariate predictive value of survival [16]. Among them, for example, it is worth remembering the clinical variables included in the indexes of Peel [8], Killip & Kimball [9] and Norris [10]: the pulmonary venous congestion on the chest X-ray or at the auscultation, a third sound, the NYHA class, a previous myocardial infarction; or the hemodynamic variables studied by Forrester [11] and Sanz *et al.* [12], such as de cardiac output, the pulmonary wedge pressure, the enddiastolic volum, the systemic blood pressure; or the variables related to the size of the necrosis: peak CK concentration, enzimatic curves or the QRS index.

However, when all these variables are included in the multivariate analysis the statistical model nearly always selects the *left ventricular ejection fraction* (LVEF) as the only variable with 'independent' predictive value of cardiac or SCD [12—16]. This variable then includes all the prognostic information available in the rest of the variables related to the cardiac function. The LVEF determined by means of the contrast or the radionuclide ventriculography is the left ventricular function parameter more commonly used in clinical practice, and is therefore a very suitable prognostic marker. SCD is exceptional in patients with an LVEF greater than 40% and the incidence increases proporcionally to its reduction. The annual mortality rate increases to 10—15% in patients with an LVEF of 20—40% and is higher than 40% when the LVEF is lower than 20% [2]. It has been shown by Fioretti [37], examining the 'receiving operator characteristic curves' (ROC), that cardiac death can also be predicted with the same degree of accuracy from the clinical variables (age, history of cardiac failure, and the degree of pulmonary congestion on the chest X-ray). Tibbits has also shown that the prognostic value of the radionuclide LVEF is slightly higher than that of the clinical variables (functional class of the NYHA before the myocardial infarction, pulmonary congestion and left bundle branch block), but the practical value of the added information is negligible (Figure 2) [17].

Other variables related to the ventricular function

The impairment of the left ventricular function is commonly related to the *loss of contractil mass* and the *size of the myocardial infarction*. However, the variables that quantify the infart size have not shown to have the same prognostic value than the LVEF, their lack of accuracy being one of the possible explanations.

The search of other functional variables with a more specific prognostic or physiopathological meaning has not met with much a success. White [18], however, suggested that the enlargement of the *end-systolic volume*, reflecting the degree of *left ventricular dilatation*, may be a more significant predictor of SCD than the LVEF alone. The dilatation could be related to the 'infarct expansion' associated with the stretching of the necrotic tissue

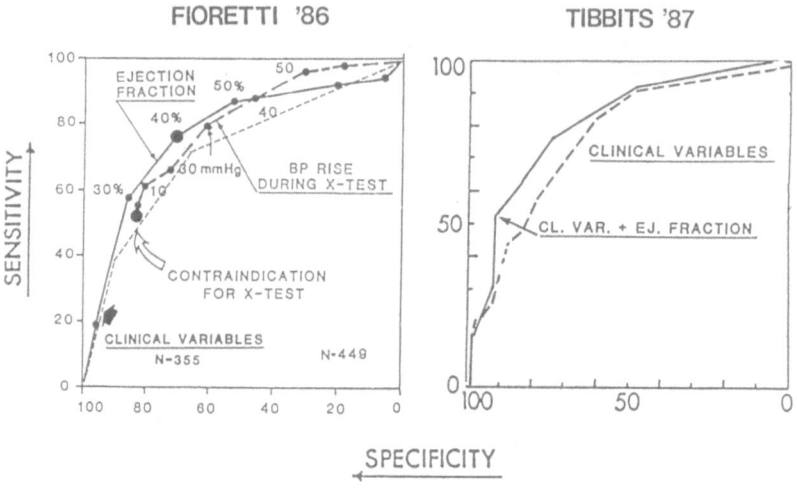

Figure 2. Sensitivity versus specificity for late mortality after myocardial infarction of variables related to ventricular function: clincial variables, EF% and exercise test ('ROC' curves). The closest curve to the upper left corner (100% sensitibity and specificity) corresponde to the variable with the largest prognostic value (Modified from Fioretti [37] and Tibbits [17]).

during the systolic contraction, leading to the progressive slippage of the necrotic fibers. The expansion usually takes place during the first two weeks, but it is not unusually that it becomes progressive and continues for months, being the leading mechanism of the functional impairment. According to this concept, the depression of the LVEF could be accounted for by two mechanisms: the initial size of the necrosis and the myocardial expansion that may follow.

A third mechanism may be the transient loss of contractility of the ischemic segment ('stunned myocardium'). In fact *acute pulmonary edema* or *cardiac failue* in the acute phase of the myocarfial infarction has shown in some studies to have a predictive value independent of the LVEF [19]. As pointed out by Rapaport [20], patients who have suffered an acute pulmonary edema are more prone to have severe coronary artery lessions and an extensive zone of myocardium at risk of transient ischemia. It seems then advisable to submit those patients to further evaluation.

According to some authors, a *left ventricular aneurism* may be a particularly ominous prognostic indicator of SCD, suggesting that aneurism is an specific anatomic substrat for ventricular fibrilation [21, 22]. Resection of the aneurism could then be advocated to prevent SCD. However the results of our prospective study on myocardial infarction ('UB/MIP', University of Barcelona/ Myocardial Infarction Project), are not in keeping with this hypothesis [23]. Although the 51 patients with aneurism diagnosed by contrast ventriculography showed a significantly higher death rate than the rest of the patients, the mortality was not different when compared with a control group of patients matched by age, LVEF and severity of coronary lessions. Furthermore, the proportion of patients dying of sudden arrhythmic death (Hinckle class I) [24] was similar in both groups (Figure 3). These data are against the aneurism being a predictor of SCD independent of cardiac function. Probably these patients have a worst prognosis because the aneurism is associated with a lower LVEF.

Moss [25] and Bigger [26] have described a significantly higher mortality rate in patients under *digitalis* (up to 38.5% at 4 months) [26]. Although it may be associated with a more pronounced depression of the cardiac function, an arrhythmogenic toxic effect can not be excluded in those patients recovering from a myocardial infarction.

Mechanism

The role of the infarct size and the depression of the left ventricular function as a substrate for SCD has a strong experimental basis. Gang *et al.* [27] have shown that the extensive necrosis is a factor leading to ventricular tachycardia in dogs [27]. Garan *et al.* [28] have also shown that the infart size and the low LVEF were the only variables to predict the appearence of sustained ventricular tachycardia elicited by programmed electrical stimulation in the animal studies [28].

However, it has not been easy to find an explanation for this relationship.

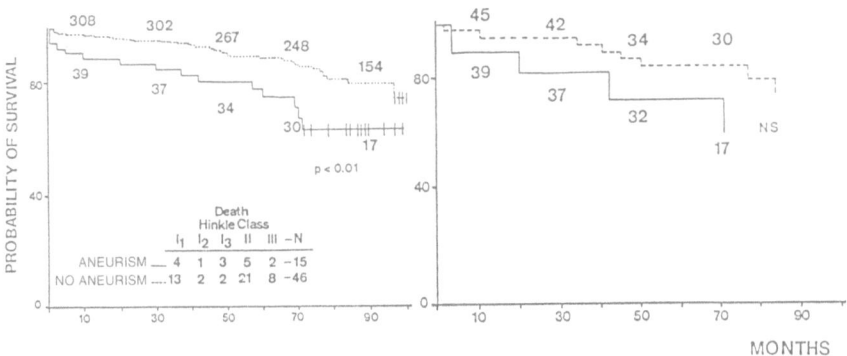

Figure 3. Kaplan-Meier survival curves of patients with ventricular aneurism studied in the 'UB/MIP'. To the left: the estimated survival of patients with anevrism (N = 51) is significantly different from the rest of the patients (p < 0.01, 'log rank test'). The table on the left lower corner shows the number of patients in each Hinckle class. To the right: the survival of patients with aneurism was not significantly different from the matched group of patients. The numbers indicate the patients followed-up.

Reentry is the accepted mechanism for the ventricular arrhythmias and the size of the myocardial scar could be a determinant factor. But the exact mechanism of the relationship between the infarct size and the pathways implicated in the induction of the ventricular tachycardia can only be speculated [28].

White *et al.* [18] raised the possibility that the global or segmental ventricular dilatation may play an important role in the induction of the ventricular fibrillation. The increase in wall stress associated with the larger radius of curvature and the elevation of the myocardial oxygen consumption that follows could favor the appearence of the ischemia and the reentry of electrical impulses between the normal and the stretched myocardial fibers of the isquemic segment.

Treatment

Unfortunatly the depression of the ventricular function due to the loss of myocardial mass is not expected to regress under treatment. This fact further stresses the need for limiting the infarct size and preserving the cardiac function in the acute phase of the myocardial infarction with the thrombolitic therapy.

The prognosis may improve, however, if the reduction of afterload can prevent or lessen the ventricular dilatation associated with the infarct expansion. Pfeffer [29] has shown that captopril is able to prevent the ventricular dilatation and to improve the survival of the experimental myocardial infarction in rats. The results of the 'CONSENSUS' Trial in patients with cardiac failure, indicating that captopril may have a preventive effect on SCD, are consistent with this hypothesis [30].

The role of surgery in preventing the transient ischemia loss of cardiac function or the resection of the aneurism still lack of definite confirmation.

Coronary artery disease and ischemia

It was soon recognized that the severity and extent of the coronary artery disease as well as the myocardial ischemia were also important risk factors as shown by the univariate analysis.

In 1975 we started in the University of Barcelona a long term prospective study (UB/MIP) to determine the catheterization variables related to survival after myocardial infarction [12]. We were able to inclue 91% of the eligible patients admited to our coronary care unit. Our data confirmed the results of previous works [31] showing that *triple vessel disease* was a prognostic factor independent of LVEF (Figure 4). Patients with a LVEF between 21 and 49% and triple vessel disease, showed a higher mortality rate than patients with single or two vessel disease. But survival was normal in patients with

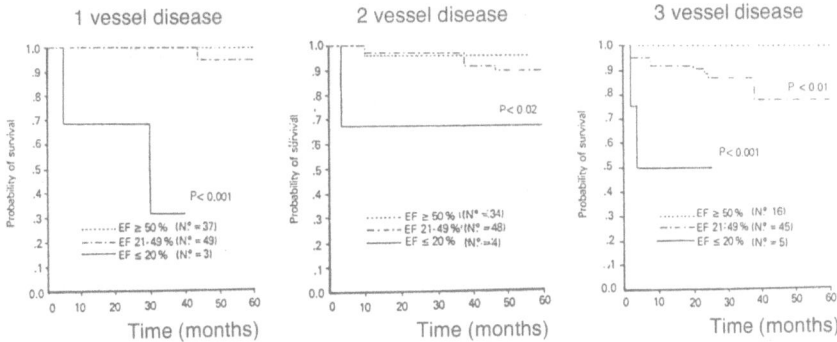

Figure 4. Kaplan-Meier survival curves in patients with single, two or triple vessel disease, stratified according to the EF% (P indicates the differences between the group with an EF% over 50% and the rest of the subgroups). N = 259 (Sans 1982 [12]).

thriple vessel disease and good ventricular function. Accordingly we suggested that profilactic surgery, usually recomended to patients with three vessel disease, should be restricted to this subgroup of patients with depressed LVEF. The benefit of this policy in patients after a myocardial infarction remains to be confirmed.

Furthermore, Sami [32] from Stanford, Theroux [33] from Montreal, and Velasco [34] from Valencia, described that early submaximal exercise testing was able to detect residual myocardial ischemia, as demonstrated by an *ischemic depression of the ST segment*, in 15—30% of the patients. The mortality ranged between 22 and 32%, significantly larger than observed in patients with normal exercise test (0—8%) (Table 2). The relationship between the ST segment depression and the coronary artery lessions has been extensively documented.

However, none of the early exercise test studies published later than 1981,

Table 2. Exercise testing after MI.

Reference	N	ST ≥ 1 mm			BP response		
		Prevalence	Mortality (%) Risk group		Prevalence	Mortality (%) Risk group	
			High	Low		High	Low
Sami '79 [32]	85	21	22	0	—	—	—
Theroux '79 [33]	210	30	27	2	—	—	—
Velasco '81 [34]	200	14	32	8	9	7	10
Weld '81 [35]	235	22	14	8	51	16	1
Krone '85 [36]	667	25	4	5	9	18	3
Fioretti '85 [37]	300	56	6	7	29	16	3

like the large studies of Weld [35], Krone [36] and Fioretti [37], have been able to confirm the prognostic value of the residual ischemia as assessed by the ST segment depression or the appearence of angina. On the contrary, they showed that *inadecuate response of the systemic arterial pressure* and reduction of the effort tolerance were specially usefull to identify a high risk group of patients, with a mortality rate of 16—18% and a low risk group with a mortality of less than 1—3%. Their results do not lend support to the ischemic hypothesis of the SCD, but rather enphasize the importance of the factors related to the ventricular function.

The exercise test is now a widely used clinical procedure to stratify the prognosis of patients after a myocardial infarction, the blood pressure response and the endurance being more useful than the electrocardiographic changes. Weld [36] reported that patients who were able to complete an early excercise test with a good blood pressure response (up to more than 110 mmHg. of systolic pressure) and showed no pulmonary congestion on the chest X-ray, had a one year mortality of 1% as compared with a 13% in the rest of the patients. Fioretti [37] arrived to similar conclusions. A rise of the systolic blood pressure greater than 30 mmHg, the lack of a previous myocardial infarction and the absence of digitalis was associated with a one year mortality of 3% (Figure 5).

Other markers of myocardial ischemia

The appearence of *myocardial perfusion defects* on Thallium-201 exercise test or of *dynamic changes in segmental wall motion analysis* on the radionuclide ventriculography under exercise may be considered a more sensitive and reliable signs of residual ischemia than the standard excercise test. Those variables showed a stronger correlation with the regional blood flow reserve estimated by digital angiographic techniques than the severity of the coronary lessions at angiography [38].

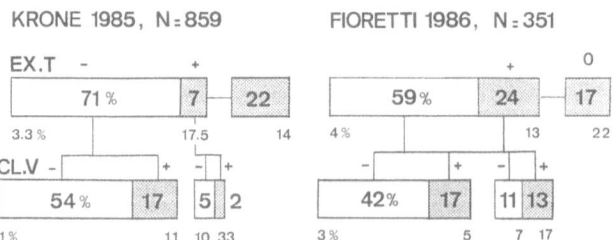

Figure 5. Step-wise stratification of the risk in post-infarction and patients, according to the clinical variables (Cl. V) and the exercise text (Ex. T). Data taken from Krone [36] a Fioretti [37]. Numbers are percentages of patients included in each group. The dark bar indictes patients with a positive response to the exercise test or with clinical variables present (+) or those who were not able to complete the test (0).

Gibson [39] has shown that multiple perfusion defects on the Thallium exercise test is a better predictor than the number of diseased vessels, electrocardiographic ischemia or angina. By means of the multivariate analysis, Hakki [40] has been able to confirm the prognostic value of the thallium-201 exercise test to be independent of the LVEF and of the ventricular arrhythmias recorded on the 24-h ambulatory Holter electrocardiographic monitoring system.

Silent myocardial ischemia has also been mentioned as a possible factor precipitating sudden arrhythmic death, since it may induce acute regional wall dynamic changes leading to segmental dilatation and arrhythmogenesis [18, 41]. This explanation suggests a link between ischemia, mechanical dysfunction and lethal arrhythmias.

Of interest is the study of Cannom *et al.* [42] which described that the incidence of SCD was higher in patients with '*non Q-wave myocardial infarction*' (30%) than in infarctions with Q-wave (15%). Those findings are in favor of the ischemic hypothesis, since a 'non Q-wave myocardial infarction' is considered an aborted or incomplete infarction due to the early spontaneous reperfusion of the coronary artery. Under these circumstances, the rate of recurrent ischemic coronary events would be understandably greater than in completed myocardial infarction. The *early post-infarction angina*, reflecting the residual ischemia, could have a similar meaning, as studied by Bosch [43].

In summary, the information available suggests that myocardial ischemia is a prognostic factor independent of LVEF, but with a weak prognostic value. The relationship of ischemia and arrhythmic death is also supported by the appearance of ventricular tachycardias after ST segment elevation in the coronary spasm [4, 44], or the independent prognostic value of tobacco and emotional stress as shown in some recent papers, pointing to sympathetic activity as a precipitating factor of ischemia and arrhythmias [18, 45, 46].

Treatment

Further support to this view [4] may be found in the results of the preventive coronary surgery or the BHAT trial. The betablockers were equally effective lowering the incidence of SCD in patients with or without ventricular arrhythmias, suggesting an anti-ischemic rather than and antiarrhythmic effect.

Ventricular arrhythmias and ventricular function

Kolter [47], Ruberman [48] and Moss [1], already described in the seventies the strong association of *complex ventricular ectopic activity* and the increase in mortality, giving rise to the arrhythmic hypothesis of the SCD. According to this hypothesis the complex ventricular extrasystole are an independent risk factor of SCD, and have a direct role in the mechanism of death, leading to ventricular tachycardia and fibrillation, through a R on T fenomenon, for example. Conversely, Califf [49] showed that there was also a good correlation between the arrhythmias detected in the 24-h ambulatory Holter electrocardiographic recordings and the radionuclide LVEF, arriving to the conclusion that the ventricular ectopic activity may be simply a marker of the more severe left ventricular disfunction.

If the predictive value of the ventricular arrhythmias were independent and additive to the ventricular disfunction, as assumed by the arrhythmia hypothesis, it would be reasonable to expect a beneficial effect of the antiarrhythmic therapy on the incidence of SCD. Otherwise the treatment could be only cosmetic if not detrimental because of the arrhythmogenic effect of the antiarrhythmic drugs.

The extensive trials of MILIS [14], with 388 patients, the MPIRP [13], that included 766 patients submitted to 24-h electrocardiographic ambulatory recordings and radionuclide ventriculography and the BHAT [50], were able to definitly establish the relationship between the presence, frequency and the complexity of the ventricular arrhythmias and the SCD (Table 3). The MILIS and the MPIRP also confirmed the association between ventricular arrhythmias and depression of LVEF. But the multivariate analysis showed without any doubt that the relationship of ventricular arrhythmia and SCD (Hinckle class I) was independent of LVEF. Nevertheless, the additive prognostic value of ventricular ectopic activity, was weak.

Since the proportion of SCD was similar in patients with and without frequent ventricular ectopic activity (3/h), this variable could be a marker of the electrical unstability of the ventricles, rather than a direct cause of the ventricular fibrillation. Figure 6, drawn with data from Bigger [13], shows the S-shape curve relating mortality rate to increasing number of ventricular

Table 3. 24-h holter monitoring after MI.

Reference	N	Mo	VPDs	Prevalence	Mortality (%) Risk group		Sudden D (%) Risk group	
					High	Low	High	Low
MILIS '82	388	14	Pairs VT	26	16	3	—	—
MPIP '84	766	24	Pairs VT	28	20	7	13	4
			≥ 10/h	20	19	9	13	5
BHAT '87	3290	25	Pairs VT	21	16	8	8	3
			≥ 10/h	13	20	8	9	4

N = Number of cases.
Mo = Months.
VPD = Ventricular premature depolarization.
VT = Ventricular tachycardia.

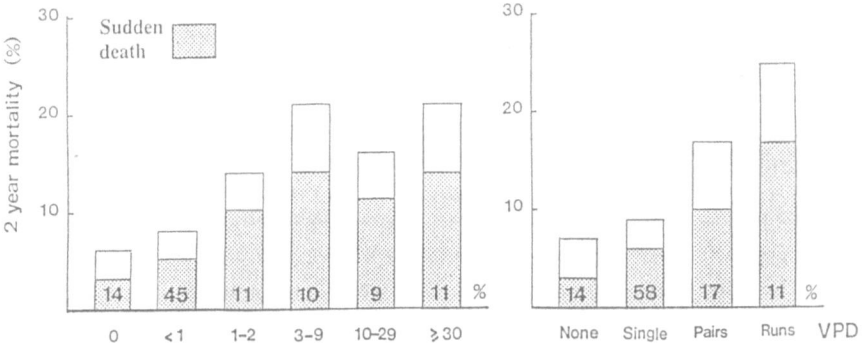

Figure 6. Two year mortality of patients surviving a myocardial infarction, according to the frequency or complexity of the ventricular ectopic activity (VPD) recorded by the 24-h Holter monitoring system. The dark area of the bar represents the % of SCD (Data taken from Bigger [13]).

premature depolarizations on the 24-h Holter recordings. The mortality increases as ectopic activity rises from one to 10/h and then reaches a 'plateau'.

Figure 7 shows that the presence of ventricular ectopic activity of 3

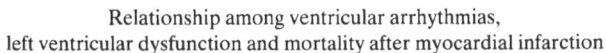

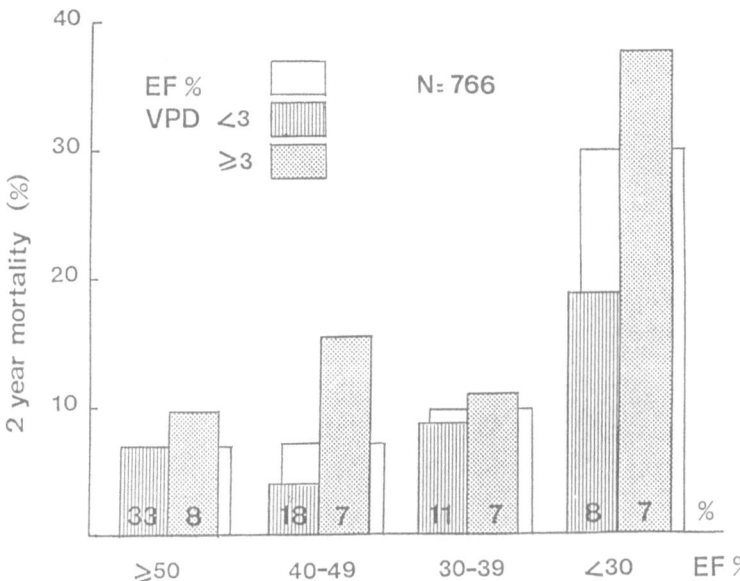

Figure 7. Two year mortality rate of patients surviving a myocardial infarction, stratified according to EF% and the presence of 3 or more VPD/h. (Data taken from Bigger [13]).

VPD/hour increases the 2 year mortality rate in patients with an LVEF of less than 30% up to 39%, significantly larger than the mortality of patients with a lesser degree of premature activity. The relation of ectopic activity and mortality is less obvious in patients with good left ventricular function. Accordingly the antiarrhythmic treatment should be restricted to patients with impaired LVEF.

Based on a study of 191 survivors of 'non Q-wave myocardial infarction' Maise [51] concluded that the ventricular ectopic activity was a significant predictor of mortality independent of LVEF, only in patients with 'non Q-wave' infarction. Mortality in patients with Q wave infarction (9%) could be related to the impairment of the left ventricular function, while death rate in patients with a 'non Q-wave infarction' (35%) might be atributed to an 'unstable ischemic state' precipitating the ventricular arrhythmias.

New parameters are presently under study in order to clarify the mecanisms of the electrical unstability in post-infarction patients: programed ventricular stimulation, post-potentials, changes in heart rate or the prolongation of the QT interval, that may reflect the dispersion of the repolarization favoring the reentry mechanism. Their prognostic value is discussed in other chapters of this symposium.

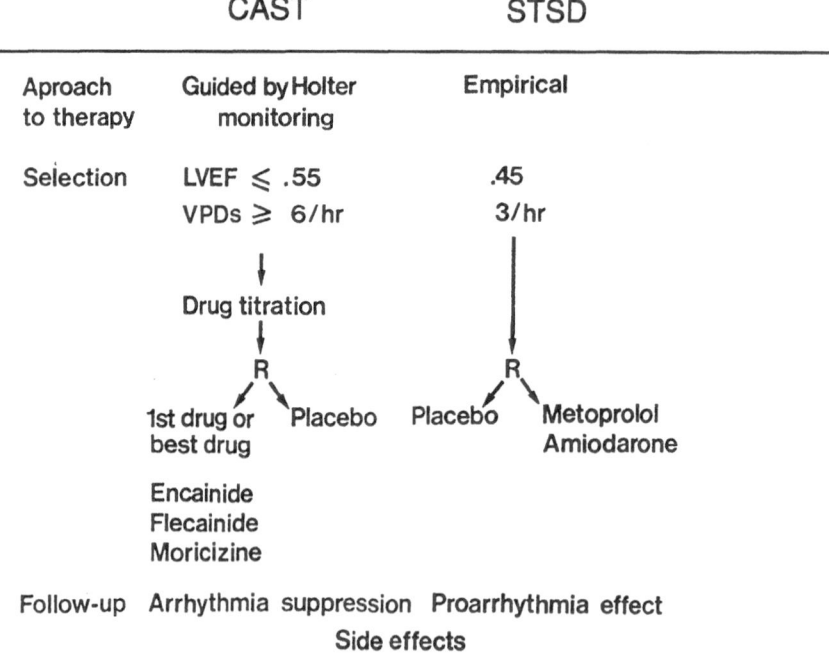

Figure 8. Essentials of the protocol design in the CAST and STSD antiarrhythmic trials.

Treatment

The definite proof of the validity of the arrhythmic hypothesis awaits the results of the clinical trials showing that antiarrhythmic treatment may be effective in preventing SCD. So far, no trial has been able to show any benefit. Recently two new clinical trials have been launched to test this hypothesis (Figure 8): the CAST [52] and the STSD (Spanish Trial on Sudden Death) [53]. Some features may distinguish these trials from the previous ones. In the first place they exclude patients with good ventricular function in order to avoid unnecessary treatment and dilution of the statistical power. And in second place a careful supervision of the arrhythmogenic effects of the drugs has been planned, since the detrimental effects of the drugs may overcome their preventive benefit. The treatment in CAST is guided by the response to the drug as monitored by the Holter recordings. The treatment is empirical in the STSD. Hopefully we will soon have a definite answer if antarrhythmic therapy to prevent SCD will be justified in patients surviving a myocardial infarction.

References

1. Moss AJ, DeCamilla J, Engstrom F, Hoffman W, Odoeroff C, Davies H: The posthospital phase of myocardial infarction. Identification of patients with increased mortality risk. Circulation 1974; 49: 460—466.
2. Multicenter Post-infarction Research Group: Risk stratification and survival after myocardial infarction. N Engl J Med 1983; 309: 331—336.
3. Moss AJ, Bigger JT, Odoroff CL: Postinfarct risk stratification. Progr Card Dis 1987; 29: 389—412.
4. Surawicz B: Prognosis of ventricular arrhythmias in relation to sudden cardiac death: therapeutic implications. JACC 1987; 10: 435—477.
5. Gottlieb SH, Ouyang P, Gottlieb SO: Death after acute myocardial infarction: interrelation between left ventricular dysfunction, arrhythmias and ischemia. Am J Cardiol 1988; 61: 7B—12B.
6. Lee ET: Statystical methods for survival data analysis. Lifetime Learning Pb. Belmont, California, 1980.
7. Diamond GA: Thallium uptake by the lungs in coronary artery disease (Letter). N Engl J Med 1988; 318: 1543.
8. Peel AAF, Semple T, Wang I, Lancaster WM, Dall JLG: A coronary prognostic index for grading the severity of infarction. Br Heart J 1962; 24: 745—760.
9. Killip T III, Kimball JT: Treatment of myocardial infarction in a coronary care unit. Am J Cardiol 1967; 20: 457—464.
10. Norris RM, Brandt PWT, Caughey DE, Lee AJ, Scott PJ: A new coronary prognostic index. Lancet 1969; 1: 275—278.
11. Forrester JS, Diamond GA, Swan HJC: Correlative classification of clinical and hemodynmaic function after myocardial infarction. Am J Cardiol 1977; 39: 137—145.
12. Sanz G, Castañer A, Betriu A, Magriña J, Roig E, Coll S, Paré JC, Navarro-Lopez F: Determinants of prognosis in survivors of myocardial infarction. A prospective clinical angiographic study. N Engl J Med 1982; 306: 1065—1070.
13. Bigger JT, Fleiss JL, Kleiger R, Miller, JP, Rolnitzky LM and MPRG: The relationship

among ventricular arrhythmias, left ventricular disfunction, and mortality in the 2 years after myocardial infarction. Circulation 1984; 69: 250—258.

14. Mukarjii J, Rude RE, Poole WK, Gustafson N, Thomas LJ, Strauss HW, Jaffe AS, Muller JE, Roberts R, Raabe DS, Crof CH, Passamani E, Braunwald E, Willerson JT and the MILIS Group: Risk factors for sudden death after acute myocardial infarction: two-year follow-up. Am J Cardiol 1984; 54: 31—36.

15. Ahne S, Gilppin E, Henning H, Curtis G, Collins D, Ross J: Limitations and advantages of the ejection fraction for defining high risk after acute myocardial infarction. Am J Cardiol 1986; 58: 872—878.

16. Moss AJ, Bigger JT, Odoroff ChL: Postinfarction risk stratification. Progr Cardiovasc Dis 1987; 29: 389—412.

17. Tibbits PA, Evaul JE, Goldstein RE, Boccuzzi SJ, Therneau TM, Parker R, Wong D and the MPRG: Serial acquisition of data to predict one year mortality rate after acute myocardial infarction. Am J Cardiol 1987; 60: 451—455.

18. White HD, Norris RM, Brown MA, Brandt PW, Whitlock RM, Wild CJ: Left ventricular end-systolic volume is the major determinant of survival after recovery from myocardial infarction. Circulation 1987; 76: 44—51.

19. Greenberg H, McMaster P, Dwyer EM and the MPRG: Left ventricular dysfunction after acute myocardial infarction: results of a prospective multicenter study. JACC 1984; 4: 867—874.

20. Rapaport E, Remedios P: The high risk patient after recovery from myocardial infarction: recognition and management. J Am Coll Cardiol 1983; 1: 391—400.

21. Josephson ME, Horowitz LN, Farshidi A, Kastor JA: Recurrent sustained ventricular tachycardia. Circulation 1978; 57: 431—439.

22. Meizlish JL, Berger HJ, Plankey M, Errico D, Levy W, Zaret BL: Functional left ventricular aneurysm formation after acute anterior transmural myocardial infarction. N Engl J Med 1984; 311: 1001—1006.

23. Heras M: Historia natural del aneurisma del ventrículo izquierdo post-infarto de miocardio. Tesis doctoral. Centro de Publicaciones. Universidad de Barcelona, 1986.

24. Hinkle LE, Thaler HT: Clinical classification of cardiac deaths. Circulation 1982; 65: 457—464.

25. Moss AJ, Davies HT, Conard DL, DeCamilla JJ, Odoroff CL: Digitalis associates cardiac mortality after acute myocardial infarction. Circulation 1983; 67: 300—334.

26. Bigger JT, Weld FM, Rolnitzky LM: Which postinfarction ventricular arrhythmias should be treated? Am Heart J 1982; 103: 660—666.

27. Gang ES, Bigger JT, Livelli FD: A model of chronic ischemic arrhythmias: the relation between electrically inducible ventricular tachycardia, ventricular fibrilation threshold and myocardial infarct size. Am J Cardiol 1982; 50: 469—477.

28. Garan H, Ruskin JN, McGobern B, Grant G: Serial analysis of electrically induced ventricular arrhythmias in a canine model of myocardial infarction. JACC 1985; 5: 1095—1106.

29. Pfeffer JM, Pfeffer MA, Braunwald E: Influence of captopril therapy on the infarcted left ventricle of the rat. Cir Res 1985; 57: 84.

30. The Consensus Trial Study Group: Effects of Enalapril on mortality in severe congestive heart failure. Results of the Cooperative North Scandinavian Enalapril Survival Study. N Engl J Med 1987; 316: 1429—1435.

31. Taylor GJ, Humphries JO, N, Mellits *et al.*: Predictors of clinical course, coronary anatomy and left ventricular function after recovery from acute myocardial infarction. Circulation 1980; 62: 960—970.

32. Sami M, Kraemer H, DeBusk RF: The prognostic significance of serial exercise testing after myocardial infarction. Circulation 1979; 60: 1238—1246.

33. Theroux P, Waters DD, Halphen C, Debaiseauux JC, Mizgala H: Prognostic value of exercise testing soon after myocardial infarction. N Engl J Med 1979; 301: 341—345.

34. Velasco J, Tormo V, Ferrer LM, Ridocci F, Blanch S: Early exercise test for evaluation

of long-term prognosis after uncomplicated myocardial infarction. Eur J Cardiol 1981; 2: 401—407.

35. Weld FM, Chu KL, Bigger JT, Rolnitzky LM: Risk stratification with low-level exercise testing 2 weeks after acute myocardial infarction. Circulation 1981; 64: 306—314.

36. Krone RJ, Gillespie JA, Weld FM, Miller JP, Moss AJ and the MPRG: Low-level exercise testing after myocardial infarction: usefulness in enhancing clinical risk stratification. Circulation 1985; 71: 80—89.

37. Fioretti P, Brower R, Simons ML, Katen H, Beelen A, Baardman T, Lubsen J, Hugenholtz P: Relative value of clinical variables, bycicle ergometry, rest radionuclide ventriculography and 24 hour ambulatory electrocardiographic monitoring at discharge to predict 1 year survival after myocardial infarction. JACC 1986; 8: 40—49.

38. Legrand V, Mancini J, Bates ER, Hodgson JMcB, Gross MD, Vogel RA: Comparative study of coronary flow reserve, coronary anatomy and results of radionuclide exercise test in patients with coronary artery disease. J Am Coll Cardiol 1986; 8: 1022—1032.

39. Gibson RS, Watson DD, Craddock GB, Crampton RS, Kaiser DL, Denny MJ, Beller GA: Prediction of cardiac events after uncomplicated myocardial infarction: a prospective study comparing predischarge exercise thalium-201 scintigraphy and coronary angiography. Circulation 1983; 68: 321—336.

40. Hakki A, Nestico PF, Heo J, Unwala AA, Iskkandrian AS: Relative prognostic value of rest thalium-201 imaging, radionuclide ventriculography and 24 hour ambulatory electrocardiographic monitoring after acute myocardial infarction. J Am Coll Cardiol 1987; 10: 25—32.

41. Amsterdam EA: Silent myocardial ischemia, arrhythmias and sudden death: are they related? Am J Cardiol 1987; 59: 919—910.

42. Cannom D, Levy W, Cohen L: The short and long term prognosis of patients with transmural and nontransmural infarction. Am J med 1976; 61: 452.

43. Bosch X, Theroux P, Waters D, Pelletier GB, Roy D: Early postinfarction ischemia: clinical, angiographic and prognostic significance. Circulation 1987; 75: 988—995.

44. Bayés de Luna A, Carreras F, Cladellas M, Oca F, Sagues F, Garcia Moll M: Holter ECG study of the electrocardiographic phenomena in Prinzmetal angina attacks with emphasis on the study of ventricular arrhythmias. J Electrocardiol 1985; 18: 265—275.

45. Ruberman W, Weinblatt E, Goldberg J, Chaudhary BS: Psychosocial influences on mortality after myocardial infarction. N Engl J Med 1984; 311: 552—559.

46. Bracket CD, Powell LH: Psychosocial and physiologic predictors of sudden cardiac death after healing of acute myocardial infarction. Am J Cardiol 1988; 61: 979—983.

47. Kolter MN, Tabatznik B, Mower MM, Tominaga S: Prognostic significanced of ventricular ectopic beats with respect to sudden death in the late postinfarction period. Circulation 1973; 47: 959—966.

48. Ruberman W, Weinblatt E, Goldberg JD, Frank CW, Chaudhary BS, Shapiro S: Ventricular premature beats and sudden death after myocardial infarction. Circulation 1981; 64: 297—305.

49. Califf RM, Wagner GS, Rosati RA: Prognostic value of ventricular arrhythmias (Abst). Am J Cardiol 1981; 47: 397.

50. Kostis JB, Byington R, Friedman LM, Goldstein S, Furberg C, for the BHAT Study Group: Prognostic significance of ventricular ectopic activity in survivors of acute myocardial infarction. J Am Coll Cardiol 1987; 10: 231—242.

51. Maisel AS, Scott N, Gilpin E, Ahne S, LeWinter M, Henning H, Collins D, Ross J: Complex ventricular arrhythmias in patients with Q wave versus non-Q wave myocardial infarction. Circulation 1985; 72: 963—970.

52. The CAPS investigators: The cardiac arrhythmia pilot study. Am J Cardiol 57; 91: 1986.

53. Grupo Investigador del Estudio Español de la Muerte Súbita (EEMS): Ensayo multicéntrico sobre la prevención de la muerte súbita con agentes antiarritmicos en el postinfarto de miocardio. Rev Esp Cardiol 1989; 42: 77—83.

21. Acute non-Q wave myocardial infarction

A summary of the diltiazem reinfarction study (DRS) and the multicenter diltiazem post-infarction trial (MDPIT)

WILLIAM E. BODEN and ROBERT E. KLEIGER

Introduction

During the last 30 years, it has been consistently observed that patients with non-Q-wave myocardial infarction (MI) have a greater likelihood of subsequent fatal and non-fatal cardiac events, particularly during long-term follow-up, than do patients with Q-wave MI. Because non-Q-wave MI is associated acutely with only a modest amount of myocardial necrosis, and because the attendant hemodynamic perturbations are less severe than in Q-wave MI patients, it is understandable why short-term survival time is decidedly greater and pump-related complications, such as congestive heart failure and shock, are decidedly fewer in patients with non-Q-wave MI [1—6].

Pathogenetic mechanisms

Data regarding the pathogenetic mechanism of acute non-Q-wave MI are not definitive. The amount of left ventricular myocardium that is presumably at risk for infarction should be the same for Q-wave or non-Q-wave MI, based on coronary angiographic and autopsy data that show that the extent of coronary artery disease and associated cardiac risk factors are nearly identical [7—16]. Moreover, if we assume that the initiating event (i.e., total coronary occlusion) in Q-wave and non-Q-wave MI is identical, it appears plausible to hypothesize that the etiology for both infarction subtypes is identical. However, in the course of Q-wave MI without intervention, thrombosis alone or that superimposed on critical coronary artery disease, results in total and sustained coronary arterial obstruction, with resulting transmural necrosis, more extensive creatine kinase (CK) release, and the evolution of Q-waves in the majority of patients. In contrast, in patients with non-Q-wave MI, the evolving infarction is aborted prematurely due to early thrombolysis (spontaneous or through intervention), cessation of acute vasospasm, or both. Such patients may have an endogenously more active

A. Bayés de Luna et al. (eds.): *Sudden Cardiac Death*, 239—253.
© 1991 Kluwer Academic Publishers, Dordrecht.

fibrinolytic system that promotes spontaneous clot lysis during the early course of evolving acute MI [17, 18].

Thus, while the degree of underlying coronary narrowing may be identical in both types of infarct, and thrombosis may be the inciting event, most patients with non-Q-wave MI exhibit nonsustained or subtotal coronary obstruction. The result is some degree of early myocardial salvage (particularly the subepicardium), predominantly subendocardial necrosis, less CK release, and the absence of evolutionary Q waves.

Role of reinfarction and early recurrent ischemia

It appears that the unexpectedly high long-term mortality rate of patients with non-Q-wave MI is due either to recurrent myocardial ischemia culminating in reinfarction [19, 20] or to arrhythmogenic sudden death [21, 22]. Cannom et al. [23] found that the incidence of sudden cardiac death was higher after non-Q-wave MI (33%) compared with Q-wave MI (15%).

Further, Theroux et al. found that the incidence of reinfarction and postinfarction angina during hospitalization was higher after non-Q-wave MI than after Q-wave MI [24]. Lekakis et al. [25] demonstrated convincingly that not only was reinfarction after non-Q-wave MI more common than after Q-wave MI, but was also associated with an additional decrement in left ventricular function and survival [25]. Other non-fatal cardiac events, including early recurrent ischemia, unstable angina, and the need for myocardial revascularization with bypass surgery or angioplasty, are more likely to occur after non-Q-wave MI [26, 27].

Importance of post-infarction angina

The frequency of early post-infarction angina and its prognostic significance was determined recently from the Diltiazem Reinfarction Study [28] of the 576 non-Q wave MI patients, 330 (57%) exhibited one or more episodes of spontaneous angina ≥ 24 hours after the index non-Q wave MI. The patients with post-infarction angina were further dichotomized on the basis of the presence (n = 115) or the absence (n = 131) of associated ischemic ST-T wave changes. The combined endpoints or early reinfarction, death prior to hospital discharge, or a combination of reinfarction or death for the subgroup of post-infarction angina alone vs. post-infarction angina with ECG changes (early recurrent ischemia) were examined. In the subgroup of patients with early recurrent ischemia, there was a *four-fold* increased incidence of reinfarction and a *ten-fold* increased incidence of death within 2 weeks (11.5% vs. 1.5%). When these endpoints were combined, there was a five-fold increased incidence of reinfarction or death prior to hospital discharge in the early recurrent ischemia subgroup.

A similar analysis for *late* outcome variables was performed for the same subgroups of patients with and without post-infarction angina occurring during the period of early hospitalization after acute non-Q wave MI [29]. Using a similar format, we compared event rates for death, myocardial revascularization and any ischemic cardiac event for non-Q wave MI patients with and without early post-infarction angina. In the subgroup with early post-infarction angina, there was a two-fold increase in late mortality and the need for myocardial revascularization, while there was a 50% increased incidence of any ischemic cardiac event during the 1 year follow-up period. (Figure 1)

Of note, when the 115 patients with post-infarction angina associated with transient ischemic ECG changes were compared to the 461 patients without post-infarction angina and ischemic ECG changes, there was an even higher comparative cardiac event rate for 1 year death (20% vs. 9%), late reinfarction (27% vs. 18%), need for myocardial revascularization (25% vs. 13%) and any ischemic cardiac event (33% vs. 16%) (Figure 2) [29].

The role of ST segment depression in non-Q wave MI

One year follow-up data on 515 patients from the Diltiazem Reinfarction Study who survived hospitalization with MB-CK confirmed acute non-Q-wave myocardial infarction were analyzed for factors related to mortality events (N = 57) and late reinfarction events (N = 64). Twelve of 24 analyzed variables were significantly associated with mortality. Those factors which were independently predictive of mortality by Cox regression analysis were persistent ST depression (p = 0.0009), a history of congestive heart failure (CHF, p = 0.0069), — older age (p = 0.0128), and ST elevation at hospital

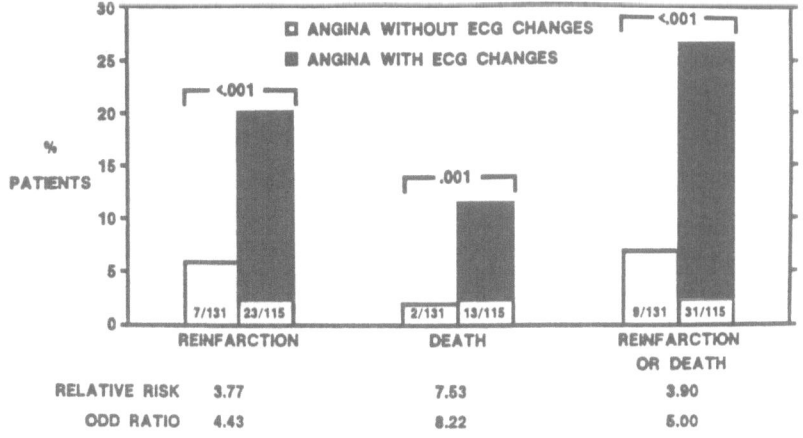

Figure 1.

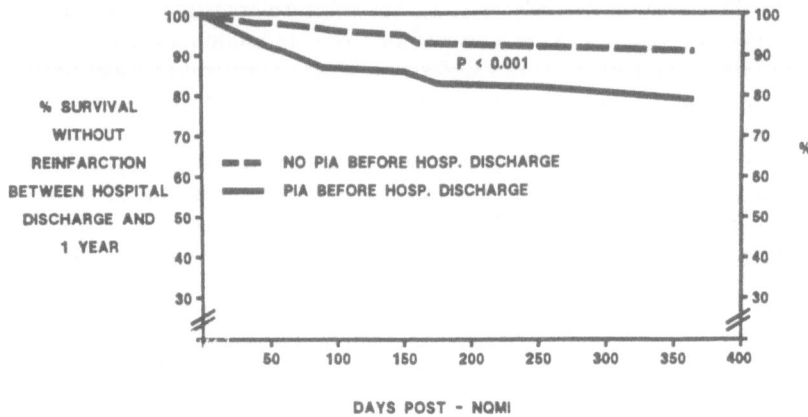

Figure 2. Cumulative mortality.

discharge (p = 0.0173). In-hospital reinfarction achieved borderline significance (p = 0.0512).

Mortality during the follow-up period was 5.5% in patients with no ST depression, 10.1% in those with ST depression at baseline *or* discharge, and 22.2% in patients with ST depression at baseline *and* discharge (i.e. 'persistent' ST depression) (Figure 3). When compared to the lower risk patients who had no ST depression at either time point, no CHF, and no discharge ST elevation, age-adjusted risk ratios for mortality ranged from a low of 1.82

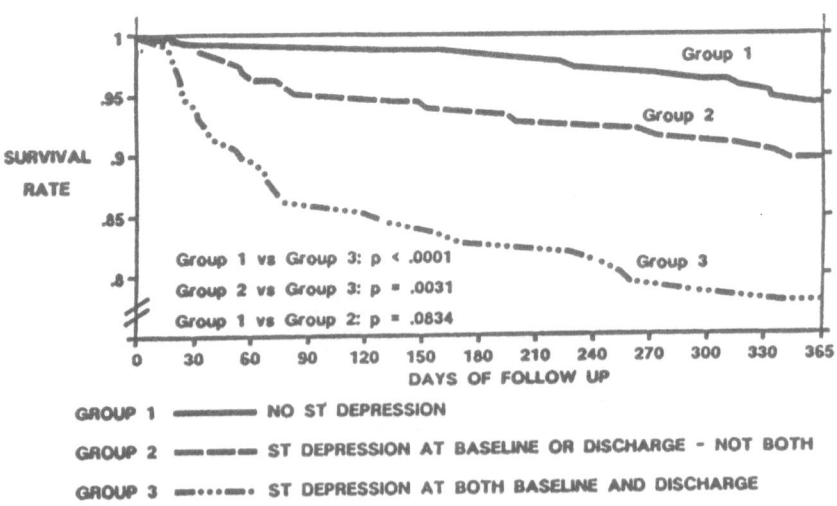

Figure 3. Mortality by category of ST depression.

(patients with ST depression at baseline or discharge but not at both time points and who had no discharge ST elevation or CHF) to a high of 13.99 (patients with persistent ST depression, discharge ST elevation, and CHF) (Figure 4). of the 483 patients with complete ECG data at both baseline and discharge, 203 (42%) could be stratified into a high risk population with a risk ratio for one year mortality more than 7 times that of patients with no risk factors. Although persistent ST depression was significantly associated with several measures of structural left ventricular damage, the independent significance of ST depression persisted even after adjusting for these factors. The independent predictors of late reinfarction were persistent ST depression, p = 0.0058; Killip Class II or III, p = 0.0106, and left ventricular hypertrophy, p = 0.0470. This analysis permitted a similar risk stratification (Figure 5).

These data indicate that:

(1) easily identified clinical and electrocardiographic factors permit stratification of patients with non-Q-wave infarction into high risk subsets who may benefit from aggressive therapy;

(2) ST depression is a highly significant and independent predictor of poor prognosis which appears to be associated with chronic left ventricular damage;

(3) the powerful predictive value of persistent ST depression in non-Q-wave MI, even after adjusting for measures of structural damage, suggests that such ST depression may reflect large areas of hypoperfused and ischemic (or 'hibernating') myocardium predisposing to reinfarction, malignant arrhythmias, and deterioration of left ventricular function.

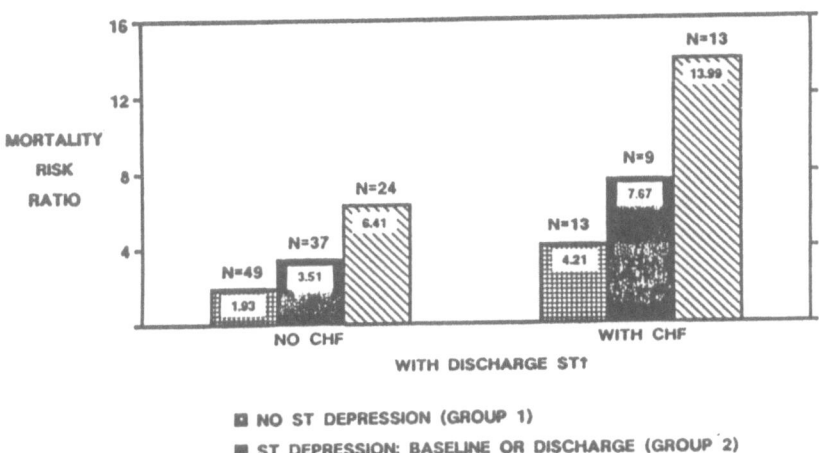

Figure 4. Age adjusted risk ratio of one year mortality.

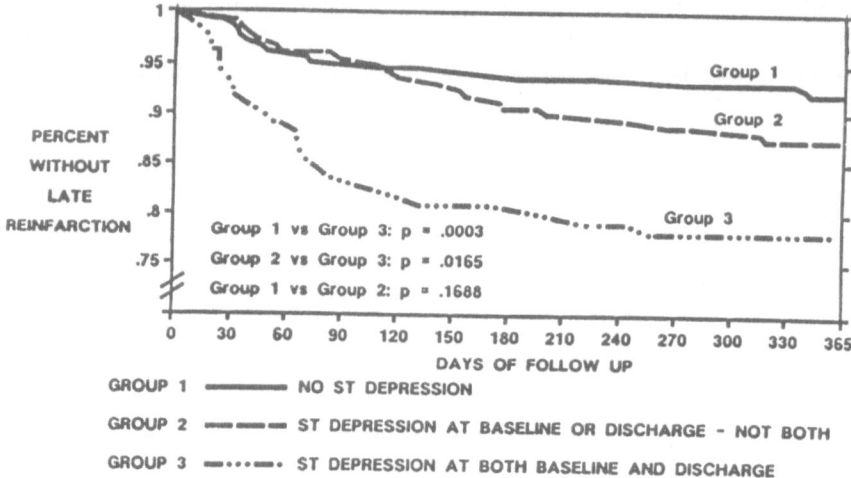

Figure 5. Late reinfarction by category of ST depression.

Role of left ventricular hypertrophy in non-Q wave MI

Left ventricular (LV) hypertrophy is known to be an independent risk factor for cardiac death, but its significance in non-Q wave MI has not been assessed previously. In a randomized diltiazem-placebo-controlled therapeutic trial of non-Q wave MI confirmed by creatine kinase-MB (CK-MB), 126 of 544 patients (23%) exhibitd LV hypertrophy using standard voltage criteria. Compared to patients without LV hypertrophy, patients with LV hypertrophy were significantly older (65 vs. 60 years, p < 0.0001) and had smaller peak adjusted CK levels (490 ± vs. 666 ± 726 IU/1, p < 0.001) than patients without LV hypertrophy [30]. Patients with and without LV hypertrophy did not differ significantly in acute mortality during hospitalization, progression to Q waves, reinfarction by CK-MB criteria or angina associated with transient electrocardiographic changes. Compared with patients without LV hypertrophy, those patients with non-Q-wave MI and LV hypertrophy had a 2-fold higher incidence of reinfarction (24 vs. 12%, p < 0.005) (Figure 7) and death (19 vs. 9%, p = 0.044) (Figure 6) during the first year of follow-up [30]. Multivariate regression analysis revealed that the relative risk of death and reinfarction during the initial year after AMI was increased by a factor of 1.7 and 2.1 among patients with LV hypertrophy, respectively [30]. It was therefore concluded that, although patients with LV hypertrophy and non-Q-wave MI have smaller enzymatic infarcts and the same short-term prognosis as do patients without LV hypertrophy, their reinfarction and mortality rates are significantly increased during the first

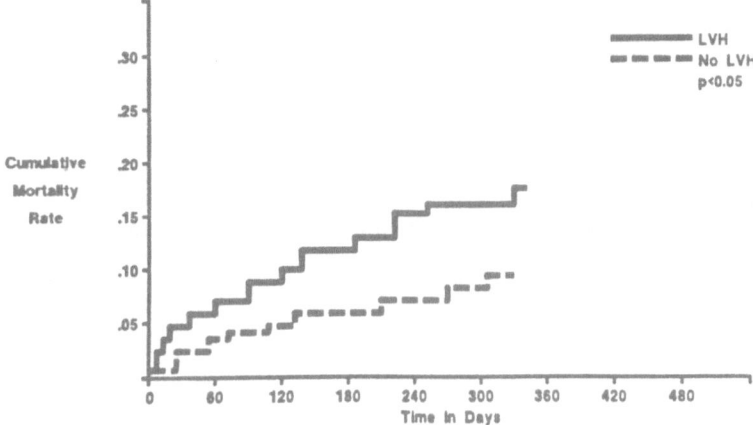

Figure 6. First-year mortality in survivors of non-Q wave AMI with and without LVH.

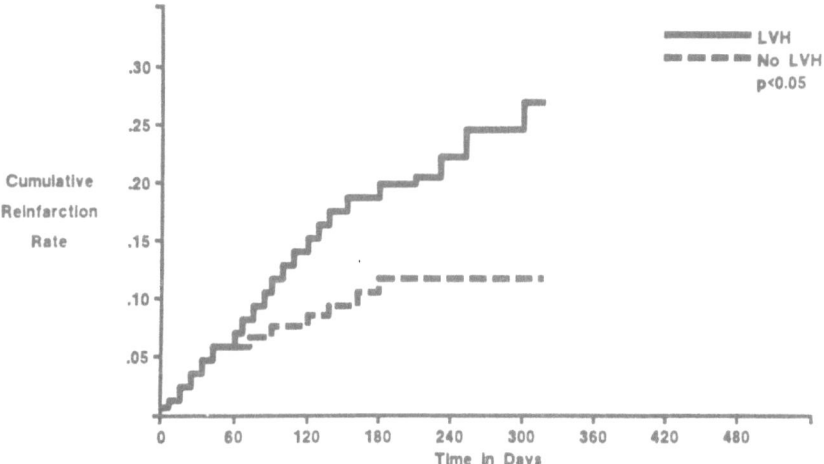

Figure 7. First-year reinfarction in survivors of non-Q wave AMI with and without LVH.

year of follow-up. Thus, patients with LV hypertrophy may warrant more intensive diagnostic evaluation and management during the recovery phase of non-Q-wave MI.

Risk assessment after non-Q wave MI

Stratification of post MI patients into low and high risk subgroups is vitally important in the overall investigation and management of patients, both acutely and long-term. Risk stratification is particularly important during the first year after acute MI, the period during which the risk of recurrent infarction and sudden death is greatest. Previous studies which have identified high risk subsets of patients with acute MI have included both Q-wave and non-Q wave infarction [31—34].

Given these short and long-term risks associated with non-Q-wave MI, many cardiologists advise that all patients with non-Q-wave MI have cardiac catheterization before hospital discharge. Before accepting this recommendation as a routine management strategy, physicians should consider several important concepts, including:

(1) The pathophysiologic basis for the greater clinical instability after non-Q-wave infarction may be related to 'incomplete infarction,' with a mass of viable myocardium that continues to be jeopardized after the infarction.
(2) Noninvasive testing, particularly stress radionuclide imaging, can identify patients who have residual ischemia.
(3) Although coronary angiography can identify an anatomic basis for ischemia, it cannot determine with certainly that a specific stenosis, or 'culprit lesion', is 'functionally significant,' i.e., that it will result in ischemia involving viable myocardium.

It should also be emphasized that patients with non-Q-wave MI make up a highly heterogeneous group. Although some patients will manifest residual peri-infarction ischemia, others (about 30—50%) will not. This latter group will have a very low incidence of recurrent ischemic events (i.e., reinfarction or unstable angina) in the year after hospital discharge, and a mortality rate of 2—5%. Whether such patients should undergo routine diagnostic coronary angiography remains controversial in the absence of findings from prospective studies. On the other hand, it appears reasonable for patients with early postinfarction angina, especially if it is associated with transient ST-T wave changes, to be considered or prompt cardiac catheterization and myocardial revascularization. This seems even more appropriate if the patients has been refractory to anti-ischemic and antiplatelet drug therapies.

Thus, it would appear that the highest risk subsets of patients with non-Q wave MI are those who develop spontaneous angina ≥ 24 hours after their index event, and those patients who have inducible ischemia during predischarge stress testing. Intermediate risk groups would likely include the remainder of non-Q wave MI patients who have congestive heart failure, those who exhibit persistent ST segment depression on review of serial ECG's obtained during hospitalization for the acute non-Q wave MI (even in the absence of symptoms), and those patients with LVH. Non-Q wave MI patients *without* any of the above clinical or electrocardiographic abnormalities would likely be considered low risk, and could be considered candidates for prophylactic secondary prevention with diltiazem (see below) together with close follow-up surveillance.

Medical management

Effect of beta blockers on reinfarction

The usefulness of long-term treatment with beta-adrenergic blocking agents has been evaluated in many large randomized clinical trials. Pooled data show that both mortality and recurrent infarction during follow-up are reduced by approximately 25% [35, 36]. None of these trials, however, was specifically designed to evaluate the subsets of patients with Q-wave and non-Q-wave infarction.

It is noteworthy that in three of the beta-blocker trials, little or no benefit with treatment in patients with non-Q-wave infarction was found. The Beta-Blocker Heart Attack Trial, [37] for example, observed reduced mortality and a lower reinfarction rate with propranolol when compared with placebo in 2858 patients with Q-wave infarction, but showed no effect on either and point in 873 patients with non-Q-wave MI. Similarly, in the Metoprolol in Acute Myocardial Infarction Trial [38] investigators found no reduction in mortality or reinfarction among the non-Q-wave patients. By comparison, the Norwegian Timolol Trial [39] showed prolonged survival in timolol-treated patients regardless of infarct type; however, the incidence of reinfarction was reduced only in patients with Q-wave MI.

Effect of calcium-channel blockers

Diltiazem reinfarction study
Changes in coronary vasomotor tone have been causally related to the prodromal syndrome of unstable angina pectoris leading to infarction, and such changes have been recognized as a potentially important etiological factor in acute myocardial infarction. Evidence has also suggested that vasomotor instability is common in the early postinfarction period and that reinfarction may result from primary changes in coronary smooth muscle tone, increased alpha-adrenergic activity, or the release of vasoactive substances from aggregating platelets. Because of the potent spasmolytic and coronary vasodilating actions of calcium channel blockers, it is reasonable to expect that these drugs might be beneficial in patients with incomplete infarctions who are vulnerable to additional ischemic insult due to transient, potentially reversible, reductions in coronary blood flow.

Currently, the Diltiazem Reinfarction Study (DRS) is the only study that has addressed the very specific problem of non-Q-wave infarction [40]. This trial, which recruited 576 patients between 1982-85 from nine medical centers in the USA and Canada, was designed to evaluate the effect of diltiazem (90 mg every 6 hours) versus placebo on the prevention of early recurrent infarction after non-Q-wave infarction Patients with non-Q-wave infarction were randomized to diltiazem (n = 287) or placebo (n = 289) between 24 and 72 hours after onset of infarction and were followed for up to 14 days. The primary endpoint, reinfarction, was defined as an abnormal reelevation of MBCK within 14 days. Secondary endpoints included post-infarction angina of any severity and refractory angina, defined as ischemic pain necessitating withdrawal from the study.

In the DRS, recurrent myocardial infarction was documented in 27 patients on placebo (9.3%) and in 15 patients on diltiazem (5.2%) [40]. Analysis of the cumulative life-table reinfarction rate showed a reduction of 51.2% (p < 0.029). Diltiazem also reduced the frequency of refractory postinfarction angina by 49.7% (p = 0.035) and the incidence of angina associated with transient ST-T wave changes by 28% (p = 0.005) [40]. Since the drug was safe and well tolerated, the authors of this multicenter study recommended prophylactic diltiazem as a valuable addition to the management of cases of non-Q-wave infarction. This certainly seems justified given the consistency of the reductions in the three prognostically important endpoints (i.e., reinfarction, angina refractory to medical therapy including intravenous nitroglycerin and angina associated with ST-T changes), and the fact that treatment with other drugs (e.g., beta-blockers, nifedipine or verapamil) is largely unproven in this subset of patients.

Other studies of calcium channel blockers can not be directly compared to the Diltiazem Reinfarction Study since no distinction was made between Q-wave and non-Q-wave infarctions. However, when the results of these studies are reviewed, the published findings are generally disappointing. For example, none of six trials of nifedipine, comprising a total of 7766 patients, showed a salutary effect on infarct size, mortality of reinfarction, and two actually suggested an increased risk for infarction or death among patients assigned to receive nifedipine versus placebo, or other trial medications. Neither of the two verapamil studies showed either a beneficial or deleterious treatment effect.

Multicenter diltiazem post-infarction trial

Clearly diltiazem has been shown to reduce the frequency of in-hospital reinfarction and refractory angina after non-Q wave myocardial infarction, but its long-term effect on reinfarction or survival has not been established. In order to address the issue of potential long-term benefit we performed a detailed prespecified subset analysis of recurrent first cardiac events (cardiac death or non-fatal reinfarctions) on a cohort of 634 non-Q wave myocardial infarction patients randomized within 3—15 days to The Multicenter Diltiazem Post-Infarction Trial [41] of prophylactic diltiazem 240 mg/day (n = 296) vs placebo (n = 338) therapy. Patients were followed for an average of 25 months (range = 12 to 52 months) and outcome was analyzed by the intention to treat principle.

Kaplan-Meier analysis showed a 43% reduction in the adjusted cumulative

1 year cardiac event rate (placebo = 15% [50/338] vs. diltiazem = 9% [25/296]); (p = 0.0296) with a Cox hazard ratio (95% confidence interval) of 0.64 (0.43—0.96) (Figure 8) [42]. There was an associated 30% reduction in total (all cause) mortality (placebo = 8% [28/338] vs. diltiazem 6% [18/296]) with a Cox hazard ratio = 0.70; 0.43—1.13. Similarly, there was a cumulative 38% reduction in cardiac mortality (plaebo = 7% [22/338] vs. diltiazem = 4% [13/296]) with a Cox hazard ratio = 0.62; 0.32—1.18. (Figure 8) The cumulative number of non-fatal reinfarctions at 6 months and 12 months was 23 and 29 in the placebo group, respectively, compared to 6 and 13 in the diltiazem group.

In addition to this main effect analysis, an interaction analysis was performed for a single prespecified covariate (the presence or absence of radiographic pulmonary congestion in the Coronary Care Unit) on outcome variables and treatment assignement on 612 patients who could be so dichotomized. For the 505 non-Q-wave infarction patients (80%) without pulmonary congestion, the adjusted 1 year rate of first cardiac events for placebo patients was 13% (34/362) compared to 6% (15/243) for diltiazem-treated patients; Cox hazard ratio = 0.62 (0.39—1.00), p < 0.05. Total cardiac mortality rates in placebo vs. diltiazem patients were 8% vs. 4% (0.54; 0.29—0.98), p < 0.05, and 7% vs. 0% (0.40; 0.19—0.86), p < 0.05, representing a 46% and 60% reduction, respectively, in the diltiazem group (Figure 9) [42].

In contrast, for the 107 patients with pulmonary congestion (20%), 1 year event rates for total and cardiac mortality in placebo vs. diltiazem patients were 10% vs. 21% (1.85%; 0.75—4.55) and 5% vs. 17% (2.11; 0.68—6.56) — and approximate 2-fold higher mortality in the diltiazem subgroup (Figure 9) [42].

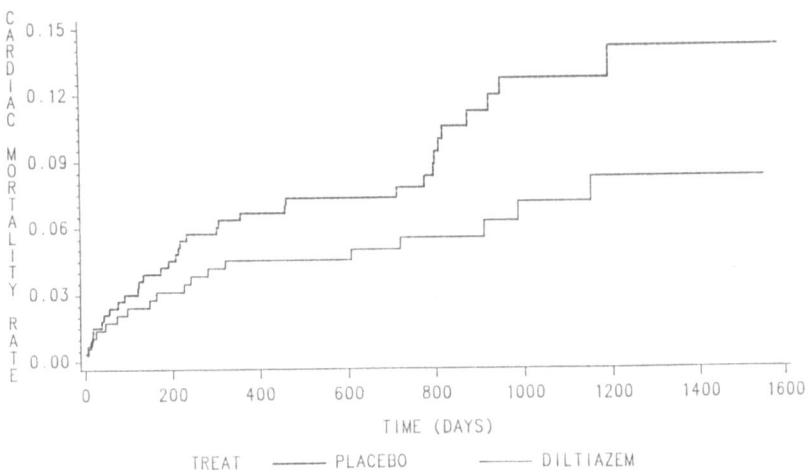

Figure 8. Non-Q patients time to cardiac death Kaplan-Meier estimates.

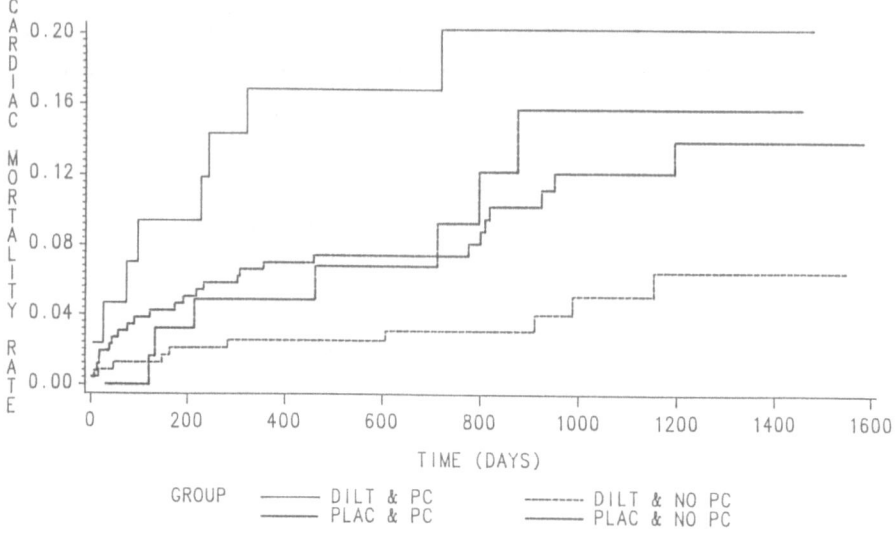

Figure 9. Non-Q patients time to cardiac death Kaplan-Meier estimates by treatment and pulmonary congestion.

Thus, diltiazem appeared effective in reducing the overall long-term cumulative first recurrent cardiac event rate after acute non-Q wave infarction; diltiazem prophylaxis was especially beneficial in the 80% of non-Q-wave infarction patients without pulmonary congestion, but was detrimental in the 20% of patients with pulmonary congestion.

Clinical implications

Non-Q wave infarction develops in approximately one-third of all patients admitted to a coronary care unit because of acute myocardial infarction, and data from three large community-wide surveys, obtained from 59 hospitals in three different geographical locations, yields a similar prevalence [43–45]. Indeed, compared to a decade ago, it appears that the prevalence of non-Q wave infarction has significantly increased.

Moreover, the pool of non-Q wave infarction patients may be expanding as a consequence of early intervention with thrombolytic therapy, which may abort an evolving Q-wave infarction and, as a consequence of improved myocardial salvage, may culminate in non-Q wave infarction. In support of this hypothesis is the preliminary data from the Thrombolysis in Myocardial Infarction Trial, in which the coronary perfusion status in patients with Q-wave was compared to those with non-Q wave infarction who presented initially with S-T segment elevation [46]. In the patients without initial Q waves (33%) had the persistence of non-Q wave infarction following successful coronary thrombolysis; moreover, in 14% of patients *with* initial Q waves prior to thrombolysis, subsequent Q waves disappeared after thrombolysis [46]. Thus, we hypothesize that 'reperfusion-induced' non-Q wave myocardial infarction may be an emerging subtype of infarction that may become increasingly more prevalent as the use of thrombolytic therapy becomes more universally available.

Summary

Since beta blockade has not been shown to be effective in non-Q wave infarction, and because dynamic changes in coronary vasomotor tone may play a role in the pathogenesis of non-Q wave infarction, and reinfarction, we believe that the data from the present study support the prophylactic use of diltiazem, in a dosage of 240 mg/day as used in this trial, in the majority of acute non-Q wave myocardial infarction patients. It appears that long-term outcome (both reinfarction and mortality) after acute non-Q wave infarction may be favorably altered by diltiazem prophylaxis in the 80% of patients without radiographic pulmonary congestion. Caution is advised, however, in the smaller subgroup of pateints with left ventricular dysfunction (20%) who may develop an increased cardiac event rate with diltiazem therapy.

Acknowledgement

The authors gratefully acknowledge the secretarial assistance of Mrs. Patricia Keddie in the preparation of this manuscript.

References

1. Norris RM, Brandt PWT, Caughey DE *et al.*: A new coronary prognostic index. Lancet 1976; 1: 274.
2. Schor S, Shani M, Modan B: Factors affecting immediate mortality of patients with acute myocardial infarction: A nation-wide study. Chest 1975; 68: 217.
3. Szklo M, Goldberg R, Kennedy HL, Tonascia JA: Survival of patients with non-transmural myocardial infarction: A population based study. Am J Cardiol 1978; 42: 648.
4. Connolly DC, Elveback LR: Comparison of hospital and post-hospital course of patients with transmural and subendocardial myocardial infarction. Am J Cardiol 1979; 43: 370.
5. Boxall J, Saltups A: A comparison of nontransmural and transmural myocardial infarction. Aust N Z J Med 1980; 10: 176.
6. Thanavaro S, Krone RJ, Kleiger RE *et al.*: In-hospital prognosis of patients with first nontransmural and transmural infarction. Circulation 1980; 61: 29.
7. Gibson RS, Beller GA, Gheorghiade M *et al.*: The prevalence and clinical significance of residual myocardial ischemia two weeks after uncomplicated non-Q-wave infarction: A prospective natural history study. Circulation 1986; 73: 1186.

8. Madias JE, Chahine RA, Gorlin A, Blocklow DJ: A comparison of transmural and nontransmural acute myocardial infarction. Circulation 1974; 49: 498.

9. Rigo P, Murray M, Taylor DR *et al.*: Hemodynamic and prognostic findings in patients with transmural and nontransmural infarction. Circulation 1975; 51: 1064.

10. Cannom D, Levy W, Cohen L: The short and long-term prognosis of patients with transmural and nontransmural infarction. Am J Med 1976; 61: 452.

11. Ahmed SS, Brancato RR: Transmural versus nontransmural myocardial infarction: Influence of location on clinical features and mortality. Angiology 1979; 30: 240.

12. Schroter H, Schulte KL, Beck OA *et al.*: Transmuraler and nichttransmuraler nyokardinfarkt. Herz 1978; 3: 185.

13. Coll S, Castaner A, Sanz G *et al.*: Prevalence and prognosis after first nontransmural myocardial infarction. Am J Cardiol 1983; 51: 1584.

14. Maisel AS, Ahnve S, Gilpin E *et al.*: Prognosis after extension of myocardial infarction: The role of Q-wave or non-Q-wave infarction. Circulation 1985; 71: 211.

15. Ogawa H, Hiramori K, Haze K *et al.*: Comparison of clinical features of non-Q-wave and Q-wave myocardial infarction. Am Heart J 1986; 111: 513.

16. Theroux P, Kouz S, Bosch X *et al.*: Clinical and angiographic features of non-Q-wave and Q-wave myocardial infarction. Circulation 1986; 74: 303.

17. Kleiman N, Goodman D, Schechtman K, Roberts R: Lack of diurnal variation in the occurrence of non-Q wave myocardial infarction: Results of a prospective study. J Am Coll Cardiol 1988; 2: 27A.

18. Gibson R: Clinical, functional, and angiographic distinctions between Q wave and non-Q wave myocardial infarction: Evidence of spontaneous reperfusion and implications for intervention trials. Circulation 1987; 75 (suppl v): V—128.

19. McQuay NW, Edwards JE, Burchell HB: Types of death in acute myocardial infarction. Arch Intern Med 1955; 96: 1.

20. Gibson RS, Young PM, Boden WE *et al.*: Prognostic significance and beneficial effect of diltiazem on the incidence of early recurrent ischemia after non-Q wave myocardial infarction: Results from the Multicenter Diltiazem Reinfarction Study. Am J Cardiol 1987; 60: 203.

21. Rigo P *et al.*: Hemodynamic and prognostic findings in patients with transmural and nontransmural infarction. Circulation 1975; 51: 1064.

22. Madias JE *et al.*: A comparison of transmural and nontransmural acute myocardial infarction. Circulation 1974; 49: 498.

23. Cannom D, Levy W, Cohen L: The short and long-term prognosis of patients with transmural and nontransmural infarction. Am J Med, 1976; 61: 452.

24. Theroux P, Kouz S, Bosh X *et al.*: Clinical and angiographic features of non-Q wave and Q-wave myocardial infarction. Circulation 1986; 74 (suppl IV): 303.

25. Lekakis J, Katosyanni K, Trichopoulos D, Tsitouris G: Q-wave versus non-Q-wave myocardial infarction: clinical characteristics and 6-month prognosis. Clin Cardiol 1984; 7: 283—288.

26. Bosch X *et al.*: Early postinfarction ischemia; Clinical, angiographic and prognostic significance. Circulation 1987; 988.

27. Richards DA *et al.*: Ventricular electrical instability: A predictor of death after myocardial infarction. Am J Cardiol 1983; 51: 75.

28. Gibson RS, Young PM, Boden WE, *et al.*: Prognostic significance and benefical effect of diltiazem on the incidence of early recurrent ischemia after non-Q-wave myocardial infarction. Am J Cardiol 1987; 60: 203.

29. Boden WE, Gibson RS, Capone RJ *et al.*: Early postinfarction angina is a predictor of poor long-term prognosis after acute non-Q wave myocardial infarction: The Diltiazem Reinfarction Study. J Am Coll Cadiol 1988; 11: 25A.

30. Boden WE, Kleiger RE, Schechtman KB *et al.*: Clinical significance and prognostic importance of left ventricular hypertrophy in non-Q-wave acute myocardial infarction. Am J Cardiol 1988; 62: 1000—1004.

31. Epstein SE, Palmeri ST, and Patterson SE: Evaluation of patients after acute myocardial infarction. N Engl J Med 1982; 307: 1487—1492.
32. The multicenter Postinfarction Research Group: Risk stratification and survival after myocardial infarction. N Engl J Med 1983; 309; 331—336.
33. Crawford MH and O'Rourke RA: The role of cardiac catheterization in patients after myocardial infarction. Cardiology Clinics 1984; 2: 105—111.
34. Beller GA, and Gibson RS: Risk stratification after myocardial infarction. Mod Concepts Cardiovasc. Dis 1986; 55: 5—10.
35. May GS: A review of long-term beta-blocker trials in survivors of myocardial infarction. Circulation 1983; 67 (suppl 1): 46.
36. Furberg CD: Effect of beta-blocker therapy on recurrent nonfatal myocardial infarction. Circulation 1983; 67 (suppl 1): 83.
37. Beta-Blocker Heart Attack Trial Research Group: A randomized trial of propranolol in patients with acute myocardial infarction. I. Mortality results. JAMA 1982; 247: 1707.
38. The MIAMI Trial Research Group: Mortality. Am J Cardiol 1985; 56 (suppl G): G-12.
39. Norweigian Multicenter Study Group: Timolol-induced reduction in mortality and reinfarction in patients surviving acute myocardial infarction. N Engl J Med 1981; 304: 801.
40. Gibson RS *et al.*: Diltiazem and reinfarction in patients with non Q wave myocardial infarction: Results of a double-blind, randomized multicenter trial. N Engl J Med 1986; 315: 423.
41. Moss AJ, Abrams J, Bigger JT, Boden WE, Bodenheimer M, Case RB *et al.*: The effect of diltiazem on mortality and reinfarction after myocardial infarction. N Engl J Med 1988; 319: 385—392.
42. Boden WE, Krone RJ, Kleiger RE, Miller JP, Hager WD, Moss AJ, and the MDPIT Research Group: Diltiazem reduces long-term cardiac event rate after non-Q wave infarction: Multicenter diltiazem post-infarction trial (MDPIT) Circulation 1988; 78 (4): II-96.
43. Szklo M, Goldberg R, Kennedy HL, Tonascia JA: Survival of patients with non-transmural myocardial infarction: a population based study. Am J Cardiol 1973; 42: 648—652.
44. Connolly DC, Elveback LR: Coronary heart disease in residents of Rochester Minnesota: Hospital and post-hospital course of patients with transmural and subendocardial myocardial infarction. Mayo Clin Proc 1985; 60: 375—381.
45. Goldberg RJ, Gore JM, Alpert JS, Dalen DE. Non-Q wave myocardial infarction: recent changes in occurrence and prognosis — a community wide perspective. Am Heart J 1987; 113: 273—279.
46. Bren GB, Wasserman AG, Ross AM. Coronary perfusion status in Q and non-Q wave infarction patients presenting with ST elevation in thrombolysis in Myocardial Infarction Study. Circulation 1987; 63 (IV): 123.

22. Treatment of heart failure

Impact on sudden death

J. GUINDO, A BAYÉS DE LUNA, P. TORNER, J. BARTOLUCCI and
R. ESTIARTE

Heart failure is the final situation in the natural history of the majority of
heart diseases. Once the first signs or symptoms appear the prognosis clearly
worsens.

In the Framingham Study [1] mortality at 4 years of having detected heart
failure was 55% in men and 24% in women. However, it is necessary to point
out that prognosis clearly depends on the first clinical manifestation of heart
failure, as it is not the same when diagnosis is made from dyspnea with
moderate effort plus a third sound or when the diagnosis is made following
acute pulmonary edema. Prognosis is also modified by the basal disease
leading to the heart failure (ischemic heart disease, valvular heart disease,
cardiomyopathy, etc.).

There is a clear relationship between heart failure and sudden death.
Approximately 50% of the deaths in these patients are sudden [2—17]. The
factors predicting poor prognosis in patients with heart failure (presence of
third sound, pulmonary rales, functional state according to the NYHA,
ejection fraction, presence of ventricular arrhythmias, etc) are discussed in
other chapters of the book. In this chapter we point out that the existence of
a vulnerable myocardium, in this case basically demonstrated by the poor
ejection fraction and premature ventricular impulses intervene in the
physiopathology of sudden death. Some modulating factors (alterations of the
autonomous nervous system, ionic and/or metabolic alterations, physical or
mental stress etc) are usually responsible for triggering the fatal event [18—
20] (Figure 1).

Value of drug therapy in the survival of patients with heart failure

Over recent years, many pharmacologic (inotropic, diuretic and vasodilator
drugs) and non-pharmacologic approaches (aortic counter pulsation pump,
heart transplant etc.) have appeared [21—31]. On continuation we are going
to focus exclusively on the value of drug therapy in the survival of patients
with heart failure, with particular regard to sudden death.

A. Bayés de Luna et al. (eds.): *Sudden Cardiac Death*, 255–265.
© 1991 Kluwer Academic Publishers, Dordrecht.

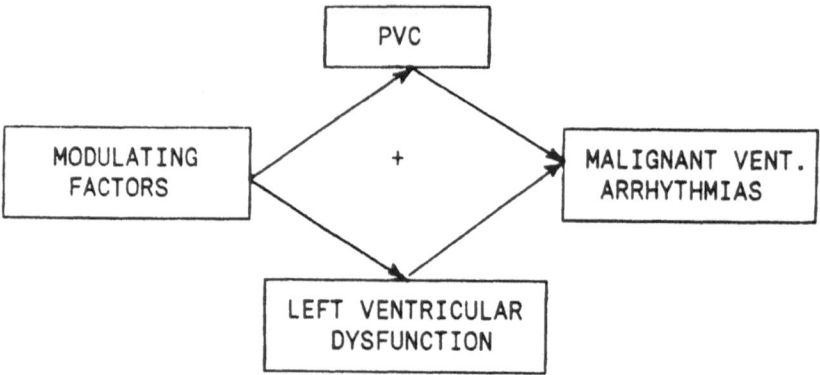

Figure 1. Physiopathology of malignant ventricular arrhythmias and sudden death in patients with dilated cardiomyopathy. PVC = premature ventricular contractions.

Inotropic drugs

Since the appearance of digoxine in the 18th century this drug has been one of the basic milestones in the treatment of heart failure. However, in recent years there has been much controversy over its efficacy in heart failure with sinus rhythm [32]. Although several studies [33—35] show that the use of digoxine is accompanied by a significative increase in the ejection fraction and a greater tolerance to exercise, there are several doubts about the beneficial influence in survival in patients with heart failure in sinus rhythm [21—32, 36]. It has even been shown that following acute myocardial infarction, its administration is accompanied by a greater mortality [37]. This is believed to be due to a proarrhythmic effect, especially when associated to electrolytic alterations which frequently appear in these patients (diuretics, renal failure, etc.).

Multiple inotropic oral drugs have appeared in recent years but none have proven superior to digoxine, although in some circumstances they may be a therapeutic alternative [38—40].

Inhibitors of phosphodiesterase have recently appeared, and as well as having positive inotropic effect they have a certain vasodilator effect [39]. To date there are no prospective trials which have evaluated their effect on survival in patients with heart failure. The PROMISE [41] study is presently underway in the United States and Canada, the aim of which is to study 750 patients with severe heart failure (class IV NYHA) refractory to conventional treatment with digitalic, diuretic and vasodilating drugs. Patients will be randomized to milrinone or placebo and will be followed up until death or until the study is considered finalized.

Diuretic drugs

Diuretic drugs are another milestone in the treatment of patients with heart failure and are indispensable in patients with hydric retention [21—31]. However, when this does not exist, their administration carries a serie of potential risks (particularly electrolytic alterations and facilitation of arrhythmias) which hardly justify their routine use. The loop diuretics are those most commonly used in patients with congestive heart failure. In initial stages of the disease adequate control of the diuresis may be obtained with the intermitent use of less potent agents such as hydrochlorotiazide.

Vasodilators

Many studies over the last decade have described the utility of vasodilators in the treatment of patients with heart failure [42—57]. They were initially considered to be indicated when diuretic or inotropic treatment was insufficient. However there is an increasing tendency to use these drugs earlier, to the point that we today believe they should be used as first line agents. The hemodynamic effect basically depends on their preferencial action upon the venous or arterial system. Within the venodilators, that most widely used in the chronic treatment of heart failure is isosorbide dinitrate [45—46]. The arterial vasodilators most commonly used are hydralazine [47] and the converting enzyme inhibitors (especially captopril and enalapril) [48—49].

Recent works clearly show that as well as improving the different hemodynamic parameters studied (cardiac output, ejection fraction, ventricular filling pressure, etc.) and the quality of life (e.g. exercise tolerance) of individuals with heart failure, vasodilators prolong survival [50—56].

In the Veterans Administration Cooperative Study [50] the efficacy of treatment with hydralazine (300 mg/day) associated with isosorbide dinitrate (160 mg/day) was compared with prazosin (20 mg/day) or placebo. A total of 642 patients with mild moderate heart failure (ejection fraction below 30%) was studied. Mean follow-up was of 2.3 years (range 6 months—5.7 years). During this period there were 120 deaths in the placebo group (44.0%), 91 in the group with prazosin (49.7%) and 72 in the group hydralazine + isosorbide dinitrate (38.7%). Of these deaths, 45% were sudden, although there were no differences between the three groups. As shown in Table 1 and Figure 2 the survival of patients treated with prazosin and placebo was similar, while the association of hydralazine and isosorbide dinitrate reduced mortality 38% in the first year, 25% in the second year and 23% in 3 years. Over the total follow-up period the reduction of mortality in the group treated with hydralazine was statistically significant (p < 0.05). Nevertheless, accumulated mortality in the two years of follow-up decreased 34% in respect to placebo (p < 0.028).

Regarding the converting enzyme inhibitors of angiotensine, there is evidence that both enalapril [52] and captopril [56] reduce mortality in patients with congestive heart failure. The Cooperative North Scandinavian Enalapril Survival Study (CONSENSUS) [57] included 253 patients with

Table 1. Veterans administration. Cumulative mortality rates at each anniversary of randomization in the placebo and hydralazine-isosorbide dinitrate (Hyd-Iso) groups (from Cohn *et al.* [50]).

Year	Alive at start		Cumulative mortality		Mortality reduction in Hyd-Iso group[a]
	Placebo N	Hyd-Iso N	Placebo %	Hyd-Iso %	(%)
1	273	186	19.5	12.1	38
2	201	147	34.3	25.6	25
3	134	108	46.9	36.2	23
4	82	70	53.6	49.7	7
5	40	36	—	—	—

[a] Based on life-table point estimate of mortality rates at the anniversary. Mortality-risk reductions that yielded an estimate of overall difference between survival curves up to the anniversary were 34% at two years and 36% at three years.

grade IV NYHA congestive heart failure who were randomized into placebo (n = 126) or enalapril (n = 127), in addition to conventional treatment. The doses of enalapril oscilated between 2.5 and 40 mg/day. Mean follow up was 188 days (range betweeen 1 day and 20 months). At 6 months total mortality was 44% in the placebo group and 26% in the enalapril group, meaning a

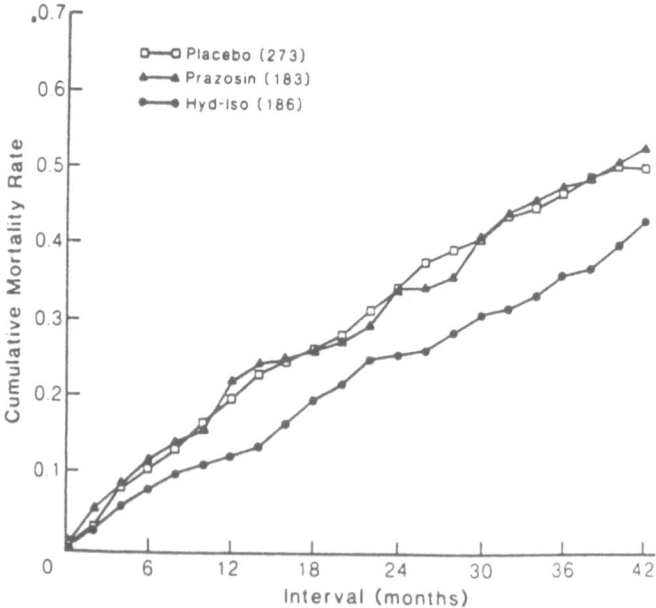

Figure 2. Veterans Administration Cooperative Study. Cumulative mortality from the time of randomization in the three treatment groups (From Cohn *et al.* [50]).

reducting of 40% (p < 0.002) (Figure 3). After the first year mortality was 52% in the placebo group and 36% in the group with enalapril (p = 0.001). At the end of the study a total of 118 patients had died, 68 in the placebo group and 50 in the enalapril group (reduction of 27%, p < 0.003). On analyzing the type of death (Table 2) it was seen that 28 patients (23%) died suddenly and 66 (56%) due to progression of the heart failure. There were no differences regarding the incidence of sudden death between the two groups. In conclusion, the CONSENSUS study shows that enalapril improves survival in grade IV NYHA congestive heart failure patients, although it does not modify the risk of sudden death.

As regards Captopril, several studies [53—56] have shown its efficacy both in improving the hemodynamic parameters and symtoms of heart failure and also in prolonging survival. Along these lines, the initial works of Pfeffer *et al.* [53, 54] showed experimentally that in rats with heart failure secondary to myocardial infarction and treated with captopril, survival was significatively prolonged in a follow-up of 1 year. The benefit of this drug appears to be particularly important in infarctions of a moderate size (involving between 30 and 45% of the circumference of the left ventricle). Newman *et al.* [56] have reaffirmed these results in the clinic. They studied 105 patients with moderate heart failure (mean ejection fraction 23%) who were randomized to captopril (n = 53) or placebo (n = 52). In a follow up of 90 days there were 11 deaths in the placebo group (21%) and only 2 in the group treated with captopril (4%) (p <0.01) (Table 3, Figure 4). Further-

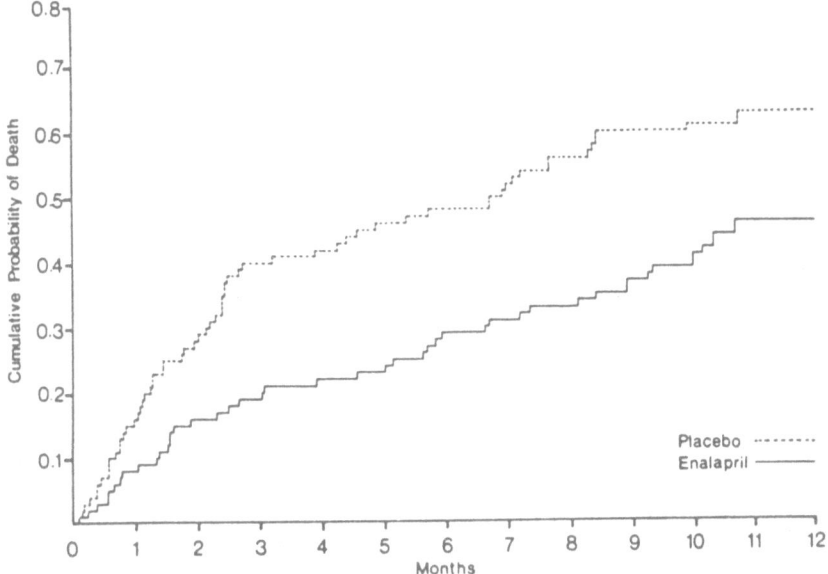

Figure 3. CONSENSUS. Cumulative probability of death in patients treated with placebo or enalapril (from CONSENSUS Trial Study Group [52]).

Table 2. Causes of death in CONSENSUS (from CONSENSUS Trial Study Group [52]).

Cause	Treatment group		p-value
	Placebo (N = 126)	Enalapril (N = 127)	(Life-table analysis)
Any cardiac death	64	44	0.001
Cardiac death within 24 hours of new symptoms	19	20	> 0.25
Sudden cardiac death (within 1 hour of new symptoms)	14	14	> 0.25
Progression of congestive heart failure	44	22	0.001
Other cardiac death	1	2	
Stroke	2	1	
Other cardiovascular deaths[a]	2	4	
Noncardiovascular death (perforated ulcer)	0	1	
Total mortality	68	50	0.003

[a] Includes deaths from renal-artery thrombosis, endocarditis, pulmonary emboli after leg amputation, bronchitis and concomitant heart failure, occlusion of femoral arterial graft, and heart failure in relation to melena (gastric ulcer).

Table 3. Ninety-day mortality status by New York heart association score at entry (Newmann *et al.* [56]).

	Captopril		Placebo	
Score	Died	Survived	Died	Survived
IIs	0	1	0	2
IIm	1	19	2	18
III	1	29	8	19
IV	0	2	1	2
Totals	2	51	11	41

more, 8 of the 11 deaths in the placebo group were sudden, while in the group treated with captopril only one patient died suddenly (p < 0.05).

Antiarrhythmic treatment

It is evident that ventricular arrhythmias are risk marks in patients with heart

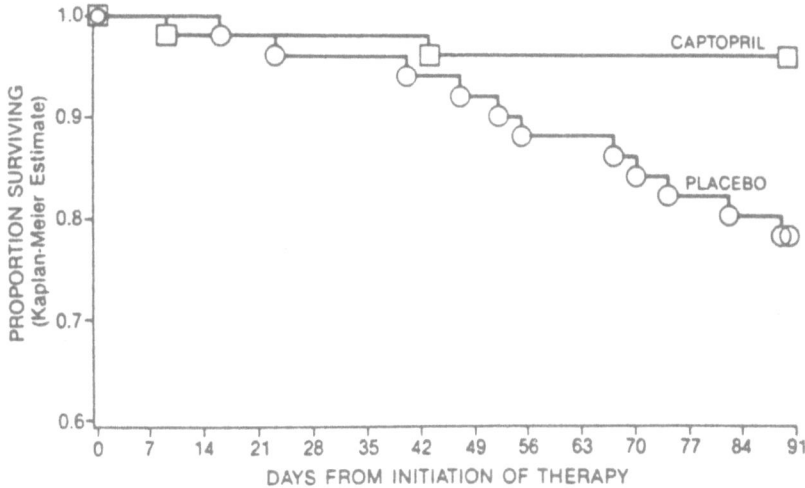

Figure 4. Patient survival as a function of time in patient treated with captopril versus placebo (from Newman *et al.* [56]).

failure, independent of the degree of severity [16–18, 58–62]. Converting enzyme inhibitors have proved to decrease the plasmatic concentration of catecholamines and increase the kaliemia [62] which, from a theoretical point of view, may have a certain beneficial effect on the arrhythmias of these patients. However, it presently seems that although vasodilator drugs prolong survival, this is probably due more to the improvement in heart failure than to a reduction in sudden death although in a short follow-up some decrease in sudden death has been demonstrated [56]. Nevertheless, it is necessary to develop large scale trials in order to confirm the beneficial effects of converting enzyme inhinitors in decreasing sudden death.

It seems necessary to know whether antiarrhythmic treatment may improve survival of patients with congestive heart failure. Although in some studies results have been favourable [63], no benefits have been demonstrated in others [15, 64–65]. It should be kept in mind that in these patients the antiarrhythmics are often poorly tolerated due to the fact that all present some degree of a negative inotropic effect, clearly limiting its use [66]. The risk of arrhythmogenesis is therefore much greater in these patients than in individuals with good ventricular function. This is due not only to the presence of a more vulnerable myocardium, but also because the heart failure implies metabolic and/or ionic alterations of the autonomous nervous system which facilitate the arrhythmogenesis. On the other hand, the treatment used in these patients (especially digitalic and diuretic drugs) may alter these anomalies and interactions in the metabolism of antiarrhythmics, even further making them even most dangerous. Flecainide and disopiramide are the more dangerous antiarrhythmics due to their depressant effect on contractility. They should not be used in patients with a low ejection fraction.

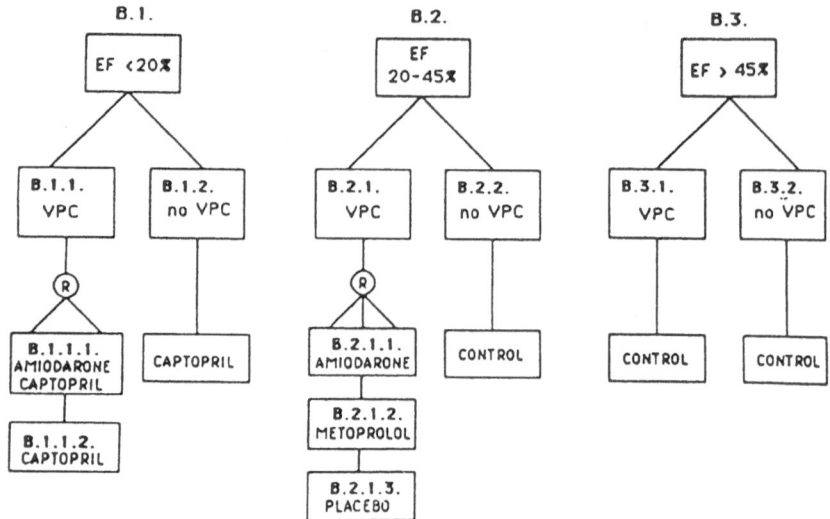

Figure 5. Algorhythm of Spanish Trial on Sudden Death (STSD). B Groups: acute myocardial infarction.

As a matter of fact, flecainide has been withdrawn from the CAST study due to its arrhythmogenic effect [67]. Propapenone also depresses left ventricular function and in some papers it has induced severe complications. In our opinion, amiodarone is the antiarrhythmic with low depressant effects.

In an attempt to determine whether antiarrhythmic treatment with amiodarone may be beneficial in patients with depressed contractility following myocardial infarction, in the Spanish Study of Sudden Death (STSD) [68] the patients with an ejection fraction below 20% and ventricular arrhythmias (group B 2.1, Figure 5) are randomized to captopril or captopril plus amiodarone. Due to the limited number of patients studied to date and the short follow-up time conclusive results are not yet available. Besides, with antiarrhythmic agents it will be necessary to carry out large scale trials to demonstrate whether an antiarrhythmic has beneficial or adverse effects. This is the conclusion of CAST in which flecainide has shown to be arrhythmogenic in a large scale trial with postinfarction patients, but not in the pilot trial (CAPS).

References

1. Kannel WB, Plehn JF, Cupples LA: Cardiac failure and sudden death in the Framingham study. Am Heart J 1988; 115: 869.
2. Likoff MJ, Chandler SL, Kay HR: Clinical determinats of mortality in chronic congestive heart failure secondary to idiopathic dilated or to ischemic cardiomyopathy. Am J Cardiol 1987; 59: 634.

3. Cohn JN: Current therapy of the failing heart. Circulation 1988; 78: 1099.
4. Packer M: Sudden unexpected death in patients with congestive heart failure: A second frontier. Circulation 1985; 72: 681.
5. Bigger JT: Why patients with congestive heart failure die: arrhythmias and sudden cardiac death. Circulation 1987; 75: IV-28.
6. Maskin CS, Siskind SJ, LeJemtel TH: High prevalence of nonsustained ventricular tachycardia in severe congestive heart failure. Am Heart J 1984; 107: 896.
7. Sakurai T, Kawai C: Sudden death in idiopathic cardiomyopathy. Jpn Circ J 1983; 47: 581.
8. Massie B, Ports T, Chatterjee K, Parmley W, Ostland J, O'Young J, Haughom F: Long-term vasodilator therapy for heart failure: clinical response and its relationship to hemodynamic measurements. Circulation 1981; 63: 269.
9. Lee WH, Packer M: Prognostic importance of serum sodium concentration and its modification by converting-enzyme inhibition in patients with severe chronic heart failure. Circulation 1986; 73: 257.
10. Wilson JR, Schwartz JS, Sutton MS-J, Ferraro N, Horowitz LN, Reichek N, Josephson ME: Prognosis in severe heart failure: relation to hemodynamic measurements and ventricular ectopic activity. J Am Coll Cardiol 1983; 2: 403.
11. Von Olshausen K, Schafer A, Mehmel HC, Schwartz F, Senges J, Kubler W: Ventricular arrhythmias in idiopathic dilated cardiomyopathy. Br Heart J 1984; 51: 195.
12. Franciosa JA, Wilen M, Ziesche SM, Cohn JN: Survival in men with severe chronic left ventricular failure due to either coronary heart disease or idiopathic dilated cardiomyopathy. Am J Cardiol 1983; 51: 831.
13. Huang SK, Messer JV, Denes P: Significance of ventricular tachycardia in idiopathic dilated cardiomyopathy: observations in 35 patients. Am J Cardiol 1983; 51: 507.
14. Francis GS: Development of arrhythmias in the patient with congestive heart failure: pathophysiology, prevalence and prognosis. Am J Cardiol 1986; 57: 3B.
15. Chakko CS, Gheorghiade M: Ventricular arrhythmias in severe heart failure: incidence, significance, and effectiveness of antiarrhythmic therapy. Am Heart J 1985; 109: 497.
16. Meinertz T, Hofman T, Kasper W, Treese M, Bechtold H, Stienen U, Pop T, Leitner E-RV, Andersen D, Meyer J: Significance of ventricular arrhythmias in idiopathic dilated cardiomyopathy. Am J Cardiol 1984; 53: 902.
17. Holmes J, Kubo SH, Cody RJ, Kligfield P: Arrhythmias in ischemic and non-ischemic dilated cardiomyopathy: prediction of mortality by ambulatory electrocardiography. Am J Cardiol 1985; 55: 146.
18. Bayés de Luna A, Guindo Soldevila J: Muerte súbita de origen cardiaco. Ed Doyma, Barcelona 1989.
19. Bayés de Luna A, Guindo J. Muerte súbita de origen cardiaco. Med Clin 1989; 92: 630.
20. Guindo J, Bayés de Luna A: Muerte Súbita en la cardiopatia isquémica. Rev Esp Cardiol 1989; 42: 116.
21. Cohn JN: Current therapy of the failing heart. Circulation 1988; 78: 1099.
22. Cohn JN: Current therapy for heart failure. Am J Med 1988; 84: 51.
23. Packer M: Therapeutic options in the management of chronic heart failure. Circulation 1989; 79: 198.
24. Francis GS: Heart failure management: the impact of drug therapy on survival. Am Heart J 1988; 115: 699.
25. Timmis A: Modern treatment of heart failure. Br Med J 1988; 297: 83.
26. Packer M: Physiologic determinants of survival in congestive heart failure. Circulation 1987; 75 (supp IV): 1—3.
27. Cohn JN: New concepts in the mechanisms and treatment of congestive heart failure. Am J Cardiol 1985; 55: 1A.
28. Cohn JN, Swedberg K, Kjekshus J: Advances in congestive heart failure. Am J Cardiol 1988; 62: 1A.

29. Parmley WW, Ryden L: Congestive heart failure. Advances in treatment. Am J Cardiol 1989; 63: 1D.
30. Riegger AJG, Kochsiek K, Robertson JIS: New aspects of therapy in heart failure. Eur Heart J 1988; 9 (supp H): 1.
31. Prati PL, Tavazzi L: Scompenso cardiaco 1988. G Ital Cardiol 1988; 18: 1045.
32. Cohn JN: Indications for digitalis therapy — a newlook. JAMA 1974; 229: 1911.
33. Captopril-digoxin multicenter research group: Comparative effects of therapy with captopril and digoxin in patients with mild or moderate heart failure. JAMA 1988; 259: 539.
34. Guyatt, GH, Sullivan MJJ, Fallen EL, Tihal H, Rideout E, Halcrow S, Nogradi S, Townsend M, Taylor W: A controlled trial of digoxin in congestive heart failure. Am J Card 1988; 61: 371.
35. Lee DC-S, Johnson RA, Bingham JB, Leahy M, Dinsmore RE, Goroll AH, Newell JB, Strauss W, Haber E: Heart failure in outpatients. N Engl J Med 1982; 306: 699.
36. Cohn JN: Inotropic therapy for heart failure. N Engl J Med 1989; 320: 729.
37. Moss AJ, Davis HT, Conard DL, DeCamilla JJ, Odoroff, ChL: Digitalis-associated cardiac mortality after myocardial infarction. Circulation 1981; 64: 1150.
38. DiBianco R, Shabetai R, Kostuk W, Moran J, Schlant RC, Wright R. A comparison of oral milrinone, digoxin, and their combination in the treatment of patients with chronic heart failure. N Engl J Med 1989; 320: 677.
39. Sonnenblick EH: The role of phosphodiesterase III. Inhibitors in Contemporary cardiovascular medicine Am J Cardiol 1989; 63: 1A.
40. Packen M: Vasodilator and inotropic drugs for the treatment of chronic heart failure: distinguishing type from hope. J Am Coll Cardiol 1988; 12: 1299.
41. Packer M: Effect of phosphodiesterase inhibitors on survival of patients with chronic congestive heart failure. Am J Cardiol 1989; 63: 41A.
42. Packer M: Do vasodilators prolong life in heart failure? N Engl J Med 1987; 316: 1471.
43. Furberg CD, Yusuf S: Effect of vasodilators on survival in chronic congestive heart failure. Am J Cardiol 1985; 55: 1110.
44. Domingo E, Lupón Rosés J: Vasodilatadores e insuficiencia cardiaca. Med Clin 1988; 90: 110.
45. Parker JO, Fung H-L, Ruggirello D, Stone JA: Tolerance to isosorbide dinitrate: rate of development and reversal. Circulation 1983; 68: 1074.
46. Franciosa JA, Cohn JN: Sustained hemodynamic effects without tolerance during long-term isosorbide dinitrate treatment of chronic left ventricular failure. Am J Cardiol 1980; 45: 648.
47. Pierpont GL, Cohn JN, Franciosa JA: Combined oral hydralazine-nitrate therapy in left ventricular failure: Hemodynamic equivalency to sodium nitroprusside. Chest 1978; 73: 8.
48. Sharpe DN: Clinical evidence of benefit from angiotensin converting enzyme inhibitors in heart failure. Cur Opin Cardiol 1988; 3 (suppl 1): S83.
49. Magnani B: Converting enzyme inhibition and heart failure. Am J Cardiol 1988; 84 (suppl 3A): 87.
50. Cohn JN, Archibald DG, Ziesche S, Franciosa JA, Harston WE, Tristani FE, Dunkman, WB, Jacobs W, Francis GS, Flohr KH, Goldman S, Cobb FR, Shah PM, Saunders R, Fletcher RD, Loeb HS, Hughes VC, Baker B: Effect of vasodilator therapy on mortality in chronic congestive heart failure. N Engl J Med 1986; 314: 1547.
51. Levine TB, Olivari MT, Garberg V, Sharkey SW, Cohn JN: Hemodynamic and clinical response to enalapril, a long-acting converting-enzyme inhibitor, in patients with congestive heart failure. Circulation 1984; 69: 548.
52. CONSENSUS Trial Study Group: Effects of enalapril on mortality in severe congestive heart failure, N Engl J Med 1987; 316: 1429.
53. Pfeffer MA, Pfeffer JM, Steinberg C, Finn P: Survival after an experimental myocardial

infarction: beneficial effects of long-term therapy with captopril. Circulation 1985; 72: 406.

54. Pfeffer JM, Pfeffer MA, Braunwald E: Hemodynamic benefits and prolonged survival with long-term captopril therapy in rats with myocardial infarction and heart failure. Circulation 1978; 75 (suppl I): I-149.

55. Pfeffer MA, Lamas GA, Vaughan DE, Parisi AF, Braunwald E: Effect of captopril on progressive ventricular dilatation after anterior myocardial infarction. N Eng J Med 1988; 319: 80.

56. Newman TJ, Maskin CS, Dennick LG, Meyer JH, Hallows BG, Cooper WH: Effects of captopril on survival in patients with heart failure. Am J Med 1988; 85 (suppl 3A): 140.

57. Packer M, Lee WH, Yushak M, Medina N: Comparación entre captopril y enalapril en pacientes con insuficiencia cardíaca crónica severa. N Engl J Med 1986; 315: 847.

58. Unverferth DV, Magorien RD, Moechsberger ML *et al.*: Factors influencing one year mortality of dilated cardiomyopathy. Am J Cardiol 1984; 54: 147.

59. Meeting of the minds: Treatment of arrhythmias in congestive heart failure. Am Heart J 1987; 114: 1265.

60. Bigger JT: Management of Ventricular arrhythmias in patients with congestive heart failure. Am J Car 1986; 57: 1B.

61. Meinertz T, Hofmann T, Hohnloser, SH: Zehender M, Just H. Arrhythmias and left ventricular dysfunction. J Amb Mon 1989; 2: 66.

62. Cleland JGF, Dargie HJ: Arrhythmias, catecholamines and electrolytes. Am J Cardiol 1988; 62: 55A.

63. Parmley WW, Chatterjee K: Congestive heart failure and arrhythmias: an overview. Am J Cardiol 1986; 57: 34B.

64. Gomes JAC, Hariman RI, Kang PS, El-Sherif N, Chowder Lyons J: Programmed electrical stimulation in patients with high grade ventricular ectopy: electrophysiological findings and prognosis for survival. Circulation 1984; 70: 43.

65. Poll DS, marchlinksi FE, Buxton AE, Doherty JU, Waxman HL, Josephson ME: Sustained ventricular tachycardia in patients with idiopathic dilated cardiomyopathy: electrophysiologic testing and lack of response to antiarrhythmic drug therapy. Circulation 1984; 70: 451.

66. Wilson JR: Use of antiarrhythmic drugs in patients with heart failure: clinical efficacy, hemodynamic results and relation to survival. Circulation 1987; 75 (suppl IV): IV-64.

67. CAST Investigators. Preliminary Report: effect of encainide and flecainide on mortality in a randomised trial of arrhythmia supression after myocardial infarction. N Engl J Med 1989; 321: 406.

68. Grupo investigador del EEMS: Ensayo clínico multicéntrico sobre la prevención de la muerte súbita con agentes antiarrítmicos en el postinfarto de miocardio. Rev Esp Cardiol 1989; 42: 77.

23. Can sudden death be avoided by timely revascularization of obstructed coronary arteries?

PAUL G. HUGENHOLTZ and J.R.T.C. ROELANDT

Introduction

The phenomenon of Sudden Cardiac Death (SCD) has interested physicians for many centuries [1]. Its clinical and morbid features were recognized and described by Leonardo da Vinci in the 15th century. In his monograph *De Subitaneis Mortibus* published in 1709, Lancisi reported on the multi-causality of the SCD syndrome, the influence of risk factors and the difficulties of identifying the patient who is at risk. Despite intensive clinical investigations into its prediction and many therapeutic trials on its prevention, the SCD syndrome remains one of the major challenges of contemporary cardiology. It appears that further research and information on the clinical setting in which SCD occurs is needed and, more particularly, on its pathologic and electrophysiologic mechanisms for a better understanding of the nature of the syndrome and for establishing a basis for rational preventive measures. Most studies have demonstrated that virtually all individuals who die suddenly have pre-existing pathology including coronary artery disease, forms of endstage heart disease, significant hypertension, cerebral disorders or chronic obstructive pulmonary disease. Patients who have suffered a myocardial infarction carry the highest risk. Of survivors of a transmural myocardial infarction, approximately 10% die within one year and about half of these die suddenly. However, the presence of a myocardial infarction alone does not define the highest risk group. Infarct survivors who have depressed left ventricular ejection fraction, frequent and/or complex premature ventricular complexes (PVCs), or a prolonged QT interval have a two to six times higher risk of sudden death when compared with survivors without these risk factors. Current information suggests a common pathophysiologic process underlying both sudden and non-sudden death in such patients. The exact nature of this 'high risk' state continues to elude us although recent research into the presence of 'after-potentials' has suggested that this may be the common marker.

Yet today, sudden cardiac death is no longer an unavoidable occurrence that strikes like an Act of God. The essential new message is that, although

A. Bayés de Luna et al. (eds.): *Sudden Cardiac Death*, 267–284.

based on incomplete and often anecdotal evidence, the major efforts world-wide over the past 20 years to achieve adequate reperfusion of human myocardium immediately before, during or after an obstructive episode has occurred, now indicate that because of such revascularization efforts the occurrence of sudden cardiac death in carefully followed series has dramatically decreased.

The purpose of this article is to discuss, on the basis of the available evidence, the current management of patients with coronary artery disease, which accounts for > 90% of all SCD, an approach which may eventually require a large-scale clinical trial to prove that unnecessary cardiac death can be avoided altogether, or at least reduced. The hypothesis underlying sudden cardiac death in the past three decades has usually been one of an electrical derangement of sufficient severity that a fatal cardiac arrhythmia would ensue. Thus efforts have largely been directed towards combatting such an arrhythmic episode, either in the prevention of their supposed precursors, or with long-term therapy aimed at avoiding cardiac arrhythmias altogether or by increasing the threshold to ventricular fibrillation, which was usually the presumed mechanism.

Evidence from multiple trials, however, has shown that even with the most efficacious anti-arrhythmic agents, capable of suppressing ventricular arrhythmias of all types, the occurrence and incidence of subsequent cardiac death was not decreased. Also trials with anti-ischemic drug therapy have so far failed to make a major impact, although beta-blockers have led to a decrease in some series.

On the other hand, from observations on surgically revascularized patients with procedures which have become widespread, such as coronary artery bypass grafting (CABG), percutaneous transluminal coronary angioplasty (PTCA), or dissolution of coronary artery thrombi by thrombolytic therapy (LYSIS), it has become evident that the observation of sudden cardiac death has markedly decreased.

Toward rational prophylactic therapy

If one takes the position that sudden cardiac death is a definition applicable to people dying within one hour, and one accepts the general evidence that 20% of these show asystole versus 80% ventricular fibrillation or other tachycardia, the essence of the approach lies in whether one believes in anti-arrhythmic therapy only or supports the thesis that a myocardial ischemic episode actually has preceded the ultimate fatal arrhythmia in up to 80% of all cases.

From the autopsy evidence carefully collected by Davies *et al.* [2—4], in cases of sudden death, confirming the earlier work of Falk [5, 6] and supported by von Dantzig and Becker [7], acute myocardial ischemia is usually the sequel to sudden plaque fissure and rupture, which, in turn with superimposed mural thrombus formation leads to sudden and complete vascular obstruction. Indeed, in nearly 70% of cases of sudden cardiac death, the underlying coronary pathology is one of plaque rupture and rapid platelet aggregation as demonstrated in Figure 1 [8—10].

If this underlying concept is accepted as being the real dominant mechanism, with the fatal cardiac arrhythmia only as its consequence, rational prophylactic therapy would have to include anti-aggregating substances (say aspirin) and mechanical (say PTCA or CABG) or pharmacological (say Lysis) measures as means of revascularization. Nowhere is this more clearly demonstrated than in the studies by Lewis *et al.* [11] and by Cairns *et al.* [12] who observed a marked decrease in sudden death rates in patients given aspirin after survival from their initial unstable angina episode. Equally, a subset in ISIS-II testifies to this concept [13]. Secondly, if established ischemia is the cause of the fatal arrhythmia, one might expect beta blockade to be useful. These compounds have, in fact, been demonstrated to play a beneficial role in sudden cardiac death, either by slowing cardiac frequency or by dampening the circadian rhythm with a reduction in early morning sudden cardiac deaths. This has been seen after administration of timolol [14], propranolol [15], atenolol [16], and similar non ISA compounds [17]. Furthermore, independently of the heart rate effect, beta blockers blunt the response of the heart to exercise or stress. This antiischemic protective action has been held responsible for the reduced occurrence of sudden death in the ISIS I study [16] (where a 15% reduction in initial vascular mortality was observed with atenolol, a benefit seen almost entirely during days 0 to 1 with a 30% reduction in mortality during that period). Another explanation of that beneficial action has been ascribed to a reduced occurrence of cardiac rupture [17]. In the MIAMI metoprolol trial a similar reduction in these different modes of death was seen [18].

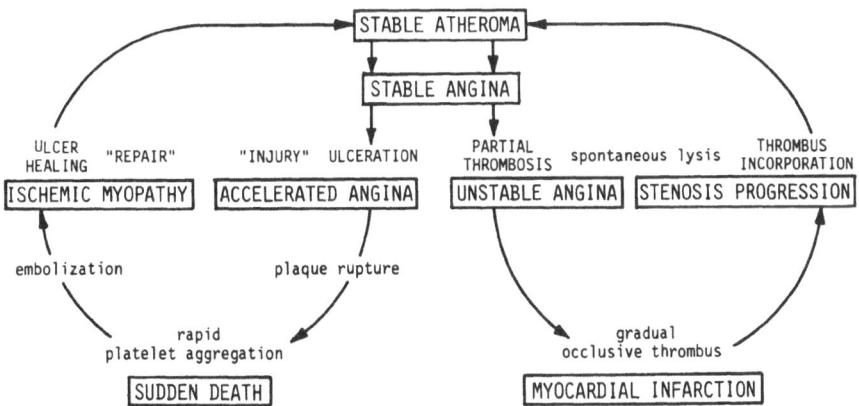

Figure 1. The ulceration-thrombosis cycle of coronary disease
(Modified after Falk, Davies, Forrester).

Indeed Fitzgerald [19], in reviewing these data, has argued: 'Patients dying of sudden ischemic cardiac death are now believed to have characteristic pathological abnormalities in their coronary vessels. Such patients have acute coronary arterial lesions characterized by: (1) plaque fissure, (2) intra intimal thrombus, and (3) intraluminal thrombosis. It is postulated that the thrombotic process is triggered by the fissuring of rupture of an atherosclerotic plaque with varying amounts of thrombus formation acompanied by micro-emboli distal to the affected segment [2—10]. The clinical sequelae will depend upon the resultant of a number of factors including, the degree of fixed stenosis in relation to the ruptured plaque, the degree of endogenous fibrinolytic acivity, the responsiveness of the coagulation cascade to thrombogenic stimulus, the extent of concomitant coronary arterial disease and the degree of previous ischemic damage to the ventricle. A frequent outcome would be transmural infarction secondary to a large intraluminal thrombus. The immediate events preceding plaque rupture are not known but they must relate to events that will destabilize the plaque within the vessel associated with alterations in the conformation of the heart during the cardiac cycle and the 'activity' of the cellular processes associated with plaque progression.' He also asked: 'If sudden death or myocardial infarction is preceded by plaque rupture and both these are reduced by long term beta blockade, then how might beta blockers reduce the incidence of plaque fissure/rupture in coronary vessels?'

He continues: 'It is proposed that beta blockade attenuates or postpones plaque rupture by reducing the *net wall strain* associated with each cardiac cycle and also reduces *peak wall strain* associated with emotion and strenuous physical activity. A coronary vessel may be subjected to differing stresses including bending, torsional, circumferential as well as shear forces. Stress as an expression of force exerted per unit area and strain, within a vessel, is the extension of the segment per unit length, this being proportional to the tension. A normal vessel has visco-elastic properties and as these are uniformly distributed around the circumference of the vessel, then shear stress will not arise. If there is inhomogeneity of the elastic properties around the circumference of the vessel due to pathological changes, such as eccentric atheromatous lesions, then tension applied to the segment may result in inequalities in force per unit area [10]. Lesions in coronary vessels tend to be distributed along regions of low wall shear which occur in that part of the coronary vessel in close contact with the myocardial wall [4, 9]. This eccentric distribution of coronary atheromatous lesions is well established from histopathological studies [10]. The atherosclerotic vessel, being tethered to the wall of the contracting ventricle, undergoes cyclic compression and expansion stress. Eccentric subintimal lesions will rupture when the resultant between progressive deterioration of the plaque and concomitant mechanical strain leads to plaque destabilization.' In fact, Davies has found that the majority of plaque fissures occur there where the plaque inserts into the normal coronary vascular wall [2—4]. 'Prolonged beta blockade reduces both peak strain and total strain per 24 hour because the heart rate is chronically reduced and the maximal strain associated with systolic contraction is attenuated because peak systolic pressure is reduced.

'This hypothesis is termed 'gating hypothesis' [19], gating being an engineering term used to describe a mechanism that prevents a mechanical engine exceeding a certain work performance. If gating reduces wall strain then it could also reduce plaque rupture and hence both sudden death and myocardial reinfarction. Some evidence to support the gating hypothesis comes from the retrospective analysis of the relationship between heart rate reduction and cardiac mortality in the Norwegian Timolol Multicenter study [14]. In this trial, 945 patients were treated with the beta blocker and 939 received placebo. Timolol (10 mg bd) was started between days 7 and 28 and the mean treatment period was 17 months. Logistic regression analysis showed that resting heart rate, measured one month after treatment, was *the* predictive variable determining the clinical outcome. A more extensive analysis by Kjeksjus [20] suggests that there is a good correlation between the reduction in heart rate and the reduction in mortality and infarction in several studies (Figure 2). This author again speculates that the mechanism may be related to the metabolic protection or antiischemic mechanisms of beta blockers. Such an explanation would fit easily into the current understanding of the pathology of sudden death and reinfarction as described by Falk and Davies [2—6]. 'Whilst beta blockers might account for amelioration of some of the downstream ischemia secondary to thrombosis and platelet

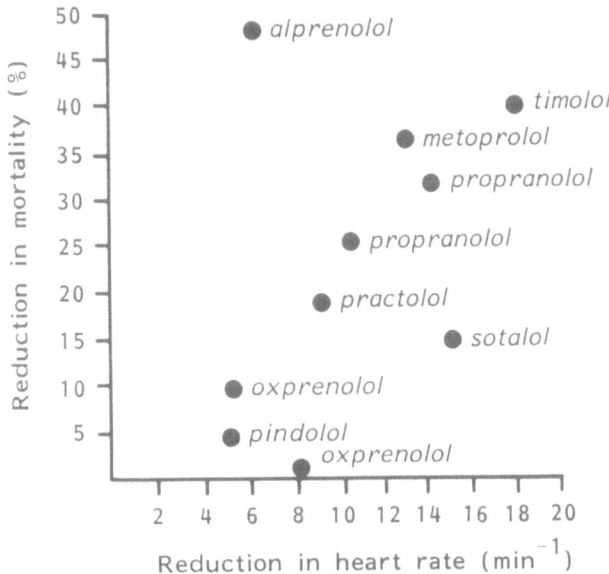

Figure 2. Correlation between reduction in heart rate and the reduction in mortality (Kjekshus [20]).

embolization, it is suggested that a more probable explanation which takes all the clinical findings into account is prevention or, more probably postponement of rupture of an unstable plaque. A further facet of this hypothesis is that prolonged beta blockade might buy time for the plaque to become stable if the cellular mechanisms leading to plaque instability are self-limiting.'

'On the other hand, the gating hypothesis might also explain why beta blockers with partial agonist properties appear to be less effective since they will have less effect in reducing the net wall strain per 24 hours because they do not reduce heart rate so effectively. A similar explanation might explain why calcium antagonists appear to be less effective. One of the major differences between beta blockers and calcium antagonists is that the latter cause little change in resting and exercise heart rate and neither do they reduce ventricular contractility at the doses used clinically. Additionally the vasodilator action of calcium antagonists may enhance sympathetic reflexes, including tachycardia, whose cardiac actions will not be opposed in the absence of beta blockade.'

These opinions are entirely consistent with those expressed in an earlier editorial by several experts on Ca^{2+} antagonists [21].

Thus, as is also argued by Clusin [22]: 'A general strategy for prophylaxis against sudden death can be discerned. To be effective, prophylactic therapy must diminish the electrophysiological consequences of acute ischemia and must be directed at the large number of patients at risk for ischemia and *not* at patients with a history of non-fatal arrhythmias. Measures with the clearest efficacy in alleviating ischemia have in common their ability to reduce the influx and accumulation of calcium within the myocardial cell. Anti-ischemic efficacy may correlate directly with the ability of a drug to prevent calcium overload during (temporary, ED) coronary artery occlusion. However it is important to remember that there are many different pathways for calcium handling within the cells and that the ability of a drug to exert calcium dependent protective effects cannot be equated with effects of the drug on calcium ion channels.'

Clusin goes on to argue that: 'Several observations suggest that calcium channel blockers also exert at least some protective effect in man, in particular, diltiazem [22, 23]. However, in large scale trials, a beneficial effect of calcium channel blockers on sudden death has not been demonstrated. In particular with nifedipine, a drug which has been most extensively studied, if anything a slight excess in mortality has occurred in the nifedipine treated group [21].' Indeed, recent evident with the SPRINT I, SPRINT II (both with nifedipine) and MDPIT (diltiazem) trials have not shown a beneficial overall action of either drug. The reasons for the apparent non-efficacy of these compounds to influence sudden cardiac death occurrence in contrast to beta blockers must be ascribed in large measure to the gating hypothesis alluded to earlier by Fitzgerald [19], despite the theoretical advantage of blocking the excess calcium influx in ischemic tissues.

Thus as far as pharmacological therapy is concerned at present, we are forced to conclude that anti-arrhythmic therapy as a general strategy is not efficacious (except in a few isolated instances where drug responsiveness has been demonstrated), nor is therapy with calcium antagonists (with the exception of diltiazem in the retrospective analysis of a subset of the MDPIT data). Only aspirin, and to a lesser extent beta blockade, has proven to reduce the cardiovascular mortality by a modest 15—20%. Yet the concept stays alive.

Much more enticing therefore is to follow the logic of complete revascularization of the coronary artery system on the hypothesis that the reduction of the ischemic episodes can only be achieved by a proper restoration of the vascular supply. Indeed from the European Coronary Surgery Study (ECSS) [24] as well as from the non-randomized part of the Coronary Artery Surgery Study registry (CASS) [25], it appears that the survival benefit of early surgery is nearly entirely due to its ability to prevent cardiac death, either non-sudden or sudden. As shown in Figure 3, in the ECSS there was a marked reduction of sudden cardiac death over the 8-year follow-up period that entailed this study design. As this study included men aged under 65 with angina pectoris of more than 3 months duration, a 50% or greater intraluminal diameter narrowing in at least two major coronary arteries, and good left ventricular function with an ejection fraction of 50% or more, the

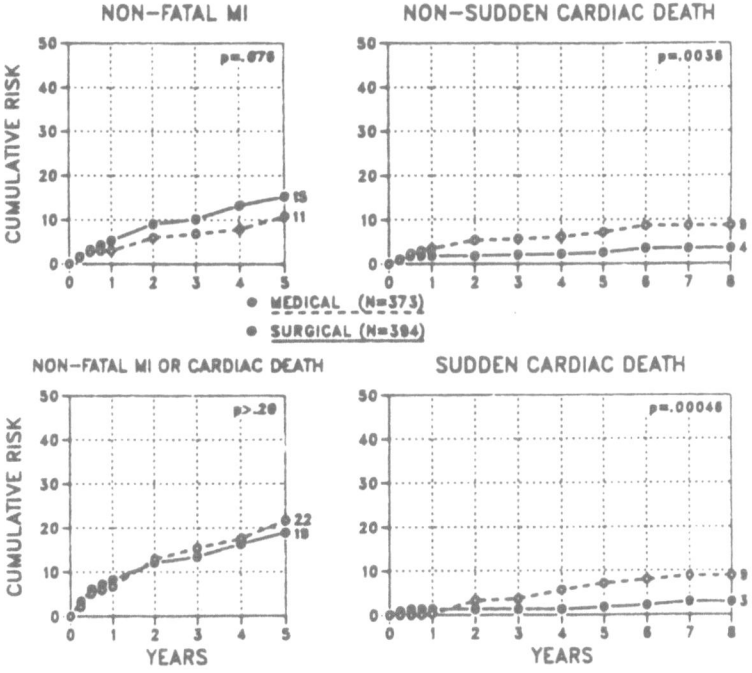

Figure 3. Non-fatal MI and cardiac death (Varnauskas, ECSS [24]).

results imply that coronary bypass surgery should be considered — in particular when there are ischemic abnormalities in the resting ECG, or marked ST-segment depression during exercise testing. Also in the CASS study, where the effect of medical versus surgical treatment on subsequent sudden cardiac death was assessed in 13,467 patients in the CASS registry, it was observed that cardiac death occurred in 452 (3.4%) of patients during a mean follow-up of 4.6 years. Of these sudden deaths occurred in 257 (4.9%) of 5258 medically treated but in only 101 (1.6%) of 6250 surgically treated patients. In a high risk patient subset with 3-vessel disease and a history of congestive heart failure 91% of surgically treated patients did survive compared to 69% of pharmacologically treated patients. After Cox's analysis was employed to correct for baseline variables, it was found that surgical treatment had an independent effect on sudden death p < 0.0001 [25]. In a later analysis of 13,476 patients with angiographically prove CAD, 323 cases of sudden death were found among 6260 patients receiving medical (i.e. drug) therapy — 5.2% over 5 years. The corresponding number for those treated surgically was 129 of 7216 just (1.8%), giving a highly significant difference of p < 0.001 [26] (Figure 4).

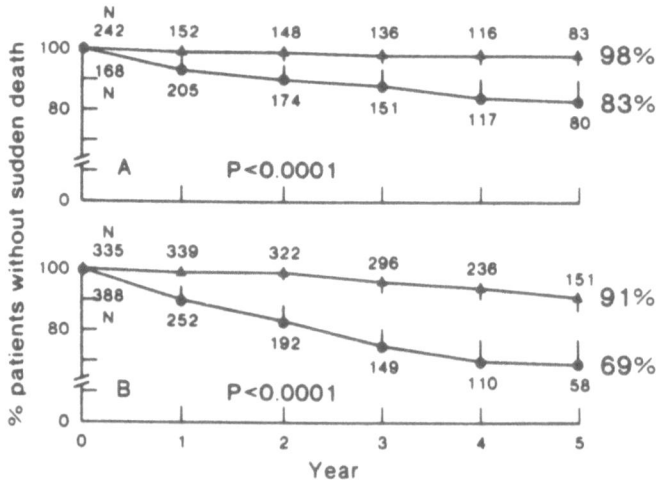

Figure 4. Patients with history of CHF (Holmes [25]).

The 'high risk' state

In this conceptual paragraph the hypothesis is argued that there must be a 'high risk state'. Here, the fact that ischemic heart disease exists can be defined as an 'ischemic' risk. Similarly, a 'mechanical' risk exists in all other forms of heart disease with impaired left ventricular function. Finally, an 'electrical' risk occurs when the primary instability is in the conduction system. These three different high risk states by themselves already call for a different approach, which also applies to the various precipitating events that might occur against the background of the three basic different elements constituting the 'high risk state' of the substrate.

In coronary heart disease the 'ischemic risk' is the dominant feature. A further precipitating event such as an increase in the extent of the arterial occlusion, for example when thrombosis becomes complete after plaque rupture, will make a hitherto ischemic myocardium into infarcted myocardium. Subsequent ventricular fibrillation on an ischemic basis will then lead to sudden death. Conversely in a normally perfused heart with an 'electrical risk', such as occurs in patients with repeated ventricular tachycardia or ventricular fibrillation triggered by a nonspecific and ubiquitous PVC sudden death may not follow. Thus, the latter condition requires a completely different therapeutic approach. In Table 2 the various precipitating events are further delineated with their recommended intervention(s).

An integral approach can now be proposed. We would like to conclude that recent onset stable as well as the varying forms of unstable angina pectoris or prior myocardial infarction, when complicated by left ventricular dysfunction and complex PVCs, or prolongation of the QT interval *always* contain an increased risk of SCD. Their combination constitutes truly, the 'high risk state'. The ubiquitous PVC is now only a partial indicator of increased risk for sudden death. Although ambulatory electrocardiography appears to offer a versatile means for demonstrating their presence, as may the detection of after-potentials, exercise testing at discharge would at present appear to be the best test and, therefore mandatory for all patients with an antecedent history of whatever form of coronary artery disease. It

Table 1. Profile of sudden cardiac death (from Oliver [40]).

Factors more associated with sudden cardiac death than acute myocardial infarction

Relative youth
Physical inactivity
Excessive cigarette smoking
Ventricular premature beats
Sustained tachycardia
QRS conduction defects
Cardiomegaly
Triple-vessel disease

Factors equally associated with sudden cardiac death and acute myocardial infarction

Hypercholesterolemia
Hypertension
Diabetes mellitus
Obesity

Table 2. Precipitating events leading to sudden cardiac death and possible intervention.

Event	Intervention
Neurophysiologic factors	Exercise, attitude manipulation
Platelet agglutination	Platelet active drugs, aspirin, lysis
Coronary vasospasm	Calcium antagonists
Rupture of atheroma	Manipulation of HDL/LDH transport, beta-blocker
Metabolic desequilibrium	Diet, ionic supplements
Electrolyte abnormalities	Diet, pure diuretics
Electrical disarray	Pacemaker, antiarrhythmic agents
Increased oxygen demand	Beta-blockers
Combination of above	PTCA or CABG ('reperfuse') combined therapy

(Roelandt & Hugenholtz [1]).

Table 3. Comparison of incidences of sudden cardiac, nonsudden cardiac, and noncardiac death in 13,476 medically and surgically treated patients.

	Group					
	Medical		Surgical		Total	
	n	%	n	%	n	%
Sudden death	323	5.2	129	1.8	452	3.4
Nonsudden cardiac death	598	9.6	380	5.3	978	7.3
Noncardiac death	122	1.9	173	2.4	295	2.2
Alive at last follow-up						
≤ 5 yr	2709	43.3	3054	42.3	5763	42.8
> 5 yr	2508	40.1	3480	48.2	5988	44.4
Total	6260		7216		13476	

(Holmes *et al.* [25]).

Table 4. Beta-blocker therapy 1985–1987.

	Number	Drugs	Cardiac events	Diastolic pressure (mmHg)
MRC trial (P1)	17354	Propranolol bendrofluaride	No reduction	98
Elderley (60–79)	855	Atenolol ± diuretic	No difference	99.7
IPPSH (PI)	6357	Oxprenolol ± other drugs	No reduction	108
HAPPY	6569	Atenolol/metoprolol vs. diuretic	No difference	107

(Fitzgerald 1987 [19]).

will remain a matter of extensive debate to what extent the complex PVCs represent an independent risk factor particularly when the extent of left ventricular dysfunction is minimal. This opinion is further supported by Hammermeister *et al.* [27] who used a detailed statistical analysis in 733 medically treated and 1870 surgically treated patients with coronary artery disease in order to identify the variables most predictive of survival. Of 46 variables, again the left ventricular ejection fraction was most predictive of survival in the medically treated patients, followed by age, degree of coronary artery disease and presence or absence on the ST segment depression on the ECG. Unfortunately they did not use exercise testing as advocated and practiced by us. This would, in our view, have facilitated the stratification process. For the surgically treated patients, the absence of PVCs proved to be the best further predictor of non-sudden death. Also, as is evident from all the cited literature, when exercise is neither feasible nor practiced, the resting LV ejection fraction supersedes PVCs in its predictive capacity. In the setting of depressed LV function, however, PVCs retain their significance [1, 28—32].

The value of exercise testing

In fact, these findings led us to investigate our own patients in detail with systematic exercise testing just prior to discharge after surviving their infarction [28]. We summarized this recently as follows: 'The relative merits of resting ejection fraction measured by radionuclide angiography and predischarge exercise stress testing were compared for predicting prognosis in hospital survivors of myocardial infarction. Two hundred and fourteen survivors of myocardial infarction out of 338 consecutive patients with acute myocardial infarction were studied over a 14 month period. Hospital mortality was 13% (45 of 338) whereas 19 additional patients out of 214 died in the subsequent year (9%). High, intermediate and low risk groups could be identified by resting left ventricular ejection fraction measurement. Mortality was 33% for nine patients with an ejection fraction less than 20%, 19% for 58 patients with an ejection fraction between 20 and 39%, and 3% for 147 patients with ejection fraction higher than 40%. Mortality was high (23%) in 47 patients who were unable to perform the stress test because of heart failure or other limitations. The patients could be stratified further into intermediate and low risk groups according to the increase in systolic blood pressure during exercise: six deaths occurred in 46 patients with a blood pressure increase of ≤ 30 mmHg while only two deaths occurred in 121 patients with an increase of ≥ 30 mmHg. Maximum workload, angina, ST segment changes, and ventricular arrhythmias were less predictive than were blood pressure changes. It was concluded that the prognostic value of radionuclide angiography at rest and of symptom limited exercise testing is similar. The latter investigation should be the method of choice since it provides more specific information for patient management and is the cheaper test to execute.

Patients with prolonged Q-T interval

The relationship of a prolonged Q-T interval to SCD is well established in several clinical settings including the primary (idiopathic) types. Secondary types can be associated with coronary artery disease or may be drug-induced of which antiarrhythmic agents lead the list. In a group of myocardial infarction survivors, the incidence of a prolonged Q-T interval was 18%. Of all sudden deaths during the first 1½ years, 57% occurred in the myocardial infarction survivors, and their risk was twice that of patients with a normal Q-T interval [29]. The interpretation of these data is somewhat confounded by the fact that some patients received antiarrhythmic drugs. Nonetheless, the statistical relevance of the prolonged QT interval as a predictor of sudden death seems a valid one, albeit often difficult to detect in practice.

Patients with exercise-induced ventricular arrhythmias

The general relationship between the presence of coronary artery disease and exercise induced ventricular ectopy has been recognized for many years. The fact that increases in sympathetic neural tone may provoke PVCs even in structurally 'normal' hearts, has been demonstrated, yet complex arrhythmias are more frequently documented during 24-hour ambulatory monitoring as compared to exercise testing [30]. A small subset of malignant ventricular arrhythmias can be provoked only by exercise testing. Thus, exercise testing may complement ambulatory monitoring as was shown by Ivanova *et al.* [31].

Management steps in avoidance of SCD

Thus, in terms of therapy and in keeping with Goldstein [32], we would recommend that the following steps be undertaken to reduce unnecessary (sudden) deaths after myocardial infarction.

General measures

Reduction in weight to ±10% of ideal, sufficient energetic and regular exercise as is commensurate with age and personality, complete cessation of all forms of smoking and reduction of total fat and the fraction of animal fats in the diet to the extent that serum cholesterol remains below 220 mg% with a favourable HDL/LDL fraction. These are the recommendations made by the WHO Task Force in 1983, concepts which we recommend to our patients upon discharge after acute myocardial infarction. Their modification was shown in a recent Finnish study to reduce SCD [33] (Figure 6).

Reduction of 'electrical risk'

Extensive short and long term trials with a wide range of antiarrhythmic agents, while demonstrating significant reductions in PVCs as well as in more severe forms of ventricular arrhythmia, have failed to reduce the incidence of sudden death. Accordingly we would limit the use of such modern agents as mexiletine, flecainide, sotalol, amiodarone and propafenone (to name but a few of the more effective ones) to those patients in whom the high electrical risk has been verified by electro-physiological testing and in whom the efficacy of the specific drug in suppressing induced ventricular arrhythmias has been proved. In certain specific cases, implantable devices, such as programmable pacemakers and defibrillators, can be considered. They are very promising in carefully selected circumstances and may ultimately well

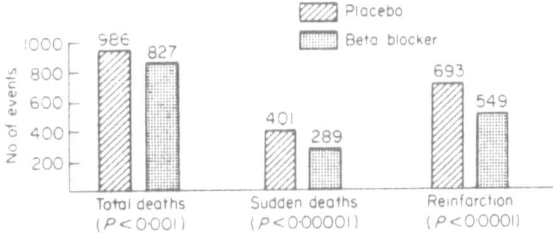

Figure 5. Effect of beta blocker therapy (Yusuf [17]).

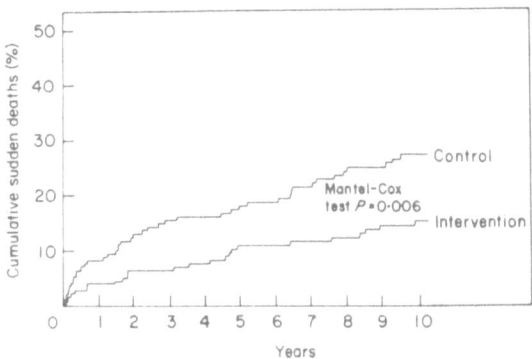

Figure 6. Cumulative sudden deaths. (Luurila [33]).

prove more effective in these relatively rare numbers of patients than drugs. General treatment of all patients will PVCs is certainly not indicated.

Reduction of 'mechanical risk'

Generally little is to be offered to those who have severely impaired mechanical function of the heart. Primarily correctable lesions such as valvular insufficiency, aneurysm, etc., present themselves logically for surgical therapy. For the remainder with very poor ejection fractions, little can be offered other than eventually cardiac transplantation, which currently is enjoying a second vogue. Even so, one year survival rates of 80% declining to 70% over 5 years are a considerable step forward compare with the natural history which would indicate death within a few months. Even temporary mechanical devices now appear on the horizon. For the interim, such patients should be treated with vasodilating agents, whose efficacy is, at best, short term and for which no long term results have yet been reported.

Reduction of 'ischemic risk'

This is the category where currently most hope can be offered. Of course, it depends on the extent to which the myocardium has previously been damaged and the size of the area under ischemic risk. The approaches separate themselves into three categories: reperfusion of the ischemic heart, protection against subsequent ischemic episodes, and avoidance of subsequent coronary obstruction.

Reperfusion of ischemic heart: of the three approaches against further ischemic risk, the most appealing is that of reperfusion with O_2 rich blood. After all, that is what the myocardial cell needs most to survive. Reperfusion can be achieved, classically by CABG, but recently it has been proved that the combination of intravenous and intracoronary administration of streptokinase (or other thrombolytic agents) followed by balloon dilatation of the underlying atheromatous lesion can reduce mortality after acute myocardial infarction by reperfusion of the infarct related vessel [34, 35]. The same message follows from CABG with or without a previous acute event from the data from the CASS and ECSS studies earlier alluded to. Our own experience in Rotterdam has shown an annual mortality of only 1% over 10 years following CABG, which by itself carried an operative mortality of approximately 1% [36]. Since 50% of the 1041 patients reported in that study had a previous infarction, these non-randomized data show, like those from other centers, that timely reperfusion by whatever route will reduce unnecessary (sudden) death. Certainly, when 'ischemic risk' is evident and the patient's coronary anatomy allows this type of intervention, this is the route to follow. Similar non-randomized data are now becoming available in follow-up studies after PTCA.

Protection against subsequent ischemic episodes, other than by reperfusion, can be carried out by several pharmacological approaches. These are indicated when the 'ischemic risk' is less or not obviously evident and yet the suspicion of future ischemic episodes remains. Here, the best evidence has been supplied by the beta-blockade trials (propranolol, timolol, metoprolol, atenolol) probably via the earlier discussed gating hypothesis. These should be given early after the survival of myocardial infarction to avoid a second episode. Such therapy would exclude those who have had an uncomplicated recovery after myocardial infarction (that is to say no complications of any kind, such as no arrhythmia, no signs of failure and no angina upon reactivation), as well as those with contraindications (hypotension, AV-block, bronchial asthma, etc.) and leave this therapy to those in whom ischemia is suspected in the near future although perhaps not evident at the time of discharge. This leaves beta-blockade for a relatively small group indeed, but at least for one in which the physician suspects, but cannot yet prove, a subsequent event (Figure 5). The same line of reasoning applies to calcium antagonists, the major benefit of which is to increase coronary blood flow by reducing vascular resistance in the coronary system in particular and in the arterial system in general, whilst also reducing cardiac oxygen consumption. Here, nifedipine, particularly in combination with a beta-blocker such as propranolol or acebutolol, has proved to be of particular benefit [37—39], against subsequent ischemic episodes although long term efficacy in terms of reduction in SCD is lacking.

It is clear that large scale investigations with combination therapy of calcium blockers and beta-blocker, to prove reduced post-myocardial infarction and eventually SCD, have yet to be carried out.

Avoidance of subsequent coronary obstruction

Since the mechanism of subsequent 'ischemic', 'mechanical' or 'electrical' instability is most likely related to new obstruction in a suspected semi-obstructed artery, or more likely yet, in a hitherto unsuspected or undetected vessel or capillary bed, any approach which could stop subsequent arterial or capillary thrombosis would seem more ideal. Since anticoagulants of the classical types have yet to be shown to have a real prophylactic value, attention has been devoted to anti-aggregatory agents of which aspirin in the latest large studies [11—13] has shown much more promise than had earlier trials with the same agent.

Summary

In conclusion it would seem that no method at present can predictably detect every individual at increased risk after myocardial infarction. However, a stratification procedure can be followed which should allow proper prophylactic therapy for most individual patients who manifest themselves to the medical community, be it after stable or unstable angina pectoris or after myocardial infarction. As Oliver has pointed out already in 1981, the time has long ceased that we can proceed with therapy in a random fashion [40]. The moment is here to use the proper stratification scheme with the specific therapy for the specific problem [28]. Of all the current options, those which properly restore coronary blood supply (CABG [25], PTCA [35] and timely Lysis [13, 34]) at present offer the best chance of a good outcome, supported by agents which reduce (re)occlusion [11—13] and reduce the net wall strain on the heart [16—20].

References

1. Roelandt J, Hugenholtz PG: Sudden death: prediction and prevention. Eur Heart J 1986; 7 (suppl. A): 169—180.
2. Davies MJ, Thomas AC: Plaque fissuring — the cause of acute myocardial infarction, sudden ischemic death and crescendo angina. Br Heart J 1985; 53: 363—73.
3. Davies MJ, Thomas AC: Thrombosis and acute coronary artery lesions in sudden cardiac ischemic death. N Eng J Med 1984; 310: 1137—40.
4. Davies MJ, Thomas AC, Knapman PA, Hangartmer JR: Intramyocardial platelet aggregation in patients with unstable angina suffering sudden ischemic cardiac death. Circulation 1986; 73: 418—427.
5. Falk E: Plaque rupture with severe pre-existing stenosis precipitating coronary thrombosis: characteristics of coronary atherosclerotic plaques underlying fatal occlusive thrombi. Br Heart J 1983; 50: 127—34.
6. Falk E: Unstable angina with fatal outcome: Dynamic coronary thrombosis leading to infarction and/or sudden death. Circulation 1985; 71: 699—708.
7. van Dantzig JM, Becker AE: Sudden cardiac death and acute pathology of coronary arteries. Eur Heart J 1986; 7: 987—91.
8. Solid mechanics and the properties of blood vessel walls. In: Caro CG, Pebley TJ, Schroter RC, Seeb WA (eds), The mechanics of the circulation. London: Oxford University Press, 1978; 86—105.
9. Sabban HN, Khaja F, Hawkins ET *el al.*: Relation of atherosclerosis to arterial wall shear in the left anterior descending coronary artery of man. Am Heart J 1986; 112: 453—8.
10. Roberts WC: Coronary arteries in coronary heart disease. Morphologic observations. Pathobiol Annu 1975; 5: 249—82.
11. Lewis HD, Davis JW, Archibald DG et al.: Protective effects of aspirin against acute myocardial infarction and death in men with unstable angina. N Engl J Med 1982; 306: 885.
12. Cairns JA, Gent M, Singer J et al.: Aspirin, sulfinpyrazone or both, in unstable angina: results of a Canadian multicenter trial. N Engl J Med 1985; 313: 1369.
13. ISIS-II Collaborative Group: Randomized trial of intravenous streptokinase, oral aspirin, both, or neither among 17187 cases of suspected acute myocardial infaction: ISIS-I. Lancet 1988 (2): 349—360.
14. Gundersen T, Grottun P, Petersen T, Kjekshus JK: The effect of timolol on mortality and reinfarction after acute myocardial infarction: prognostic important of heart rate at rest. Am J Cardiol 1986 (2): 20—24.
15. Snow PJD: Effect of propranolol in myocardial infarction. Lancet 1965 (2): 551—3.
16. ISIS I Collaborative Group: Randomized trial of intravenous atenolol among 16027 cases of suspected acute myocardial infarction: ISIS-I. Lancet 1986 (2): 57—65.

17. Yusuf S, Peto R, Lewis J, Collins R, Sleight P: Beta-blockade during and after myocardial infarction: an overview of the randomized trials. Prog Cardiovasc Dis 1985; 26: 335—71.

18. The MIAMI Trial Research Group: Metoprolol in acute myocardial infarction (MIAMI). A randomized placebo-controlled international trial. Eur Heart J 1985; 6: 199—226.

19. Fitzgerald JD: By what means might beta blockers prolong life after acute myocardial infarction? Eur Heart J 1987; 8: 945—951.

20. Kjekshus J: Comments — beta blockers: heart rate reduction, a mechanism of benefit? Eur Heart J 1985; 6 (Suppl. A): 29—30.

21. Hugenholtz PG, Serruys PW, Fleckenstein A, Nayler W: Why calcium antagonists are most useful before or during early myocardial ischemia and not after infarction has been established. Eur Heart J 1986; 270—278.

22. Clusin WT: What is the solution to sudden cardiac death: calcium modulation or arrhythmia clinics? Cardiovascular Drugs & Therapy 1; 1987: 335—342.

23. Gibson RS, Boden WE, Theroux P et al.: Diltiazem and reinfarction in patients with non-Q-wave myocardial infarction. N Engl J Med 1986; 315: 423—9.

24. Varnauskas E: European Coronary Surgery Study (ECSS). Z Kardiol 1985, 74; Suppl. 6: 73—78.

25. Holmes DR Jr, Davis KB, Mock MB et al.: The effect of medical and surgical treatment on subsequent sudden cardiac death in patients with coronary artery disease: a report from the Coronary Artery Surgery Study (CASS). Circulation June 1986; Vol. 73, No. 6: 1254—63.

26. Ryan TJ: Personal communication 1989.

27. Hammermeister KE, Derouen TA, Dodge HT: Variables predictive of survival in patients with coronary disease. Selection by univariate and multivariate analyses from clinical, electrocardiographic, exercise, arteriographic, and quantitative angiographic evaluations. Circulation 1979; 59: 421.

28. Fioretti P et al.: Prediction of mortality in hospital survivors of myocardial infarction. Comparison of predischarge exercise testing and radionuclide ventriculography at rest. Br Heart J 1984; 52: 292.

29. Schwartz RJ, Wolf S: QT interval prolongation as predictor of sudden death in patients with myocardial infarction. Circulation 1978; 57: 1074.

30. Problete PF, Kennedy HL, Caralis DG et al.: Detection of ventricular ectopy in patients with coronary heart disease and normal subjects by exercise testing and ambulatory electrocardiography. Chest 1978; 74: 402.

31. Ivanova LA, Mazur NA, Smirnova TM et al.: Electrocardiographic exercise testing and ambulatory monitoring to identify patients with ischemic heart disease at high risk of sudden death. Am J Cardiol 1980; 45: 1132.

32. Goldstein S: Mechanisms and prevention of sudden death in coronary heart disease. 1989 Sudden death conference, Barcelona.

33. Hämäläinen H, Luurila OJ, Kallio V et al.: Long-term reduction in sudden deaths after a multifactorial intervention programme in patients with myocardial infarction: 10-year results of a controlled investigation. Eur Heart J 1989; 10: 55—62.

34. Simoons ML, Serruys PW, vanden Brand M, et al.: Early thrombolysis in acute myocardial infarction: limitation of infarct size and improved survival. JACC April 1986; Vol. 7, No. 4: 717—28.

35. Serruys PW, Simoons ML, Surapranata H et al.: Preservation of global and regional left ventricular function after early thrombolysis in acute myocardial infarction. J Am Coll Cardiol 1986; 7: 729—42.

36. Laird-Meeter K: Thesis: Result of ten years art-coronary bypass surgery at the Thoraxcenter, Rotterdam, 1983.

37. Pfisterer M, Brand JM, Burhart F: Combined acebutolol/nifedipine therapy in patients with chronic coronary artery disease: additional improvement of ischemia-induced left ventricular dysfunction. Am J Cardiol 1982; 49: 259.

38. De Jong JW, Harmsen E, de Tombe PP *et al.*: Energy conservation in ischemic rat heart by nifedipine plus propranolol. Eur Heart J 1983; 49: 259.
39. Wolffenbuttel BHR, Verdouw PD: Nifedipine and myocardial performance in the presence and absence of beta-blockade with propranolol. Arch Int Pharmacodyn Ther 1983; 266: 83.
40. Oliver MF: Sudden cardiac death. In: Yu PN, Goodwin JF (eds), Progress in cardiology. Philadelphia: Lea & Febiger 1981: 127.

24. Sudden cardiac death: A multifactorial problem

HEIN J. J. WELLENS and PEDRO BRUGADA

Introduction

In the USA 400,000 people die suddenly each year or one person every minute! In an important number of them, the sudden demise is the first presentation of cardiovascular disease. Although, as discussed by Roberts [1], many different causes can lead to sudden death; in the majority of victims, coronary artery disease is the culprit. In this article we will therefore concentrate on the role of coronary artery disease and its consequences.

What do we know about sudden cardiac death in 1989 and what can we possibly do to prevent this dramatic and unwanted event from occurring?

Recognition of high risk groups

Although (as shown in Table 1) sudden death can be the first manifestation of coronary disease, sudden death victims are frequently known as cardiac patients [2—4]. They should be the group of patients therefore to whom our efforts should be primarily directed especially because in recent years it has become clear that among these patients, risk stratification in predicting those who may die suddenly is possible.

Table 1. Background of patients with sudden cardiac death and possibility of identifying high risk patients.

	Incidence	Recognition
1. Not preceded by symptoms	45%	not possible
2. Short-lasting premonitory symptoms (hours to weeks, specific, unspecific)	20%	partially
3. Longer lasting angina pectoris	15%	possible
4. Myocardial infarction survivor	20%	possible

A. Bayés de Luna et al. (eds.): *Sudden Cardiac Death*, 285–296.
© 1991 Kluwer Academic Publishers, Dordrecht.

The patient with known coronary artery disease

The literature on sudden death in the patient with coronary artery disease points to the importance of myocardial ischemia, left ventricular function, and ventricular arrhythmias. As shown in Figure 1 these three factors-ischemia, hemodynamic dysfunction, and electrical instability are closely interrelated. Each of these three main factors is affected by dynamic changes such as changes in degree of ischemia, triggers, blood platelet function, influence of the autonomic nervous system (ANS), etc. The importance of all these different contributing factors may vary, depending upon the stage of coronary artery disease. For example, sudden death in the previously asymptomatic patient is frequently the result of acute myocardial ischemia leading to the lethal cardiac arrhythmia. The mechanism of sudden death can be totally different in the patient with an old myocardial infarction and a large scar. Our knowledge of all the factors contributing to sudden death is far from complete. We believe that in this multifactorial complex situation, a practical approach to the problem requires the analysis of the contributing factors, which are known and can be recognized.

The easiest group to start with are patients who have *suffered from a*

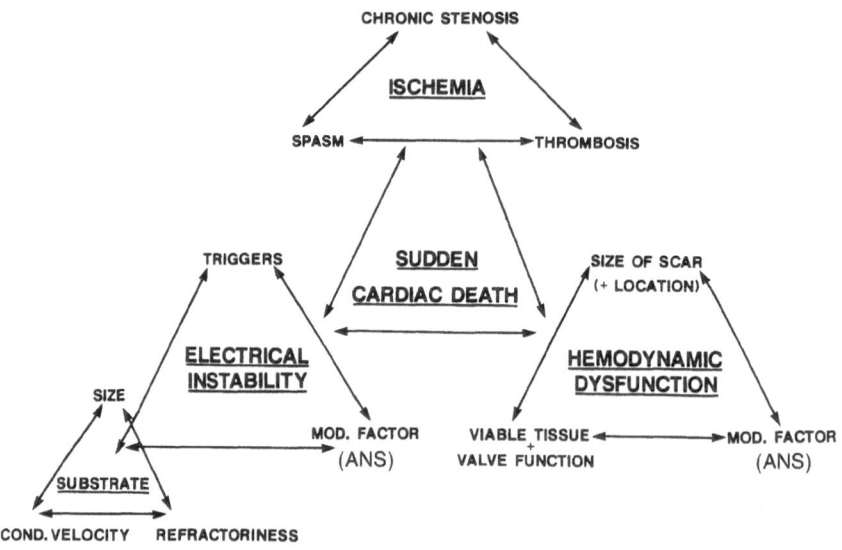

Figure 1. Model showing the factors that play a role in sudden cardiac death in the patient with coronary artery disease. As shown, ischemia, hymodynamic dysfunction, and electrical instability are the three components closely interrelated in producing sudden cardiac death. Several known (and probably other unknown) factors play a role in each of the three main components of the model. Not shown in this figure is the role of time, for example, the age of a myocardial infarction or the duration of ischemia. ANS = autonomic nervous system.

myocardial infarction in the past. In these patients, the degree of impairment of left ventricular function has emerged as the most important factor determining prognosis.

The patient with a left ventricular ejection fraction of 20—30% has a 30% 1-year mortality rate as compared to a 5% value in patients with a left ventricular ejection fraction of 50% or more [5]. A critical analysis of the independent value of left ventricular ejection fraction has been published [6]. Patients requiring treatment for congestive failure after myocardial infarction have a particular ominous prognosis [7, 8]. It is of interest that about half of the patients with symptomatic pump failure after myocardial infarction die suddenly [7].

Residual ischemia outside the infarcted area is also of prognostic significance. Painful and silent ischemia in rest or during exercise are markers for an increased risk of dying suddenly. Several methods have been advanced to obtain information about the presence or absence of residual ischemia, such as the resting ECG, 24-hour Holter recordings, exercise ECG testing alone or combined with radionuclide techniques, and recently also dobutamine infusion [9].

Within the residual ischemia group, risk is inversely related to duration of exercise before the onset of complaints or ST segment depression and also inversely related to the rise in blood presue during exercise [10, 11]. The high risk post-MI patient can therefore be recognized by performing an exercise test.

An important area of discussion is the significance of ventricular arrhythmias. There is no question that the occurrence of spontaneous sustained ventricular tachycardia after the acute phase of myocardial infarction worsens prognosis [12]. Discussion centers around the independent prognostic significance of other expressions of ectopic ventricular activity, including frequency of ventricular premature beats, couplets, and nonsustained ventricular tachycardia. While on one hand investigators such as Bigger [13] found prognostic significance of nonsustained ventricular tachycardia independent from left ventricular function, other investigators could not come to the same conclusion [6, 14, 15]. Studies in which incidence, time of occurrence, and characteristics of ventricular ectopy are carefully related to site and size of infaction and extent of the residual ischemic area are required to give a more definite answer to this question.

The information obtained in patients who have suffered from a myocardial infarction that extent of muscle loss is the prime determinant of the future indicates the extreme importance of reducing infarct size as much as possible when the patient presents *with impending or early myocardial infarction.* Recent data have shown that infarct size can be reduced by early administration of thrombolytic therapy [16], indicating the importance of the shortest possible time interval between onset of complaints and treatment. Reduction in infarct size is not only of importance for left ventricular function, but also reduced the substrate for malignant ventricular arrhythmias [17].

The patient unknown to have coronary heart disease

As described, many sudden cardiac death victims have no previous cardiac history [2, 18—20], although somewhat different conclusions were recently reported [20]. In that study it was found that in only a minority of patients resuscitated out of hospital no previous cardiac history was present [21].

The asymptomatic patient

It is possible to recognize groups at higher risk for sudden death in the asymptomatic population. Although risk factors can be identified as smoking, high blood pressure, lipid abnormalities, a familial history of coronary artery disease, and an abnormal rest or exercise electrocardiogram, the predictive value of these abnormalities is too low to justify large scale expensive investigations such as thallium stress testing studies or coronary angiography in the asymptomatic population. It remains to be shown what impact lowering of the cholesterol value will have on the incidence of sudden death. Until that information is available wide spread prescription of cholesterol lowering drugs should be discouraged.

Present therapeutic strategies

Depending on the setting and background, different steps have to be taken to reduce sudden death in patients with coronary heart disease.

Sudden death outside the hospital

As indicated in Table 2, in the patient dying suddenly outside the hospital, resuscitation has to be started immediately followed by rapid admission to hospital. Resuscitation outside the hospital can be very effective. In areas such as Seattle where a well-organized resuscitation system incorporating citizen-initiated rescue efforts is operative, approximately 1/3 of patients who are resuscitated outside the hospital are discharged alive from hospital [22]. Prehospital resuscitation can therefore lead to a sizable reduction in the number of sudden death victims. This becomes even more important, when one realizes that the outlook for the successfully resuscitated patient has improved considerably in recent years. Risk statification in these patients is possible [23].

The coronary heart disease patient reaching hospital

In the patient reaching the hospital with chest pain and developing

Table 2. Steps in reducing sudden cardiac death.

Known CAD population

Early phase (out of hospital): Resuscitation
Required: Personnel and facilities for resuscitation followed by rapid transportation to hospital.
Early phase (in hospital): Aggressive treatment of impending and early myocardial infarction.
Required: Awareness by laymen and first line physician of the importance of the shortest possible hospital delay. In hospital knowledge and facilities to recognize high risk subsets.
Late phase (in hospital): Risk stratification
Required: Information about pump function, residual ischemia, and spontaneous ventricular tachycardia. This should be followed by appropriate therapy (if possible!).
Late phase (out hospital): Recognition of changes in previously stable condition followed by appropriate action.
Required: Education of patient and first line physician.

Unknown CAD population
— Identification of high risk groups (smokers, hypertension, hyperlipemia, familial incidence CAD) followed by counseling.
— General advise on diet (fat, salt, etc.) and exercise.

---

myocardial infarction, evidence has been presented that infarct size is the most important prognostic predictor in the myocardial infarction survivor [5]. Measures to prevent myocardial infarction or interventions as early as possible after myocardial infarction to reduce infarct size are therefore an important target to reduce sudden death later. Recently much emphasis has been placed on early risk stratification in patients with unstable angina. Questions involving the proper determination of the size of the area at risk [24], possible profits of thrombolytic therapy, PTCA, or early surgery have only partially been answered. As shown in the study of the Interuniversity Cardiology Institute of the Netherlands (ICIN), 20% of patients admitted with unstable angina develop a myocardial infarction with 48 hours [25]. Regarding the patients admitted to the hospital with an acute myocardial infarction, another study from ICIN demostrated that thrombolytic therapy is especially useful when electrocardiographic evidence is present of an extensive anterior or inferior wall infarction and the patient is treated within 4 hours after onset of chest pain [26, 27].

If the damage is done, our presently available therapeutic measures for the patient left with limited left ventricular function are disappointing. Approximately 15% of myocardial infarction survivors fall into that category. No randomized studies are available on the effects of inotropic durgs or vasodilators in patients with poor pump function after myocardial infarction, nor are data known on the effect of reconstructive surgery of the left ventricle.

If the combination of poor left ventricular function and residual ischemia is present, revascularization procedures improve prognosis and reduce the incidence of sudden cardiac death [28, 29]. It is essential therefore to determine residual ischemia in the myocardial infarction survivor with poor pump function.

Much controversy exists about the value of treating ventricular arrhytmias after myocardial infarction. Secondary prevention trials of antiarrhythmic therapy have thus far been unable to demonstrate a beneficial effect [30]. The problems with these studies include: (1) the absence of stratification according to risk, (2) the absence of individualization of antiarrhythmic drug dose, and (3) the absence of knowledge of the true value of tests used to determine drug efficacy. The CAST study, presently in progress, in which about 4500 survivors of myocardial infarction will be enrolled, will hopefully answer the question of whether effective control of potentially malignant ventricular arrhythmias will improve survival.

In contrast to antiarrhyhtmic drug therapy, treatment with a beta-blocking agent has been shown to reduce sudden cardiac death [31]. A 25% reduction in sudden death has been demonstrated in the first 2 years after myocardial infarction. The beneficial action seems to be based upon amelioration of ischemia and elimination or blunting or sympathetically mediated modulation in heterogeneity of myocardial repolarization and refractoriness. Presence of cardioselectivity, intrinsic sympathomimetic activity, or membrane depressant action do not seem to play an important role in the protective action of the beta-blocking agent. Since beta-blocking agents after myocardial infarction have been used primarily in patients with reasonable left ventricular function, 100 patients of that type have to be treated for 2 years in order to prevent death in two of them. This suggests that better selection of patients likely to benefit from beta-blocking therapy is necessary. Patients with overt and silent ischemia and/or hypertension seem to be prone candidates for treatment with a beta-blocking drug. An important question is the value of beta-blocking therapy in the patient with mechanical and electrical complications. Furberg et al. [32] suggest beneficial action but more work is needed to define the exact value of beta-blocking therapy in these patients.

While in the whole group of myocardial infarction surviviors, antiarrhythmic drug therapy so far has not been shown to be beneficial, antiarrhythmic drug therapy does save lives in patients with spontaneously occurring ventricular tachycardia or ventricular fibrillation. Also the experience with the implantable defibrillator indicates that subgroups with life-threatening ventricular arrhythmias can be recognized who will profit from that device.

A special group at high risk of dying suddenly are those patients, having ventricular tachycardia or ventricular fibrillation following myocardial infarction.

In a recent prospective study we have evaluated the predictive value of different parameters for cardiac events in these patients. Seventy parameters from the clinical history, the electrocardiogram, exercise testing, 24 hour ECG recording, hemodynamic and angiographic findings and results of programmed electrical stimulation of the heart were studied in 200 patients with an old myocardial infarction developing ventricular tachycardia or ventricular fibrillation thereafter. All patients were followed for two years as to the incidence of sudden and non-sudden cardiac death while they were treated with antiarrhythmic drugs.

We found that four clinical questions can be of help in assessing risk for non sudden and sudden cardiac death in patients with documented ventricular tachycardia or ventricular fibrillation having one or more episodes of a myocardial infarction. These questions are:

1) What is the New York Heart Association classification outside the arrhythmia?
2) Did the patient loose consciousness during the arrhythmia?
3) Did ventricular tachycardia or ventricular fibrillation occur in between day 3 to day 60 after myocardial infarction or later?
4) Did the patient have more than one myocardial infarction in the past?

As shown in Figure 2 presence or absence of a positive answer to 1 or

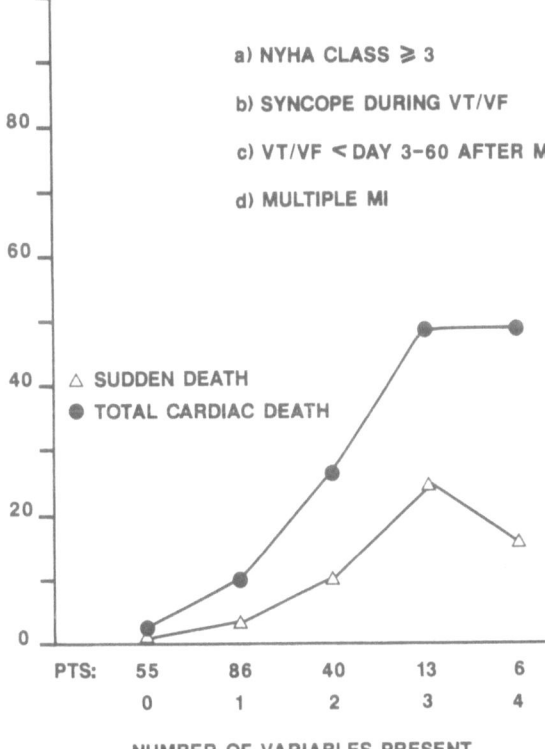

Figure 2. Incidence of total cardiac death (●) and sudden cardiac death (△) in relation to presence or absence of 4 clinical variables (listed in upper right hand corner) during a 2 year follow-up in 200 patients with VT (169 patients) or VF (31 patients) after myocardial infarction. As shown, information from the clinical history can be very helpful in risk stratification after VT/VF.

more of these 4 questions allows differentiation between patients having a very small chance of dying a cardiac death and patients having a very poor change to survive the 2 year period.

In evaluating the value of other non-invasive parameters we found that a VT rate (on the electrocardiogram) above 200/min was a poor prognostic sign. When the value of 24 hour ECG recordings and exercise testing was studied we found like others [33] that patients showing persistence of Lown 4b (non sustained ventricular tachycardia) during antiarrhythmic drug treatment did less well as compared to those showing disappearance of ventricular ectopic activity. Occurrence of appearance of sustained ventricular arrhythmias during exercise predicted a greater chance of a poor outcome.

Presence of three vessel disease and a left ventricular ejection fraction of 30% or less was (not surprisingly) a predictor of a poor survival chance. Programmed electrical stimulation gave helpful information when, as reported previously by other group [34—36] induction of ventricular tachycardia was still possible during antiarrhythmic drug therapy. This indicates poor prognosis especially in terms of recurrences of sustained ventricular arrhythmias.

The coronary heart disease patient after discharge from hospital

As pointed out, risk stratification and appropriate therapeutic measures should take place before discharge. In the post-hospital phase, attention should be focused on changes in the stability of the condition. Coronary artery disease is usually a progressive disease and patient and first line physician should be knowledgeable about the necessity of seeking cardiological advice when changes in condition occur. The cardiologist will then perform the necessary investigation to establish its significance and take appropriate action.

The unknown coronary artery disease population

In several countries including the USA and the Netherlands, mortality figures for coronary heart disease are decreasing. It is not quiet clear which factors are responsible: changes in diet, smoking, or exercise habits, treatment of high blood pressure or the advent of coronary care, bypass surgery, and medication such as beta-blocking and calcium antagonists.

In a large epidemiologic study of employees of the DuPont Company, Pell and Fayerweather reported a fall in incidence of myocardial infarction, sudden death, and total mumber of cardiac deaths over a 26-year period (1957—1983) [37]. The authors conclude that general measures like diet, discontinuation of smoking, etc. contributed more to the decreasing mortality than medication or interventions in the known coronary heart dieasse

Table 3. Evaluation of value of therapeutic and preventive measures in reducing sudden death in known and unknown CAD population.

---

1. Determine incidence of sudden death in
   A) Known CAD population
   B) Unknown CAD population
2. Repeat the study 10 years later
3. Draw conclusions:
   A) Reduction in sudden death incidence in group A suggests effect of therapy of CAD.
   B) Reduction in sudden death incidence in group B suggests effect of preventive measures.

Table 4. Guidelines of deciding on community screening programs in coronary heart disease according to Cadman *et al.* [38].

---

1. Has the program's effectiveness been demonstrated in a randomized trial?
2. Are efficacious treatments available and financially affordable?
3. Is there a good screening test?
4. Does the program reach those who could profit from it?
5. Can the health system cope and financially afford the screening program?
6. Will those with positive screening comply with subsequent advice and interventions?
7. Are psychological and socio-economic consequences of positive screening overcome by efficacious treatment?

---

patient. For future planning, it seems to be important to be better informed about the role of general versus more specific measures. This could be studied in the following way (Table 3). Determine the number of sudden deaths in the population and divide them into those occurring in known cardiac patients (group A) and those in whom suddem death was the first manifestation of cardiac disease (group B). If the same is repeated 10 years later, a decrease in the size of group B will indicate effectiveness of general measures. A decrease in size of group A points to a beneficial effect of specific measures related to individualized information of the cardiac status of the patient.

Epidemiologic studies indicate that in the Western world, 60% of patients suffering from a myocardial infarction fall in 20% of the population, having one or more risk factors including smoking, elevated cholesterol level, or elevated blood pressure. Therefore, 40% of myocardial infarction patients come from 80% of our population without any high risk factor. But even in the asymptomatic patient high risk group, techniques such as exercise testing do not fulfill the requirements for community screening programs discussed by Cadman *et al.* [38] shown in Table 4.

Conclusion

Sudden cardiac death is a multifactorial problem. At the present time, only one-third of patients dying suddenly can be identified as likely candidates prior to the event. In patients with known coronary artery disease, every possible effort should be made to reduce myocardial damage during acute ischemia. In the patient who has suffered from myocardial damage, appropriate risk stratification should be performed and therapeutic measures taken. So far, only beta-blocking agents have been shown to be effective in preventing sudden death after survival from a myocardial infarction. Studies are urgently needed to establish the value of antiarrhythmic drugs in relation to risk. In those studies, value of the presently available tests to predict success or failure of drug therapy should be critically evaluated.

References

1. Roberts WC: Sudden cardiac death: Definition and causes. Am J Cardiol 1986; 57: 1410—1413.
2. Doyle JT, Kannel WB, McNamara PM, Quickenton P, Gordon T: Factors related to suddenness of coronary death: combined Albany-Framingham studies. Am J Cardiol 1976; 37: 1073—1078.
3. Kulbertus HE, Wellens HJJ (eds): Sudden death. The Hague: Martinus Nijhoff, 1980.
4. Greenberg HM, Dwyer EM (eds): Sudden coronary death. Ann NY Acad Sci 1982; 382: 1—484.
5. Moss AJ, Bigger TJ, Case RB, Gillespie JA, Goldstein RE, Greenberg HM, Kronc R, Marcus FJ, Odoroff CL, Oliver GC: The Multicenter Postinfarction Research Group: Risk stratification and survival after myocardial infarction. N Engl J Med 1983; 390: 331—336.
6. Ahnve S, Gilpin E, Henning H, Curtis G, Collins D, Ross J: Limitations and advantages of the ejection fraction for defining high risk after acute myocardial infarction. Am J Cardiol 1986; 58: 872—878.
7. Packer M: Sudden unexpected death in patients with congestive hart failure: a second frontier. Circulation 1985; 72: 681—685.
8. Dwyer EM, Greenberg H, Case RB, and the Multicenter Postinfarction Research Group: Association between transient pulmonary congestion during acute myocardial infarction and high incidence of death in six months. Am J Cardiol 1986; 58: 900—905.
9. Berthe C, Piérard LA, Hiernaux M, Trotteur G, Lempereur P, Carlier J, Kulbertus HE: Predicting the extent and location of coronary artery disease in acute myocardial infarction by echocardiography during dobutamine infusion. Am J Cardiol 1986; 58: 1167—1172.
10. Fioretti P, Brower RW, Simoons ML, Bos RJ, Baardman T, Beelen A, Hugenholtz PG: Prediction of mortality during the first year after acute myocardial infarction from clinical variables and stress test at hospital discharge. Am J Cardiol 1985; 55: 1313—1318.
11. Akhara F, Upward J, Keates J, Jackson G: Early exercise testing and elective coronary artery surgery after uncomplicated myocardial infarction. Effect on morbidity and mortality. Br Heart J 1984; 52: 413—417.
12. Wellens HJJ, Brugada P, de Zwaan, C Bendermacher P, Bär FW: Clinical characteristics, prognostic significance and treatment of sustained ventricular tachycardia following acute myocardial infarction. In Kulbertus H, and Wellens HJJ, eds. Mount Kisco, NY: Futura Publishing Co., The First Year after a Myocardial Infarction. 1983; 227—237.
13. Bigger JTH, Fleiss JL, Rolnitzky LM, and the multicenter Post-infarction Research Group: Prevalence, characteristics and significance of ventricular tachycardia detected by

24 hour continuous electrocardiographic recordings in the late hospital phase of acute myocardial infarction. Am J Cardiol 1986; 58: 1151—1160.

14. Lichtlen PR, Bethge KP, Platiel H: Incidence of sudden death in relation to left ventricular anatomy and rhythm profile. Z Kardiol 1980; 69: 639—648.

15. Edlin DE, Morganroth J, Iskiandran AS, Spielman SR, Horowitz LN, Kay H: Ischemia at rest is independent of the extent of ventricular dysfunction and arrhythmias in patients with coronary artery disease. Am Heart J 1985; 190: 228—231.

16. Simoons ML, Van de Brand M, de Zwaan C, Verheugt RWA, Remme W, Serruys PW, Bär FW, Res J, Krauss XH, Vermeer F: Improved survival after early thrombolysis in acute myocardial infarction. Lancet 1985 (2): 578—582.

17. Kersschot I, Brugada P, Ramentol M, Zehender M, Waldecker B, Geibel A, de Zwaan C, Wellens HJJ: Effects of early reperfusion in acute myocardial infarction on arrhythmias induced by programmed stimulation. A prospective radomized study. J Am Coll Cardiol 1986; 7: 1234—1242.

18. Madsen JK: Ischemic heart disease and prodromics of sudden cardiac death. Br Heart J 1985; 54: 27—32.

19. Goldstein S, Freidman L, Hutchinson R, Canner P, Romhilt D, Schlant R, Sobrino R, Verter J, Wasserman A, and The Aspirin Myocardial Infarction Study Research Group: Timing, mechanism, and clinical setting of witnessed deaths in postmyocardial infarction patients. JACC 1984; 3: 1111—1117.

20. Mikharji J, Rude RE, Poole WK, Gustafson N, Thomas LJ, Strauss HW, Jaffe AS, Miller JE, Roberts R, Raabe DS, Croft CH, Passamani E, Braunwald E, Willerson JT and the MILIS Study Group: Risk factors for sudden death after acute myocardial infarction: two year follow-up. Am J Cardiol 1984; 54: 31—36.

21. Goldstein S, Vanderbrug Medendorp S, Landis JR, Wolfe RA, Leighton R, Ritter G, Vasu M, Acheson A: Analysis of cardiac symptoms preceding cardiac arrest. Am J Cardiol 1986; 58: 1195—1198.

22. Cobb LA, Hallstrom AP: Community-based cardiopulmonary resuscitation. What have we learned? New Engl J Med 1983; 390: 330—341.

23. Golstein S, Landis JR, Leighton R, Ritter G, Vasu CM, Wolfe RA, Acheson A, Medendorp SV: Predictive survival models for resuscitated victims of out-of-hospital cardiac arrest with coronary heart disease. Circulation 1985; 71: 873—880.

24. de Zwaan C, Bär FW, Wellens HJJ: Characteristic electrocardiographic pattern indicating a critical stenosis high in the left anterior descending coronary artery in patients admitted because of impending myocardial infarction. Am Heart J 1982; 103: 730—735.

25. Holland Interuniversity Nifedipine/Metoprolol trial (HINT) Research Group: Early treatment of unstable angina in the coronary care unit: a randomized, double blind, placebo controlled comparison of recurrent ischemia in patients treated with Nifedipine or Metoprolol or both. Lancet 1986; 56: 400—413.

26. Vermeer F, Simons, ML, Bär FW, Tijssen JGP, Van Domburg RT, Serruys PW, Verheugt FWA, Res JCJ, de Zwaan C, van der Laarse A, Krauss XH, Lubsen J, Hugenholtz PG: Which patients benefit most from early thrombolytic therapy with intracoronary streptokinase? Circulation 1986; 74: 1379—1389.

27. Bär FW, Vermeer F, de Zwaan C, Ramentol M, Braat S, Simoons ML, Hermens WT, Krauss XH, Wellens HJJ: Value of admission electrocardiogram in predicting outcome of thrombolytic therapy in acute myocardial infarction. Am J Cardiol 1987; 59: 6—13.

28. Passamani E, Davis KB, Gillespie MJ, Killip T, and the CASS principal investigators and their associates: A randomized trial of coronary artery bypass surgery. Survival of patients with a low ejection fraction. N Engl J Med 1985; 312: 1665—1671.

29. Holmes DR, Davis KB, Mack MB, Fisher LD, Gersh BJ, Killip T, Pettinger M: The effect of medical and surgical treatment on subsequent sudden cardiac death in patients with coronary artery disease: a report from the coronary artery surgery study. Circulation 1986; 73: 1254—1263.

30. May GS, Eberlein KA, Furberg CD, Passamani ER, Demets DL: Secondary prevention after myocardial infarction: a review of long term trials. Progr Cardovasc Dis 1982; 24: 331—352.
31. Yusuf S, Peto R, Lewis J, Collins R, Sleight P: Beta-blockage during and after myocardial infarction: an overview of the radomized trials. Progr Cardiovasc 1985; 27: 335—371.
32. Furberg CD, Moton-Hawkins C, Lichtstein E for the Beta-blocker Heart Attack Trial Study Group: Effect of propranolol in post-infarction patients with mechanical and electrical complications. Circulation 1984; 69: 761—767.
33. Kim SG: The management of patient with life-threatening ventricular arrhytmias: programmed stimulation or Holter monitoring (either or both?). Circulation 1987; 76: 1—5.
34. Fisher JD, Cohen HL, Hehra R, Altschuler H, Escher DJW Furman S: Cardiac pacing pacemakers. II Serial electrophysiologic-pharmacologic testing for control of recurrent tachyarrhythmias. Am Heart J 1977; 93: 658—668.
35. Mason JW, Winkel RA: Electrode-catheter arrhythmia induction in selection and assessment of antiarrhythmic drug therapy for recurrent ventricular tachycardia. Circulation 1978; 58: 971—985.
36. Horowitz LN, Josephson ME, Farshidi A, Spielman SR, Michelson EL, Greenspan AM: Recurrent sustained ventricular tachycardia. 3. Role of the electrophysiologic study in selection of antiarrhythmic regiments. Circulation 1978; 58: 986—997.
37. Pell S, Fayerweather WE: Trends in the incidence of myocardial infarction and in associated mortality and morbidity in a large employed population, 1957—1983. N Engl J Med 1985; 312: 1005—1011.
38. Cadman D, Chambers L, Feldman W, Sackett D: Assessing the effectiveness of community screening program. JAMAS 1984; 251: 1580—1580.

25. Final conclusions

P. PUECH

Sudden death is presently one of the greatest challenges facing public health and international cardiology due to its high incidence and dramatic appearance, particularly because it is often totally unpredictable and affects individuals who appear to be not only active community members but also in good health.

However, in many cases, the sudden death candidate has some potentially dangerous heart disease which should be evaluated and treated.

As the pathogenesis of sudden death is plurifactorial. A unilateral approach to prevention it is insufficient.

From the patients who have presented sudden death during Holter monitorization we have learnt that sudden death is usually due to ventricular fibrillation, often preceded by ventricular tachycardia. The proarrhythmic effect of antiarrhythmic drugs, particularly 'torsades de pointe' ventricular tachycardia, contributes considerably to death in subjects on antiarrhythmic treatment, and could annul the expected beneficial effect of this treatment in individuals at risk. On the other hand, deaths due to bradyarrhythmia have become more rare since the development of pacemakers.

The factors implied in sudden death (less than one hour after the appearance of the first symptoms) appear to vary in order of importance.

The significance of vulnerable myocardium and impact of left ventricular function on global mortality and sudden death has been clearly demonstrated. The role of ischemia is controversial and the circumstances preceding sudden death are considered as most important, while Holter findings (seen by the ischemic modifications of repolarization before the final arrhythmic event) tend to minimize its influence.

The elements which intervene in the final arrhythmia are grouped into a trilogy which includes the arrhythmogenic substrate, the trigger factor and modulating factors. The arrhythmic substrate is a reentry circuit, in most cases, due to a defined anatomic lesion (e.g. myocardial scar) or local electrophysiologic disorders which favour anisotropy. The most frequent trigger factor is the presence of premature ventricular contraction which may, in several circumstances increase the danger of unbalancing the substrate,

A. Bayés de Luna et al. (eds.): *Sudden Cardiac Death*, 297–298.

penetrating the critical zone of the circuit. However, the extrasystole is not the only trigger factor, and acceleration of heart rate, long cycle-short cycle sequences, are also trigger factors which Holter recordings have revealed.

Among the modulating factors we find that variations in the neurovegetative tone appear to play an important role. These include variations in heart rate (absolute or relative tachycardia, reduction of circadian variability of heart rhythm) without forgetting the variations in ionic balance (K and Mg), and the role of psychological stress or physical stress, QT interval modifications and the therapeutic influences.

Evaluation of risk factors should encompass both invasive and non-invasive approach. Holter recordings allow the study of the trigger factor (PVC), of the autonomous nervous system (variations in heart rate) and ischemia (ST–T).

Effort tests occasionally associated to examination with radioisotops explore the ischemia and the presence of arrhythmias due to effort. The electrocardiogram of high amplification and signal averaging study the presence of late potentials, non-invasive markers of a reentry substrate. The invasive approach, using programs of ventricular stimulation, studies the arrhythmogenic substrate and is useful to select the subjects who respond to antiarrhythmic treatment.

Although all methods of evaluation are limited, it is possible to define the individual at risk of sudden death, particularly after myocardial infarction. Such a person may present:
— poor ventricular function with an ejection fraction < 40%
— frequent or complex premature ventricular contractions in the Holter tapes
— poorly tolerated, recidivant spontaneous ventricular tachycardia
— late potentials with a duration of over 40 ms in the signal averaging ECG
— sustained ventricular tachycardias reproducible by programmed stimulation which remain inducible after antiarrhythmic therapy.

The inefficacy of antiarrhythmic treatment (including amiodarone) on ventricular extrasystoles and/or ventricular tachycardias of patients with these characteristics or antecedents of one or multiple cardiac arrests, shows the need for non-pharmacologic options such as surgery, catheter ablation techniques and implantable electrical device.

The highly recurrent character of malignant ventricular arrhythmias may, in a few well-selected cases, include the therapeutic possibility of heart transplant, particularly if there is a severe myocardic alteration limiting life expectancy.

Index

308

Developments in Cardiovascular Medicine

1. Ch.T. Lancée (ed.): *Echocardiology*. 1979   ISBN 90-247-2209-8
2. J. Baan, A.C. Arntzenius and E.L. Yellin (eds.): *Cardiac Dynamics*. 1980
   ISBN 90-247-2212-8
3. H.J.Th. Thalen and C.C. Meere (eds.): *Fundamentals of Cardiac Pacing*. 1979
   ISBN 90-247-2245-4
4. H.E. Kulbertus and H.J.J. Wellens (eds.): *Sudden Death*. 1980   ISBN 90-247-2290-X
5. L.S. Dreifus and A.N. Brest (eds.): *Clinical Applications of Cardiovascular Drugs*.
   1980   ISBN 90-247-2295-0
6. M.P. Spencer and J.M. Reid: *Cerebrovascular Evaluation with Doppler Ultrasound*.
   With contributions by E.C. Brockenbrough, R.S. Reneman, G.I. Thomas and D.L.
   Davis. 1981   ISBN 90-247-2384-1
7. D.P. Zipes, J.C. Bailey and V. Elharrar (eds.): *The Slow Inward Current and Cardiac
   Arrhythmias*. 1980   ISBN 90-247-2380-9
8. H. Kesteloot and J.V. Joossens (eds.): *Epidemiology of Arterial Blood Pressure*. 1980
   ISBN 90-247-2386-8
9. F.J.Th. Wackers (ed.): *Thallium-201 and Technetium-99m-Pyrophosphate. Myocardial Imaging in the Coronary Care Unit*. 1980   ISBN 90-247-2396-5
10. A. Maseri, C. Marchesi, S. Chierchia and M.G. Trivella (eds.): *Coronary Care Units*.
    Proceedings of a European Seminar, held in Pisa, Italy (1978). 1981
    ISBN 90-247-2456-2
11. J. Morganroth, E.N. Moore, L.S. Dreifus and E.L. Michelson (eds.): *The Evaluation of
    New Antiarrhythmic Drugs*. Proceedings of the First Symposium on New Drugs and
    Devices, held in Philadelphia, Pa., U.S.A. (1980). 1981   ISBN 90-247-2474-0
12. P. Alboni: *Intraventricular Conduction Disturbances*. 1981   ISBN 90-247-2483-X
13. H. Rijsterborgh (ed.): *Echocardiology*. 1981   ISBN 90-247-2491-0
14. G.S. Wagner (ed.): *Myocardial Infarction*. Measurement and Intervention. 1982
    ISBN 90-247-2513-5
15. R.S. Meltzer and J. Roelandt (eds.): *Contrast Echocardiography*. 1982
    ISBN 90-247-2531-3
16. A. Amery, R. Fagard, P. Lijnen and J. Staessen (eds.): *Hypertensive Cardiovascular
    Disease*. Pathophysiology and Treatment. 1982   IBSN 90-247-2534-8
17. L.N. Bouman and H.J. Jongsma (eds.): *Cardiac Rate and Rhythm*. Physiological,
    Morphological and Developmental Aspects. 1982   ISBN 90-247-2626-3
18. J. Morganroth and E.N. Moore (eds.): *The Evaluation of Beta Blocker and Calcium
    Antagonist Drugs*. Proceedings of the 2nd Symposium on New Drugs and Devices,
    held in Philadelphia, Pa., U.S.A. (1981). 1982   ISBN 90-247-2642-5
19. M.B. Rosenbaum and M.V. Elizari (eds.): *Frontiers of Cardiac Electrophysiology*.
    1983   ISBN 90-247-2663-8
20. J. Roelandt and P.G. Hugenholtz (eds.): *Long-term Ambulatory Electrocardiography*.
    1982   ISBN 90-247-2664-6
21. A.A.J. Adgey (ed.): *Acute Phase of Ischemic Heart Disease and Myocardial
    Infarction*. 1982   ISBN 90-247-2675-1
22. P. Hanrath, W. Bleifeld and J. Souquet (eds.): *Cardiovascular Diagnosis by
    Ultrasound*. Transesophageal, Computerized, Contrast, Doppler Echocardiography.
    1982   ISBN 90-247-2692-1

23. J. Roelandt (ed.): *The Practice of M-Mode and Two-dimensional Echocardiography.* 1983   ISBN 90-247-2745-6

24. J. Meyer, P. Schweizer and R. Erbel (eds.): *Advances in Noninvasive Cardiology.* Ultrasound, Computed Tomography, Radioisotopes, Digital Angiography. 1983
                                                  ISBN 0-89838-576-8

25. J. Morganroth and E.N. Moore (eds.): *Sudden Cardiac Death and Congestive Heart Failure.* Diagnosis and Treatment. Proceedings of the 3rd Symposium on New Drugs and Devices, held in Philadelphia, Pa., U.S.A. (1982). 1983   ISBN 0-89838-580-6

26. H.M. Perry Jr. (ed.): *Lifelong Management of Hypertension.* 1983
                                                  ISBN 0-89838-582-2

27. E.A. Jaffe (ed.): *Biology of Endothelial Cells.* 1984   ISBN 0-89838-587-3

28. B. Surawicz, C.P. Reddy and E.N. Prystowsky (eds.): *Tachycardias.* 1984
                                                  ISBN 0-89838-588-1

29. M.P. Spencer (ed.): *Cardiac Doppler Diagnosis.* Proceedings of a Symposium, held in Clearwater, Fla., U.S.A. (1983). 1983   ISBN 0-89838-591-1

30. H. Villarreal and M.P. Sambhi (eds.): *Topics in Pathophysiology of Hypertension.* 1984   ISBN 0-89838-595-4

31. F.H. Messerli (ed.): *Cardiovascular Disease in the Elderly.* 1984
                                   Revised edition, 1988: see below under Volume 76

32. M.L. Simoons and J.H.C. Reiber (eds.): *Nuclear Imaging in Clinical Cardiology.* 1984   ISBN 0-89838-599-7

33. H.E.D.J. ter Keurs and J.J. Schipperheyn (eds.): *Cardiac Left Ventricular Hypertrophy.* 1983   ISBN 0-89838-612-8

34. N. Sperelakis (ed.): *Physiology and Pathology of the Heart.* 1984
                                   Revised edition, 1988: see below under Volume 90

35. F.H. Messerli (ed.): *Kidney in Essential Hypertension.* Proceedings of a Course, held in New Orleans, La., U.S.A. (1983). 1984   ISBN 0-89838-616-0

36. M.P. Sambhi (ed.): *Fundamental Fault in Hypertension.* 1984   ISBN 0-89838-638-1

37. C. Marchesi (ed.): *Ambulatory Monitoring.* Cardiovascular System and Allied Applications. Proceedings of a Workshop, held in Pisa, Italy (1983). 1984
                                                  ISBN 0-89838-642-X

38. W. Kupper, R.N. MacAlpin and W. Bleifeld (eds.): *Coronary Tone in Ischemic Heart Disease.* 1984   ISBN 0-89838-646-2

39. N. Sperelakis and J.B. Caulfield (eds.): *Calcium Antagonists.* Mechanism of Action on Cardiac Muscle and Vascular Smooth Muscle. Proceedings of the 5th Annual Meeting of the American Section of the I.S.H.R., held in Hilton Head, S.C., U.S.A. (1983). 1984   ISBN 0-89838-655-1

40. Th. Godfraind, A.G. Herman and D. Wellens (eds.): *Calcium Entry Blockers in Cardiovascular and Cerebral Dysfunctions.* 1984   ISBN 0-89838-658-6

41. J. Morganroth and E.N. Moore (eds.): *Interventions in the Acute Phase of Myocardial Infarction.* Proceedings of the 4th Symposium on New Drugs and Devices, held in Philadelphia, Pa., U.S.A. (1983). 1984   ISBN 0-89838-659-4

42. F.L. Abel and W.H. Newman (eds.): *Functional Aspects of the Normal, Hypertrophied and Failing Heart.* Proceedings of the 5th Annual Meeting of the American Section of the I.S.H.R., held in Hilton Head, S.C., U.S.A. (1983). 1984
                                                  ISBN 0-89838-665-9

Developments in Cardiovascular Medicine

Developments in Cardiovascular Medicine

78. M.M. Scheinman (ed.): *Catheter Ablation of Cardiac Arrhythmias.* Basic Bioelectrical Effects and Clinical Indications. 1988   ISBN 0-89838-967-4
79. J.A.E. Spaan, A.V.G. Bruschke and A.C. Gittenberger-De Groot (eds.): *Coronary Circulation.* From Basic Mechanisms to Clinical Implications. 1987
ISBN 0-89838-978-X
80. C. Visser, G. Kan and R.S. Meltzer (eds.): *Echocardiography in Coronary Artery Disease.* 1988   ISBN 0-89838-979-8
81. A. Bayés de Luna, A. Betriu and G. Permanyer (eds.): *Therapeutics in Cardiology.* 1988   ISBN 0-89838-981-X
82. D.M. Mirvis (ed.): *Body Surface Electrocardiographic Mapping.* 1988
ISBN 0-89838-983-6
83. M.A. Konstam and J.M. Isner (eds.): *The Right Ventricle.* 1988   ISBN 0-89838-987-9
84. C.T. Kappagoda and P.V. Greenwood (eds.): *Long-term Management of Patients after Myocardial Infarction.* 1988   ISBN 0-89838-352-8
85. W.H. Gaasch and H.J. Levine (eds.): *Chronic Aortic Regurgitation.* 1988
ISBN 0-89838-364-1
86. P.K. Singal (ed.): *Oxygen Radicals in the Pathophysiology of Heart Disease.* 1988
ISBN 0-89838-375-7
87. J.H.C. Reiber and P.W. Serruys (eds.): *New Developments in Quantitative Coronary Arteriography.* 1988   ISBN 0-89838-377-3
88. J. Morganroth and E.N. Moore (eds.): *Silent Myocardial Ischemia.* Proceedings of the 8th Annual Symposium on New Drugs and Devices (1987). 1988
ISBN 0-89838-380-3
89. H.E.D.J. ter Keurs and M.I.M. Noble (eds.): *Starling's Law of the Heart Revisted.* 1988   ISBN 0-89838-382-X
90. N. Sperelakis (ed.): *Physiology and Pathophysiology of the Heart.* (Rev. ed.) 1988
ISBN 0-89838-388-9
91. J.W. de Jong (ed.): *Myocardial Energy Metabolism.* 1988   ISBN 0-89838-394-3
92. V. Hombach, H.H. Hilger and H.L. Kennedy (eds.): *Electrocardiography and Cardiac Drug Therapy.* Proceedings of an International Symposium, held in Cologne, F.R.G. (1987). 1988   ISBN 0-89838-395-1
93. H. Iwata, J.B. Lombardini and T. Segawa (eds.): *Taurine and the Heart.* 1988
ISBN 0-89838-396-X
94. M.R. Rosen and Y. Palti (eds.): *Lethal Arrhythmias Resulting from Myocardial Ischemia and Infarction.* Proceedings of the 2nd Rappaport Symposium, held in Haifa, Israel (1988). 1988   ISBN 0-89838-401-X
95. M. Iwase and I. Sotobata: *Clinical Echocardiography.* With a Foreword by M.P. Spencer. 1989   ISBN 0-7923-0004-1
96. I. Cikes (ed.): *Echocardiography in Cardiac Interventions.* 1989
ISBN 0-7923-0088-2
97. E. Rapaport (ed.): *Early Interventions in Acute Myocardial Infarction.* 1989
ISBN 0-7923-0175-7
98. M.E. Safar and F. Fouad-Tarazi (eds.): *The Heart in Hypertension.* A Tribute to Robert C. Tarazi (1925-1986). 1989   ISBN 0-7923-0197-8
99. S. Meerbaum and R. Meltzer (eds.): *Myocardial Contrast Two-dimensional Echocardiography.* 1989   ISBN 0-7923-0205-2

Developments in Cardiovascular Medicine

100. J. Morganroth and E.N. Moore (eds.): *Risk/Benefit Analysis for the Use and Approval of Thrombolytic, Antiarrhythmic, and Hypolipidemic Agents*. Proceedings of the 9th Annual Symposium on New Drugs and Devices (1988). 1989   ISBN 0-7923-0294-X

101. P.W. Serruys, R. Simon and K.J. Beatt (eds.): *PTCA - An Investigational Tool and a Non-operative Treatment of Acute Ischemia*. 1990   ISBN 0-7923-0346-6

102. I.S. Anand, P.I. Wahi and N.S. Dhalla (eds.): *Pathophysiology and Pharmacology of Heart Disease*. 1989   ISBN 0-7923-0367-9

103. G.S. Abela (ed.): *Lasers in Cardiovascular Medicine and Surgery*. Fundamentals and Technique. 1990   ISBN 0-7923-0440-3

104. H.M. Piper (ed.): *Pathophysiology of Severe Ischemic Myocardial Injury*. 1990
    ISBN 0-7923-0459-4

105. S.M. Teague (ed.): *Stress Doppler Echocardiography*. 1990   ISBN 0-7923-0499-3

106. P.R. Saxena, D.I. Wallis, W. Wouters and P. Bevan (eds.): *Cardiovascular Pharmacology of 5-Hydroxytryptamine*. Prospective Therapeutic Applications. 1990
    ISBN 0-7923-0502-7

107. A.P. Shepherd and P.A. Öberg (eds.): *Laser-Doppler Blood Flowmetry*. 1990
    ISBN 0-7923-0508-6

108. J. Soler-Soler, G. Permanyer-Miralda and J. Sagristà-Sauleda (eds.): *Pericardial Disease*. New Insights and Old Dilemmas. Preface by Ralph Shabetai. 1990
    ISBN 0-7923-0510-8

109. J.P.M. Hamer: *Practical Echocardiography in the Adult*. With Doppler and Color-Doppler Flow Imaging. 1990   ISBN 0-7923-0670-8

110. A. Bayés de Luna, P. Brugada, J. Cosin Aguilar and F. Navarro Lopez (eds.): *Sudden Cardiac Death*. 1991   ISBN 0-7923-0716-X

111. E. Andries and R. Stroobandt (eds.): *Hemodynamics in Daily Practice*. 1991
    ISBN 0-7923-0725-9

112. J. Morganroth and E.N. Moore (eds.): *Use and Approval of Antihypertensive Agents and Surrogate Endpoints for the Approval of Drugs affecting Antiarrhythmic Heart Failure and Hypolipidemia*. Proceedings of the 10th Annual Symposium on New Drugs and Devices (1989). 1990   ISBN 0-7923-0756-9

113. S. Iliceto, P. Rizzon and J.R.T.C. Roelandt (eds.): *Ultrasound in Coronary Artery Disease*. Present Role and Future Perspectives. 1990   ISBN 0-7923-0784-4

114. J.V. Chapman and G.R. Sutherland (eds.): *The Noninvasive Evaluation of Hemodynamics in Congenital Heart Disease*. Doppler Ultrasound Applications in the Adult and Pediatric Patient with Congenital Heart Disease. 1990
    ISBN 0-7923-0836-0

115. G.T. Meester and F. Pinciroli (eds.): *Databases for Cardiology*. 1991
    ISBN 0-7923-0886-7

116. B. Korecky and N.S. Dhalla (eds.): *Subcellular Basis of Contractile Failure*. 1990
    ISBN 0-7923-0890-5

117. J.H.C. Reiber and P.W. Serruys (eds.): *Quantitative Coronary Arteriography*. 1991
    ISBN 0-7923-0913-8

118. E. van der Wall and A. de Roos (eds.): *Magnetic Resonance Imaging in Coronary Artery Disease*. 1991   ISBN 0-7923-0940-5

Developments in Cardiovascular Medicine

Previous volumes are still available

KLUWER ACADEMIC PUBLISHERS – DORDRECHT / BOSTON / LONDON